Solving the Interstitial Cystitis Puzzle

Second Edition

A Guide to Natural Healing

Amrit K. Willis, RN, BSN

Holistic Life Enterprises
Los Angeles

Published by
Holistic Life Enterprises
9461 Charleville Boulevard
Suite 198
Beverly Hills, CA 90212-3107
Voice/Fax: (877) 682-1634

Library of Congress Control Number: 2003113672

International Standard Book Number (ISBN):

Paper: 0-9710869-2-3

Printed in the United States of America on alkaline paper.

Dedication

This book is dedicated to all those individuals who suffer from interstitial cystitis and the practitioners who help us. May you find hope and inspiration in your healing journey.

May all beings be happy.
May all beings be free from suffering.

"From one point of view, personal liberation without freeing others is selfish and unfair, because all sentient beings also have the natural right and desire to be free of suffering."

—Dalai Lama

Acknowledgements

I wish to thank God and my parents for giving me life.

I would like to thank Julian Lange and Dr. Roger Barnes in helping in my discovery and recovery from interstitial cystitis.

In this second edition, I would like to say thank you to Mark Clark, holistic pharmacist, who is always willing to give such helpful and healing information.

I wish to express my deepest love to my precious son, Hunter, who waited so patiently for me to finish this second edition.

I want to give my most profound gratitude and love to my dearest husband, Bry, without whose help this book could not have been completed. His love, patience, and devotion to my welfare is deeply appreciated. I am truly blessed.

Last but not least, I wish to express my deepest gratitude and admiration to Dr. Allen Weiner, for without his loving patience and guidance this book would have never been written.

Disclaimer

PLEASE READ THE DISCLAIMER CAREFULLY BEFORE USING THIS BOOK. By using this book, you signify your assent to this disclaimer. If you do not agree to this disclaimer, please do not use the book.

Amrit K. Willis, RN, BSN, is a holistic nurse not a medical doctor. She is a recovered IC patient. The diet and health procedures in this book are based on the training, personal experiences, and research of the author. Because each person and situation is unique, the author and publisher urge the reader to check with a qualified healthcare professional before using this diet or any procedure where there is any question as to its appropriateness. Statements made are not intended to diagnose, treat, cure, or prevent any disease. This information is not intended to replace the advice, diagnosis, or treatment of a medical doctor. The information in this book is for educational and research purposes, and neither the author nor publisher intends to provide medical diagnosis or medical treatment.

Any attempt to diagnose and treat an illness using the information in this book should come under the direction of a holistic medical physician. Because there is always some risk involved in any treatment or procedure, the publisher and author are not responsible for any adverse effects or consequences resulting from the use of any of the suggestions or procedures in this book. No guarantee or assurance is given to anyone as to the specific results that might be obtained.

Anyone seeking to take any of the supplements and therapies mentioned in this book should do so only under the care and advice of a holistic medical doctor, naturopath, or other competent, licensed health care professional. Please do not use this book if you are unwilling to assume the risks. In the event you use this information without your doctor's approval, you are prescribing for yourself, which is your constitutional right.

You can find a holistic medical doctor by visiting the American College for Advancement in Medicine at http://www.acam.org or call (800) 532-3688.

Solving the Interstitial Cystitis Puzzle

CONTENTS

INTRODUCTION

"Until man can produce a blade of grass, nature can laugh at his so called scientific knowledge. Remedies from chemicals will never stand in favor compared with the products of nature, the living cell of the plant and the final result of the rays of the sun, the mother of all life."

— Thomas A. Edison

Dear Reader,

Doctors have been saying for years, "There is no cure for interstitial cystitis." I am not proposing that I have a *cure* for interstitial cystitis, nor am I saying I have an easy answer for resolving IC. What I have learned, though, is that alkalizing is essential to healing IC. If you follow a hypoallergenic alkalizing diet and other suggestions in this book, you should be able to eliminate IC symptoms. I prefer to use the concepts *recovery* and *healing* when addressing IC. I feel that persons with IC are similar to persons who follow a 12 Step Program for alcohol and substance abuse: "It works if you work it." Alkalizing is a program we need to work on one day at a time.

I believe persons with IC are similar to persons with heart disease when they are diagnosed with a cardiac condition. Diet changes and daily activities are recommended to manage or even reverse a heart condition. Some individuals follow the health suggestions and feel well, while others struggle to comply, compromise their therapy or ignore the advice.

I am excited to be presenting the Second Edition of *Solving the Interstitial Cystitis Puzzle: A Guide to Natural Healing*. It has been over two years since the First Edition was published, and I am delighted to share with you the new insights I have gained from my own experiences and especially from my readers. Feedback resulting from the First Edition indicated that I needed to walk the reader through the first few months of alkalizing and eliminating allergens systematically. Although I was not specific in the First Edition in how to get started, many individuals greatly reduced or eliminated their IC symptoms. I also learned that some readers had the impression that as soon as their urine pH readings were alkaline, all their symptoms would disappear. This is usually not the case. In some situations, I received reports that within a few days of starting an alkalizing diet, certain individuals were comfortable during the day and sleeping through the night.

I wish to emphasize to the reader that I am proposing a diet and life style change. It is not possible to alkalize for a while and then go back to eating and living in ways that led to IC in the first place. According to Dr. Susan Lark, MD, a medical specialist on alkalizing, it can take anywhere from one to three years of alkalizing to recover from chronic disease. IC is a complex and chronic disease that can take years to manifest. Nature can heal, but she takes her time. Patience is of the essence. I have included success stories in this edition to give you hope and encouragement.

I have discovered some additional supplements that I feel might be helpful to the reader while working on their alkalizing program. I am also describing in more detail the lines of defense against disease, which are the body's pH balance, the intestinal tract (leaky gut), the liver, and the endocrine system, especially the adrenal glands.

Please note as this book goes to print I reference many resources such as addresses, Web sites, and phone numbers, which are current as of this writing. These are subject to change.

I would like to say a special thanks to several people who helped to contribute to this second edition:

Dawn Mahowald, CYI, Certified Yoga Instructor, and
Dr. Emmey A. Ripoll, MD, for their contributions for the chapters on Ayurveda, Acupuncture and Acupressure, and Yoga for interstitial cystitis.

Shira Lee, MA, herbal consultant, and her soothing contribution on the chapter entitled Nourishing Ourselves with Herbs.

Jeanne Karow, the co-moderator of my Yahoo IC Puzzle Group, for all her long hours of help and advice! Jeanne is a real "Gem" in the IC community, offering endless hours of support to those in need.

William Zeckhausen, D. Min., Pastoral Psychotherapist, for his comforting words about stress and his personal experience with Pelvic Floor Therapy.

Mary Sparacino, "The Chef," for her long hours of dedication in the kitchen to help prepare tasty alkalizing recipes.

There is much to learn, so let's get started!

Solving the Interstitial Cystitis Puzzle

PREFACE

"With regard to health or sickness, these are not 'sent to us', but are the results of keeping or not keeping the laws of God."

— Florence Nightingale

The purpose of this book is to share with those individuals who are suffering from interstitial cystitis (IC) my discoveries and recovery from this painful *dis*-ease. Briefly, through my research, studies, and my own healing process with IC, it became apparent that I had an acid-alkali imbalance—, that a person with IC is in an acidic state.

Dr. Dennis Myers, MD, a doctor who specializes in Euro-American medicine and alkalization states, "The fact is, every disease begins, at a cellular level, with those particular cells becoming acid, toxic, polluted. Since the internal environment or internal milieu the cells live in effects all diseases, this is the best place to start no matter what is wrong with you." [1] Dr. Myers calls this state of over acidity *latent acidosis* or to put it another way, we are base (alkali) deficient. With IC we have a latent or tissue acidosis. We will discuss in detail what this all means in the chapter Understanding Acid-Alkali Balance And Its Effect on Interstitial Cystitis.

Since this is the second edition of *Solving the Interstitial Cystitis Puzzle* I have revised and added information I have researched and gathered from my own continued recovery and the recovery of others using an alkalizing approach. In addition to alkalizing and eliminating allergens it became more clearly apparent after working with others that the detoxification and healing of other body systems is essential for total recovery. Dr. Henry Bieler, MD, describes three lines of defense against toxicity and disease: the *first line of defense* he states is the *digestive system*, the *second line of defense* is the *liver*, and *third line of defense* is the endocrine system, especially the *thyroid gland and adrenal glands*.

The following quote is from Catherine Simone's book *Along the Healing Path* as she describes IC.

"I believe that our differences arise out of our one major commonality, which in my opinion is this...

"IC patients have a toxic body.

"We are all toxic for different reasons and to different degrees, but I have found that IC patients have pretty much the epitome of the toxic body. The more severe the IC the more toxic and sick the rest of the body. IC patients often feel as if they are full of poison or on chemical overload. There is a feeling of too much acid in the system. (This is why antacids, baking soda and water, Prelief™, and Tummy Tamers are so helpful to many IC patients. They allow them to be able to eat and drink things they normally couldn't tolerate, providing them some relief from the pain and burning.) The stomach, the intestines, the kidneys and bladder are all burning with acid. This is what IC felt like to me and to many other IC patients I have spoken to."[2]

Reports from the medical community show that individuals with IC complain that acidic foods and beverages cause an exacerbation of symptoms, such as pain and burning in the bladder. It has also been reported by the medical community that taking alkalizing substances, such as baking soda or Prelief™ sprinkled on food, diminishes IC symptoms. What this indicates to me is that persons with IC need to decrease the body's acidity and increase alkalinity. In *Solving the Interstitial Puzzle* you will learn how to rebalance your internal milieu or inner terrain naturally through diet, simple natural supplements and some life style changes.

Most Americans are eating an inverted diet of 80% acidifying foods and only 20% alkalizing foods. In Dr. Susan Lark's book *The Chemistry of Success*, she examined the Economic Research Service of the USDA statistics of the American diet. She added up the number of pounds of highly acid-forming foods that the average American eats per year with the average yearly intake of more alkalizing foods. The ratio she discovered was 17:3 in favor of acid-forming foods. This highly acid-forming diet puts a great strain on the buffering systems of the body to neutralize all the acid that is produced by such a diet.

Dr. Lark states, "As we age, our ability to maintain a slightly alkaline balance in our cells and tissues diminishes. All too many factors in modern life, including the standard American diet, also affect acid/alkaline balance in the body. Our diet is high in acidic and acid-creating foods, and the fast pace of life today increases acidity."[3]

"Maintaining the cells and tissues of the body in their healthy, slightly alkaline state helps to prevent inflammation. In contrast, over acidity promotes the onset of painful and disabling inflammatory conditions as diverse as colds, sinusitis, rheumatoid arthritis and interstitial cystitis."[4]

"The body does not have an endless quantity of bicarbonate ions available to neutralize all irresponsible infringements on the law of alkaline-acid. The alkaline reserve is only a back-up system with limited quantity to keep you from constantly poisoning yourself with too much acid-forming food. When there is overindulgence in acid-forming foods (especially fried processed foods), the body sickens. In its marvelous wisdom, the body will make every possible effort to rebalance this transgression by expelling as quickly as possible, all the acid-forming residues. But when this alkaline reserve is depleted, death follows."[5]

It was only a matter of few days before I started to feel better on the alkalizing diet. Just as a diabetic checks their blood sugar levels and alters their diet I was able to monitor my own progress by measuring the pH of my urine and correcting my diet.

I began to recover by changing to an alkalizing diet/lifestyle, eliminating foods and environmental factors to which I was allergic. I addressed the leaky gut syndrome, cleansed and supported my liver and the adrenals. I was able to gain control over my own healing process. I continue to work on an alkalizing diet and avoid my allergens. I continue to cleanse and support my gastrointestinal tract, the liver, kidneys, and adrenals through diet, natural supplements, and treatments. I also continue to work on a gentle long term detox program.

"Modern medicine teaches that pain means sickness. It does not recognize that pain is also the body's way of informing us that we are doing something wrong. Pain can tell us that we are smoking too much, eating too much, or eating the wrong things."[6]

Solving the Interstitial Cystitis Puzzle

TESTIMONIAL

"Even one miracle cure can show the value of a therapy with the body's own healing powers. If the therapy is natural, non-invasive, and does no harm, it can be tried with confidence as a valid choice."

— Linda Rector-Page, ND, PhD

My journey of interstitial cystitis began in 1996. I experienced multiple bouts of cystitis that summer and fall, and took several courses of broad-spectrum antibiotics. In January of 1997 at the age of 44, I became pregnant.

Not long after my son's birth, I began to experience more episodes of pain and urinary frequency, usually resorting to taking more antibiotics. I sought the help of acupuncturists, herbalists, chiropractors, yoga, gynecologists, and urologists.

As is typical of most IC patients, I endured several years of suffering and seeking numerous medical consults until I was finally diagnosed with IC. I was worn out and depressed from the burning and pain in my bladder, nocturia (nighttime urinary frequency), and urinating every 10 minutes during the day.

Consulting yet another urologist's office, my urine specimen was sterile; there was no infection. He performed a cystoscopy and informed me I had interstitial cystitis. I was very upset. I was told by the urologist I could come into the doctor's office and have medications injected into my bladder on a regular basis. He said the cause and cure of IC was unknown but certain oral medications might help relieve some pain.

Then my urologist gave me my first glimmer of hope. He handed me a simple diet sheet with a few foods to avoid and said that by eliminating these certain foods I might decrease some of my symptoms. It was apparent to me that if avoiding certain foods helped diminish the symptoms of IC that the answer to its resolution was diet-related.

Returning home, I explored my holistic books and references, and I searched for an answer to my healing. I found the suggestions I had tried before, such as; uva-ursi, corn silk, marshmallow leaf, golden seal, cranberry juice, acupressure points, relaxation techniques, sitz baths, heating pads, cold packs, et cetera. These were supportive but not a cure. I turned to *Alternative Medicine: The Definitive Guide* by the Burton Goldberg Group. Something Dr. Larrian Gillespie, MD, stated about diet and cystitis struck me, "If you have an infection, taking cranberry juice, which contains hippuronic acid, makes as much sense as putting out a fire with gasoline, it only adds more acid to the urine, which in turn, increases the burning sensation. Cranberry juice may be helpful if you want to prevent an infection, but if you already have one, it only makes matters worse. Rather, try one-quarter teaspoon of baking soda in water. You should feel relief in twenty minutes." [1]

My urologist gave me instructions on diet modifications for IC. Dr. Gillespie was suggesting a dose of baking soda for cystitis that I knew would increase one's pH. These were things I could research and control. To me, this added up to examining my diet and assessing my pH or acid-alkali balance. I was intrigued. I checked my urine pH; it was 4.6. Normal urine has a pH of 4.6 to 8. Could it be my urine was burning my bladder? I recall over the years feeling as if I was "allergic" to my own urine. Urinating or getting rid of the urine gave some temporary relief.

I needed to raise the pH of my urine—but how? I needed to explore also the possibility of allergies to food and my environment. My next stop was Santa Monica Homeopathic Pharmacy where I discovered a book entitled *Acid and Alkaline* by Herman Aihara. Here are some excerpts that convinced me to experiment with an alkalizing diet: "Most proteins in food combine with sulfur and many are also combined with phosphorus. When the protein is metabolized, these elements remain as *sulfuric acid* and *phosphoric acid* and must be neutralized by ammonia, calcium, sodium, and potassium before they can be excreted by the kidneys. This is the reason high protein foods, especially animal foods, generally are acid-forming foods. This is also true of most grains because they contain much sulfur and phosphorus. In fruit and most vegetables, the organic acid (such as the acidity of an orange which you can taste) contains many elements such as potassium, sodium, calcium, and magnesium. Organic acids, when oxidized, become carbon dioxide and water; the alkaline elements (K, Na, Ca, and Mg) remain and neutralize body acid. In other words, strangely enough, acid foods reduce body acids. This is the reason that fruits and most vegetables are considered alkaline forming foods. Conversely, high protein foods and most grains, when metabolized, produce acid that must be neutralized; therefore they are generally acid forming foods." [2]

"In theory, whether a given food is acid forming or alkaline forming is determined by the proportion of acid forming and alkaline forming elements contained in the food. In practical reality, however, it is determined by test tube. This procedure is known as titration. First, the food to be measured is burned to ashes. (It is this step of burning the food that takes the place of digestion and thus gives us a picture of whether the food is acid or alkali forming.) Next, a standard amount of very pure water, say one liter, is added to 100 grams of these ashes to make a solution. This solution is tested to see whether it is acid or alkaline. Once we know whether the solution is acid or alkaline, we can measure the concentration or strength of the acidity or alkalinity of the ash solution." [3]

Solving the Interstitial Cystitis Puzzle

After assessing my diet, I realized I was eating a high protein, acid-forming diet, and probably consuming foods known to cause allergies for me. I never considered I might have had food allergies.

I eliminated coffee, spices, and other bladder irritants from my diet and made an appointment to be checked for food allergies with my holistic health care provider. I discovered I had several food intolerances and a few true allergies. I have taken allergy tests at York Labs and Immuno Labs. I discovered I had allergies to soy and yeast (IgE) and about thirty food sensitivities! (IgG).

I started a list of alkalizing foods I was not allergic or sensitive to and consumed only those foods. For the next several days, I ate only foods listed on the alkalizing hypoallergenic diet list. I kept an IC food, pain, and supplement diary. In the first forty-eight hours of converting to a hypoallergenic alkalizing diet, I did note some periods of poor concentration, but this soon passed. You may find your mental capacities to react or respond slower in the first 48 hours of switching to a hypoallergenic alkalizing diet, but this will clear. You may even want to consider starting an alkalizing program on the weekend because of this possible side effect.

Within several days of starting the diet, I noted a marked decrease in my urgency and frequency to urinate. To my amazement, my pain and burning was disappearing. I checked my urine pH. 7 is a neutral pH. My urine pH had changed from 4.6 to 5.5. This might seem like an insignificant change, but the change of one point using the pH scale indicated my urine was ten times more alkaline. I was urinating every 2 hours instead of every 10 minutes. I was only getting up at night once to urinate instead of every two hours.

It took months of trial and error of adding, assessing, and eliminating certain foods, beverages, and spices. I kept a food, bladder-symptom, and pH diary to document my findings. I lost some weight and felt more energized.

I was usually symptom-free. When I did run into a food that caused me pain or burning, I had to wait many hours to have it fade away until I discovered taking homeopathic remedies for allergies and inflammation eliminated my symptoms in 15 to 20 minutes. Taking the homeopathics for allergies and inflammation after I had an allergic reaction hastened my assessment process.

During this assessment period, I did not use perfumes and took no over the counter medications. I took no supplements, vitamins, or herbs. I used a natural organic soap and shampoo to which I was not allergic. I drank pure water and diluted apple juice.

Since much of my diet consisted of organic vegetables and some fruits, I was not worried about my nutrition score. I chose fresh organic foods whenever possible. I started with mostly vegetables because I found them to be less troublesome than fruits.

When on an allergy elimination diet and testing for allergies, one is in a state of calorie restriction. When one is in a state of calorie restriction, the urine pH will be lower, so until one can reach the daily calorie requirements for weight maintenance, the urine pH may be decreased. Do not be discouraged if your urine pH is lower in the beginning. An alkalizing program can take several years for the body to regain its balance and build an alkaline reserve again. However, you should start to feel the benefits of an alkalizing diet combined with allergy elimination diet in a few weeks.

By eating an alkalizing allergy-free diet with adequate calories, one should see the trend of the urine pH begin to rise. After several months on the alkalizing allergy-free diet, my morning urine pH trend was 6.5 to 7.

Once establishing the alkalizing allergy-free food list, one can add new foods as time passes and keep a food diary. What I discovered was that the better alkalized I became my tolerance for foods that originally bothered me improved. For example, originally I could not tolerate juices or fruits high in citric acid, such as oranges, lemons, or spicy foods. After several months on the alkalizing diet, I had no difficulty eating citrus fruits or even spicy foods. Guacamole is one of my favorite alkalizing foods since it contains tomatoes and avocados, which are high in potassium. I added natural essential oils, supplements, vitamins, herbs, one at a time, after I was comfortable and observed for any IC symptoms.

It was a time-consuming process, but I was determined to live pain-free without drugs or frequent medical intervention.

While searching for an answer to solving my interstitial cystitis puzzle, I found there was an underlying acid-alkali imbalance. However, since the body systems are interconnected I discovered that I needed to address other systems that had to be restored because they were also affecting my inflammation, discomfort, and acid-alkali imbalance.

I took multiple courses of antibiotics over the years for my history of cystitis, which in turn destroyed the normal healthy flora in my gastrointestinal tract. When the "good" bacteria are wiped out with antibiotics, one can develop what is now classified in the medical community as the leaky gut syndrome (LGS). LGS allows large food particles to leak into the blood stream, which causes the body's immune system to see these food particles as foreign and responds by releasing histamine, which causes an inflammatory response, i.e., food allergies and food sensitivities. Any inflammatory process will increase a person's acidity.

In addition, LGS causes malnutrition and pH imbalance because nutrients and minerals are not being absorbed properly. Large food particles in the blood stream create additional stress on the liver since blood-carrying nutrients from the small intestines goes directly through the blood portal system to the liver. Therefore, in resolving IC I looked holistically at my healing. To help heal LGS, I took an herbal formula Clear® by Awareness Corporation for an intestinal cleanse of harmful microbes followed with hypoallergenic non-dairy Jarrow probiotics.

To summarize, my history of cystitis was treated with antibiotics. In turn, these antibiotics eventually lead to a weakening and leakage of the intestines or LGS. LGS leads to multiple food allergies and sensitivities and contributed to inflammation, malnutrition, over-acidity, an overtaxed liver and exhausted adrenal glands. Upon initial evaluation, I discovered my diet was very acid-forming.

My first and most important step in healing IC was to switch to an alkalizing diet. LGS, food allergies and sensitivities needed to be managed. Additionally, I pursued an intestinal parastie cleansing program, a liver flush and liver support. To heal the adrenal glands, stress reduction, and overall nutrition needed to be addressed.

Hallelujah! Now I could take my son to a park even if it did not have a bathroom! I was ecstatic, and so was my husband. I decided to research these subjects further and knew I wanted to write a book explaining the IC puzzle!

Solving the Interstitial Cystitis Puzzle

ANATOMY OF THE BLADDER

"If I'd known I was going to live so long, I'd have taken better care of myself."

— Leon Eldred

The urinary bladder is a temporary storage pouch for urine. It is composed of collapsible muscle. In men, the bladder lies in the pelvis just behind the pubic bone and the urethra is approximately 8 to 9 inches long, running from the neck of the bladder to the tip of the penis. The urethra passes through the prostate gland. In women the bladder is located in front of the uterus and behind the pubic bone and the urethra is approximately 1½ inches long and is just above the opening of the vagina.

The lower portion of the bladder, continuous with the urethra, is called the neck; its upper tip, connected to the naval by a ligament, is called the apex. The region between the two openings of the two ureters and the urethra is the trigone. The trigone area is the area that signals us to urinate. The muscles consist of interlacing smooth muscle fibers.

As the bladder fills with urine, it rises into the abdomen. Under normal conditions, the bladder can distend to hold 750ml to 1,000ml (approximately one quart) of urine. When the bladder contains about 250ml (about one cup) of urine, the individual has a conscious desire to urinate. A moderately full bladder holds about 470ml (about two cups) of urine.

Two sphincters control the release of urine. The urethra is the end portion of the urinary system. A small tube carries urine by peristalsis from the bladder out of its urinary opening called the urinary meatus.

Inside the urethra and the bladder is a lining called urothelial cells. This lining is protected by a mucous layer that keeps the tissue from being burned by acidic urine. This mucous layer is called the GAG layer (sulfated glycosaminoglycan). This GAG layer protects against acids and toxic elements.

In persons with interstitial cystitis, the GAG layer is compromised making the individual more susceptible to bacterial infections, toxins, and acidic urine. In addition, it has been noted that according to the reports of Doctors Irwin and Galloway (1993) there is a relative lack of blood flow in the bladders' of IC patients compared to non-IC patients during bladder filling.

Helpful Medical Terms and Explanations Regarding a Urine Test or Urinalysis

Definition

Urinalysis is a diagnostic physical, chemical, and microscopic examination of a urine sample. Specimens can be obtained by normal emptying of the bladder or by a medical procedure called catheterization.

Voided Specimens

Urinalysis should not be performed while a woman is menstruating or having a vaginal discharge. A woman who must have a urinalysis while she has a vaginal discharge or is having her period should insert a fresh tampon before beginning the test.

Persons do not have to fast or change their food intake before a urinalysis. They should, however, avoid intense athletic training or heavy physical work before the test because it may result in small amounts of blood in the urine.

Bladder Catheterization

Bladder catheterization is sometimes used to collect urine. Collecting a urine sample from emptying the bladder takes about two or three minutes. The sample can be collected at home as well as in a doctor's office. Urine specimens are usually collected early in the morning before breakfast. Urine collected eight hours after eating and at least six hours after the most recent urination is more likely to indicate abnormalities. Some people may be asked to void into a clean container when first getting out of bed in the morning.

Specimen Containers

A sterile container is usually used for a specimen being collected for a colony count. A colony count is a test that detects bacteria in urine that has been cultured for 24 to 48 hours. It is used instead of a routine urinalysis when a person's symptoms suggest a urinary tract infection. Non-sterile containers can be used for routine specimens that will not be tested for bacteria or colony count.

Laboratory Procedures

Storage

Urine specimens should not remain unrefrigerated for longer than two hours. A urine specimen that cannot be delivered to a laboratory within two hours should be stored in a refrigerator. The reason for this precaution is that urine samples undergo chemical changes at room temperature. Blood cells begin to dissolve and the urine loses its acidity.

Visual Examination

A doctor, nurse, or laboratory technician will look at the specimen to see if the urine is red, cloudy, or looks unusual in any way. He or she will also note any unusual odor.

Testing Techniques

Urine samples are tested with a variety of different instruments and techniques. Some tests use dipsticks, which are thin strips of plastic that change color in the presence of specific substances. Dipsticks can be used to measure the acidity of the urine (its pH) or the presence of blood, protein, sugar, or substances produced during the breakdown of fatty acids (ketones).

A urinometer is used to compare the density of the urine specimen with the density of plain water. This measurement is called specific gravity.

The urine specimen is also examined under a microscope to determine whether it contains blood cells, crystals, or small pieces of fibrous material (casts).

Preparation

Voided specimens

Most urine specimens from adults or older children are collected by the patient's urinating into a suitable container. Soaps and disinfectants may contaminate urine specimens and should not be used. The doctor or laboratory may supply a special antiseptic solution that won't irritate the skin. The method for collection varies somewhat according to age and sex.

Women and girls

Before collecting a urine sample, a woman or girl should use a clean cotton ball moistened with lukewarm water to cleanse the external genital area. Gently separating the folded skin (labia) on either side of her vagina, she should move the cotton ball from the front of the area to the back. After repeating this process several times, using a fresh piece of cotton each time, she should dry the area with a clean towel.

To prevent menstrual blood, vaginal discharge, or germs from the external genitalia from contaminating the specimen, a woman or girl should release some urine before she begins to collect her sample. A urine specimen obtained this way is called a midstream clean catch.

Men and Boys

A man or boy should use a piece of clean cotton, moistened with antiseptic, to cleanse the head of his penis and the passage through which urine leaves his body (the urethral meatus). He should draw back his foreskin if he has not been circumcised. He should move the cotton in a circular motion away from the urinary opening, using a fresh piece of cotton each time. After repeating this process several times, he should use a fresh piece of cotton to remove the antiseptic. After the area has been thoroughly cleansed, he should begin urinating and collect a small sample in a container without interrupting the stream of urine.

Bladder Catheterization

Bladder catheterization is a sterile medical procedure used to collect uncontaminated urine when the person cannot urinate. A catheter is a thin flexible tube that the doctor inserts through the urethra into the bladder to allow urine to flow out. A plain rubber or latex tube is used for catheterization and is removed as soon as the specimen is collected. Be sure to inform your doctor if you have an allergy to latex or rubber.

Normal Results

Contents and Appearance

Normal urine is a clear straw-colored liquid. It has a slight odor. It contains some crystals, a small number of cells from the tissues that line the bladder, and transparent (hyaline) casts. Normal urine does not contain sugars, yeast cells, protein, ketones, bacteria, or parasitic organisms.

The time of day a urine sample is collected can make a difference in the appearance of the specimen. Some foods and medicines, including red beets, asparagus, and penicillin, can affect the color or smell of urine. Although most color variations are harmless, they sometimes indicate the presence of serious disease. A doctor, nurse, or laboratory technician should be notified if the urine is red or cloudy or looks unusual in any way.

Acidity
The pH of normal urine is 4.6-8.0. Its specific gravity is 1.0005-1.035.

Abnormal Results

Cloudiness
Urine may be cloudy (turbid) because it contains red or white blood cells, bacteria, fat, mucus, digestive fluid (chyle), or pus from a bladder or kidney infection.

Odor
Foul-smelling urine is a common symptom of urinary-tract infection. A fruity odor is associated with diabetes mellitus, starvation and dehydration, or ketone formation.

pH
A pH factor greater than 7 (more alkaline) may be due to alkalosis. A pH factor below 7 (more acid) may be due to fever or acidosis.

Blood and Tissue Cells
Red blood cells in the urine can be due to vigorous exercise or exposure to toxic chemicals. Bloody urine can also be a sign of bleeding in the genitourinary tract as a result of systemic bleeding disorders, various kidney diseases, bacterial infections, parasitic infections, obstructions in the urinary tract, traumatic injuries, and tumors.

A high number of white blood cells in the urine is usually a symptom of urinary tract infection. A large number of cells from tissue lining (epithelial cells) can indicate damage to the small tubes that carry material into and out of the kidneys.

Casts
Casts are small fibrous objects that are formed when protein and other materials settle in the kidney tubules and collecting ducts. Casts are dislodged by normal urine flow. A large number of them in a urine specimen is a sign of kidney disease.

Crystals
There are several different chemicals in body fluids that can form crystals that appear in urine. Some of these appear in normal urine, such as calcium oxalate or uric acid crystals. A large number of calcium oxalate

crystals, however, may be a sign of abnormally high levels of calcium in the blood (hypercalcemia).

Protein

Protein in the urine can be a symptom of kidney stones, inflammation of the kidneys, degenerative kidney disease, or multiple tumors.

Sugars

A high level of glucose and other sugars in the urine (glycosuria) is often a symptom of diabetes mellitus. Glycosuria can also be caused by advanced kidney disease.

Milk

Milk in the urine is normal if a woman is pregnant, has just given birth, or is breast-feeding.

Ketones

The presence of abnormally high numbers of ketones in the urine (ketonuria) usually results from uncontrolled diabetes mellitus. Ketonuria can also be caused by prolonged diarrhea or vomiting that results in starvation.

Bilirubin

Bilirubin is an orange-yellow pigment found in bile, a fluid secreted by the liver. When it is found in urine, bilirubin may be a symptom of liver disease.

Other Findings

The presence of bacteria, parasites, or yeast cells in the urine may be a symptom of urinary tract infection or contamination of the external genitalia. Other factors that may affect urinalysis results include failure to collect a specimen during the day's first voiding; frequent urination; large dietary intake of vitamin C.

Common Urinalysis Findings for Persons with IC

§ Normal findings

§ Microscopic hematuria (blood in the urine) or pyuria (white blood cells in the urine) might or might not be present

§ By definition, the urine culture must also be negative

§ Vaginal and urethral cultures must also be negative for gonorrhea, fungus, Chlamydia, and Trichomonas

§ Voided, catheterized, or bladder wash cytology is usually performed to rule out other diagnosis

Solving the Interstitial Cystitis Puzzle

DEFINING INTERSTITIAL CYSTITIS

"The best prescription is knowledge."
— Dr. C. Everett Koop, former Surgeon General of the US

Defining Interstitial Cystitis

Interstitial: Relating to or situated in the small, narrow spaces between tissues or parts of an organ

Cystitis: Inflammation of the urinary bladder

Medical Definition

"Interstitial cystitis (IC) is characterized by urgency, frequency, nocturia, and bladder pain that is generally relieved by voiding. The urine is sterile, and the urine cytology shows no evidence of malignancy. In 1915, Hunner reported on eight women with a history of suprapubic pain, frequency, nocturia, and urgency. Cystoscopically, he described either linear cracks in the bladder wall or ulcers (Hunner, 1915). At that time, he concluded 'a diagnosis of this peculiar form of bladder ulceration depends ultimately on its resistance to all ordinary forms of treatment.'

"Thus, IC was a diagnosis of exclusion in 1915 and remains so today." [1] The article continues, "The endothelial surface of the transitional cells lining the bladder has a surface mucus coat that in part contains glycosaminoglycans (GAG). The so-called GAG layer consists of mucopolysaccharides attached to a core protein that in turn is bound to a central hyaluronic acid string (Ratcliffe, 1994) Parsons et al. (1977) have shown the GAG layer to be involved in the defense mechanisms of the bladder urothelium. The glycosaminoglycans in the epithelium are distinct from those of deeper layers, implying a different function (Hurst et al., 1987). This bladder surface can be digested with *acid*, after which there is an increase in the adherence of bacteria, proteins, and calcium to the bladder epithelium. (Parsons et al., 1985, 1980)" [2]

Dr. Robert Moldwin, MD

Dr. Robert M. Moldwin, MD, in his book *The Interstitial Cystitis Survival Guide* discusses the many problems that may account for the symptoms associated with IC. He states that a decrease of blood flow to the bladder wall could directly affect the nerves of the bladder leading to hypersensitivity and inflammation.

"Doctors Irwin and Galloway (1993) were the first to report a relative lack of blood flow in the bladders' of IC patients when compared to non-IC patients during bladder filling." [3]

Dr. Theoharis Theoharides, MD & Grannum Sant, MD

According to Theoharis C. Theoharides, Department of Pharmacology and Experimental Therapeutics, Tufts University School of Medicine, and Grannum R. Sant, Department of Urology, Tufts University School of Medicine the etiology of IC is multifactorial and is better defined as a clinical syndrome. According to Theoharides and Sant, the etiologies of IC include autoimmunity, infection, genetic, neurogenic, and hormonal factors as well as the effect of toxic substances in the urine.

Dr. Theoharides suggests that activated mast cells found in the bladders of persons with IC creates many of the symptoms of IC. Dr. Theoharides is well known in the IC community for his work with the mast cell theory of IC. He theorizes that mast cell degranulation is the basic mechanism of IC, since this leads to the damaged GAG layer. Mast cells are a part of allergic reactions. It is when the mast cell degranulates and releases such irritating chemicals as histamine, tryptase, and methylhistamine that it leads to tissue damage, inflammation, and pain. Antihistamines have been used to help relieve IC symptoms. Elmiron, too, has been reported to be effective in suppressing the degranulation of mast cells and decrease histamines.

Dr. Susan Lark, MD

"To test for interstitial cystitis, a urine sample is normally analyzed for the presence of bacteria. The urine should show no sign of bacterial infection and often has an alkaline pH. As mentioned above, when bladder cells are damaged, they become more acidic. They leak their contents into the urine, losing their alkaline minerals while, at the same time, gaining acidic hydrogen ions from the surrounding environment. Thus, the cells become more acidic while the urine pH begins to rise. The overacidity of the cells makes it more difficult for the bladder tissue to repair itself." [4]

According to Dr. Lark, an aspect of allergies and mast cell degranulation that has been completely overlooked by the medical community is the fact that an overly acidic environment of the body will lead to inflammation and rapid mast cell degranulation. Dr. Lark states the severity of allergic reactions depends on the degree of acidity of the internal environment of the body. "When the body is overly acidic and mast cells are activated by an allergen, they will tend to break down more quickly and are more likely to generate histamines and other inflammatory chemicals. Overacidity can both trigger the symptoms of and lengthen the period of convalescence in allergic individuals. Unfortunately, the underlying cause is often over-acidity, which is rarely treated. Many people are unaware of the role that overacidity plays in the reactivity to allergens." [5]

Dr. John Forrest, MD

Dr. John Forrest, MD, who conducted a workshop, *Men and IC*, stated that in the late 1980s he did many cystectomies (surgical removal of the bladder) with internal pouches (diverting the urine to *intestinal* tissue pouches) with an opening to the abdomen. This is called an Indiana Pouch. Dr. Forrest had to remove every pouch because patients developed IC symptoms in the Indiana pouch.

Dr. Larrian Gillespie, MD

Dr. Larrian Gillespie, MD, uro-gynecologist, and former medical director of the Pelvic Pain Treatment Center in Beverly Hills, California, has written a book titled *You Don't Have to Live with Cystitis*. Dr. Gillespie has treated thousands of patients with interstitial cystitis.

Dr. Gillespie states, "In England, for example, it has been found in 1 of every 660 outpatients with cystitis. In Scandinavia, it has been identified in 1 in 350 patients. In the United States, some physicians believe that 1 in 20 cystitis sufferers is a victim of interstitial cystitis. If interstitial cystitis is an environmental disease, such variations in incidence are to be expected. Women in Europe are exposed to different drugs, pollution factor, and diets from American women." [6]

In describing IC, Dr. Gillespie states, "It involves...a slow destruction of the bladder by urine." [7] "Urine, with all its toxic substances and high acidity, does not burn or injure a normal bladder. But if you constantly put urine directly on skin that has no protective GAG layer, you will get a burn." [8] "Urine is indeed ulcerating and could burn away the very lining of the bladder." [9] "As I developed a model, a patient one day told me she was taking baking soda for her symptoms and found it helpful...Baking soda is alkaline. It would make the urine in the kidney less acid...In turn, urine reaching the bladder would be less acid and therefore less highly charged."[10]

Dr. Gillespie goes on to address the urine pH factor of the IC patients she has worked with. She states her patients' urine in the bladder was found to be alkaline or in other words with a higher pH. She attributes a higher urine pH to the fact that cells in the bladder leak bicarbonate to compensate for the bladder tissues being burned by acidic urine. She confirms that her IC patients had a low urine pH because the urine she evaluated by catheterization from the kidneys was 5.5. Normal urine pH is 4.6 to 8. A pH below 7 using the pH scale is acidic, while a pH above 7 is alkaline.

Dr. Susan Keay, MD

A unique protein in the urine of IC patients has been isolated by Susan Keay, MD, PhD, and her colleagues at the University of Maryland. This protein is called APF (antiproliferative factor). APF is not found in urine from patients without urologic symptoms or from those who have acute urinary tract infections or other urologic conditions. This protein may be directly responsible for preventing repair of the damaged epithelial lining in IC patients. In addition, it has been discovered that heparin-binding epidermal growth factor-like growth factor (HB-EGF), known to be important for epithelial cell proliferation and wound healing, is significantly decreased in IC patient urine specimens.

The results of further research could lead to identification of agents that will suppress the production of APF, or enhance the production of HB-EGF, both resulting in the formation of a healthy bladder lining. APF may ultimately provide a non-invasive clinical test for IC that would have a major impact on early diagnosis and treatment of the disease.

Vanderbilt Study: Chlamydia Pneumoniae

"Researchers at Vanderbilt University Medical Center, Nashville, Tennessee, have discovered a potential role of Chlamydia pneumoniae in the pathogenesis of interstitial cystitis (IC).

"The C. pneumoniae organism, first described in 1988, is an airborne organism transmitted via cough. As an obligate intracellular parasite, it is difficult to detect by routine cultures, can cause chronic infections, and may not elicit an acute inflammatory response. C. pneumoniae is commonly associated with respiratory tract infection, but has also been implicated in the development of coronary artery plaques.

"The data, using polymerase chain reaction (PCR) analysis of urine, revealed that 81% of patients with IC and 16% of controls were positive for C. pneumoniae, suggesting a potential role for this organism in the development of IC.

"Seventeen patients with IC as outlined by NIADDK criteria and six control patients underwent bladder biopsy. Selection of control patients was limited to those patients without history of irritative voiding systems, transitional cell carcinoma, or recurrent urinary tract infection. Biopsy specimens were analyzed for C. pneumoniae using standard tissue culture technique. Of those patients with IC, 82% (14/17) had tissue culture positive for C. pneumoniae. In control patients, 16% (1/6) had tissue cultures positive for C. pneumoniae.

"'We found a statistically significant correlation between IC and infection with C. pneumoniae based on tissue culture,' said Dr. Jenny J. Franke, assistant professor of Urologic Surgery at Vanderbilt. 'These results also parallel those obtained with urine PCR. The possible role of C. pneumoniae in the pathogenesis of IC remains to be determined by further analysis of tissue culture results as well as monitoring patient response to appropriate antimicrobial therapy.'

"The study of the organism has intensified as Vanderbilt and other medical centers around the country, including Johns Hopkins and The Mayo Clinic, look at the role of Chlamydia in diseases such as multiple sclerosis, rheumatoid arthritis, pyoderma gangrenosum, coronary artery disease, and IC." [11]

Defining Interstitial Cystitis (Demographics)

Interstitial cystitis (IC), a chronic pelvic pain disorder, is a condition resulting in recurring discomfort or pain in the bladder and the surrounding pelvic region. According to current medical research thus far, persons with IC do *not* have an infection; the urine is sterile. Interstitial cystitis is considered a syndrome that affects approximately one million people in the United States. This is considered a conservative estimate because many IC sufferers are misdiagnosed or undiagnosed. In a workshop on the topic of men and IC, Dr. John Forrest, stated that he strongly disagreed that IC in men is rare and that we must break out of the thinking of it as a rare disorder in order for there to be a breakthrough in treating this more effectively. Many persons with irritable bladder, chronic cystitis, and prostatitis in reality probably have interstitial cystitis. IC is diagnosed in women ten times more than men.

The demographics of this condition are as follows: from an article taken from *Campbell's Urology*, "The majority of patients with IC are female. Koziol (1994), in a survey of 565 IC patients, reported that 89 per cent were female. The age of onset is variable, with the reported median age at onset of the IC symptoms between 40 and 50 years of age, with 9% to 26% of patients under 30 at onset of symptoms. (Held, 1994) Hanash and Pool (1970) reported a peak incidence between 60 and 69 for men in their series. The IC syndrome has been reported in children and adolescents. (Farkas et al., 1977; Geist and Antolak, 1970)." [12]

The average time it takes for most persons with IC to be correctly diagnosed is about four to five years. The average age of onset is approximately 40 years old; however, 25% are now under the age of 30. Approximately 60% of persons with IC are unable to work or attend school full time.

Other illnesses commonly associated with IC

Other illnesses commonly associated with IC are sinusitis, fibromyalgia, irritable bowel, vulvodynia, systemic Candida infection, chronic fatigue syndrome, endometriosis, migraines, rheumatoid arthritis, lupus erythematous, Sjogren syndrome, and other types of immune problems such as a history of allergies and sensitivities. Many persons with IC also experience fatigue, an inability to concentrate, insomnia, and depression.

Quality of Life and IC

The quality of life for persons with IC is reported to be worse than for patients experiencing chronic renal failure and undergoing dialysis. IC takes a terrible toll in terms of human suffering, lost income, and strained intimate relationships. In reference to a landmark epidemiological study, a conservative average annual cost estimate of treating interstitial cystitis in the United States is $1.7 billion. Due to pain and a compromised quality of life with interstitial cystitis, persons with IC have suicidal thoughts three to four times above the national average. 70% of persons with IC report family relationships, and responsibilities are adversely affected.

Symptoms of IC

The symptoms of IC vary from person to person. An individual may experience mild discomfort, pressure, tenderness, or intense pain in the bladder, urethra and surrounding pelvic area before, during, and after urination. There is nocturia (frequent night time urination). According to Dr. Forrest, men may also complain of back and perineal pain (referred pain) in the same percentages of women. Men will also commonly complain of scrotal pain (referred pain). Persons with IC often describe their bladder pain as a burning sensation. Some complain of achiness in the bladder or stabbing pains. Symptoms might include urgency (an urgent need to urinate) or frequency (a need to urinate frequently). Urination patterns vary from voiding every ten minutes to every hour due to urgency, discomfort and reduced bladder capacity. Many persons express temporary relief of symptoms once the bladder is empty. Some persons with IC may leak urine from the bladder. Persons with IC experience pain during sexual intercourse and for days after intercourse.

Triggers that Exacerbate IC

Situations that generally increase IC symptoms are consuming large volumes of fluids, stress, sexual intercourse, constrictive clothing, and exercises that involve jarring motions such as running or jogging. Swimming in chlorinated, pools exacerbates symptoms. 50% of persons with IC have increased pain while riding in a car. Certain foods especially acidic foods and drinks, medications, vitamins and supplements also are IC triggers. Many persons report an increase in allergies and IC symptoms in the spring.

Diagnosing IC

Usually before a diagnosis of interstitial cystitis is given, a urologist will perform a cystoscopy with hydrodistention. The patient is usually placed under anesthesia. A cystoscopic examination is performed (where the doctor looks into the bladder with a long scope or tube). Irregularities of the bladder wall are sought. A Hunner's ulcer (or patch) might be seen, but this occurs in fewer than 10% of IC patients. The bladder is then distended with a sterile solution to a fairly high pressure. The doctor is looking for superficial bladder tears. He is also measuring bladder capacity, which is only about 600 to 700cc in an IC patient under anesthesia. Normal bladder capacity for someone without IC under anesthesia and hydrodistention would be about 800 to 1,200cc. The bladder capacity for someone with IC while awake is usually less than 350cc. In addition, the bladder is examined for glomerulations or small bleeding points on the bladder surface often seen in patients with IC. There is a reported breakdown of the GAG layer in the bladder and decreased blood flow.

When exploring the possibility of IC, make certain that you are examined by a gynecologist as well as an urologist. Other medical problems that have similar symptoms to IC need to be ruled out and/or treated such as: vaginitis or vaginal infections that can cause pain and burning from yeast, trichomonas, bacterial vaginosis, and herpes. Some other problems that can cause similar symptoms to IC include bladder infections or bacterial cystitis, radiation cystitis, surgical adhesions, ovarian tumor, ectopic pregnancy, multiple sclerosis, and benign and malignant bladder tumors. In addition, endometriosis, hernias, prostatitis, and pelvic floor dysfunction need to be ruled out. A chiropractic evaluation is a good idea since spinal misalignments can put pressure on the nerves innervating the bladder and perineum and cause pain. All these possibilities need to be considered and resolved if present.

Locus Minoris Resistentiae

Not every person who has an acid-forming diet/lifestyle has IC. However, many individuals have other disease processes related to overacidity such as irritable bowel, gastritis, colitis, arthritis, osteoporosis, heart disease, ulcers, cancer, prostatitis, cholecystitis (gall bladder disease), *et cetera*. What this suggests is that symptoms of inflammation, pain, and disease manifest differently in person to person with latent or tissue acidosis.

Dr. Dennis Myers describes overacidity of the body as a latent acidosis that leads to chronic degenerative disease. Latent acidosis leads to generic symptoms of pain, inflammation, and swelling in the body's weakest place or the *locus minoris resistentiae* or the place of least resistance. Frank organ degeneration begins to take place with latent acidosis. Dr. Myers states that this "localization in the body's place of least resistance can take the form of any of the specific, named, chronic, degenerative, diseases. Chronic degenerative disease is wholistic, it affects the whole body." [13]

Living in an acid state is not good for the human body. There appear to be other mitigating factors that may have weakened the bladder or the *locus minoris resistentiae* in persons with IC.

Children and IC

With respect to children and adolescents, the following history might predispose them to IC:

1. Overuse of antibiotics, usually related to multiple childhood ear infections and asthma or bronchitis, contributes to LGS.

2. LGS predisposes one to systemic yeast infections, food allergies, and inflammation. Food allergies and its related inflammatory state contribute to acidosis. Malnutrition from LGS can contribute to decreased absorption of essential nutrients and minerals. Poor diet choices such as high sugar intake and diets low in nutrients can contribute to latent acidosis.

3. Childhood asthma, a compromised respiratory condition, can contribute to an acidic state.

4. Immature bodies and organs are sensitive and cannot tolerate highly acidic diet/stress and lifestyle.

Each case should be evaluated individually.

Summary

Interstitial cystitis is believed to be a syndrome with perhaps a variety of origins. Certain subsets of persons may have IC as a result of one mechanism more than another or multiple mechanisms.

It is this writer's opinion that the underlying cause of *most* cases of IC is long-term overacidity along with allergies. In addition, it is also this writer's opinion that the body's lines of defense and detoxification such as the gastro-intestinal tract (leaky gut syndrome), the liver, and the endocrine system (especially the adrenals) are also compromised. With IC the kidneys and bladder are the *locus minoris resistentiae*.

Acidic urine bathes the bladder almost continuously due to the general acid-forming diet most Americans consume. In addition to an acid-forming diet, Americans also consume medications and over the counter drugs that are toxic and acidic to the bladder and tax the liver. As a rule, American life styles tend to be fast-pasted, which also leads to overacidity and toxicity.

My exacerbation of symptoms of burning, frequency, and pain were related to stress as well as the consumption of acid-forming foods, highly acidic foods, substances that were toxic and irritating to the bladder and certain allergens or irritants that I was exposed to, usually in food.

It has been well documented that the elimination of certain acidic foods and substances (like cola with a pH of 2.5) for persons with IC and the addition of an alkaline substance sodium bicarbonate (baking soda with a pH of 8.3) or Prelief can help diminish the symptoms of pain and burning. What this indicates is the need to decrease acid and increase the alkali in our bodies to relieve IC symptoms.

It is known that the bladder of a person with long time IC may be shrunken and shriveled. Damage to the susceptible bladder can be caused by strong acidic urine containing toxins and irritants such as medications, urea, irritants in foods and supplements. Allergies create mast cell breakdown in the bladder and this release of histamines damages the bladder lining and leads to related pain and inflammation. Decreased blood flow to the bladder of persons with IC has been documented, which would decrease oxygen and nutrients to the cells of the bladder and thereby increase pain. Tissue acidosis contributes to decreased circulation of nutrients and oxygen to the bladder and other organ systems.

Dr. Theoharides suggests that certain compounds and activities lead to mast cell breakdown. These include free radicals, hormones (like estradiol

Solving the Interstitial Cystitis Puzzle

and estrogen), IgE and antigen (autoimmune reaction), bacteria, neuropeptides (Substance P) neurotransmitters (acetylcholine), physical stress (cold, pressure, exercise, heat), emotional stress, radiation (including solar), toxins (bacterial, plant, and seafood toxins), virus, contrast media used in radiology, drugs (local anesthetics, morphine, high doses of non-steroidal anti-inflammatory/NSAIDS, high doses of antihistamines). Interestingly enough, most mast cell triggers that Dr. Theoharides reports are acid-forming.

Persons with IC report feeling hypersensitive to so much in their environment. I am not suggesting that one must live in a "bubble." However, it is prudent to avoid true toxins and allergens, and reduce stress. The foundation to overcoming IC is to balance our inner terrain by balancing the body's pH. In addition, one needs to strengthen the organs involved in the line of defense against toxicity and disease: gastrointestinal tract, liver, and the endocrine system (especially the adrenals). Since mast cell degranulation is such a significant part of IC, it is prudent to support the liver and the adrenals since these are the organs that produce our *natural* antihistamines. A sluggish liver and tired adrenal glands do not allow us to manufacture our own *natural* antihistamines.

By maintaining a hypoallergenic alkalizing diet/lifestyle, one will maintain the following: a healthy alkaline blood pH that provides a healthy alkaline state for all cells, tissues, and organs. Alkalinity promotes proper circulation of nutrients and oxygen that supports proper functioning of all organ systems. An alkalizing diet will produce a neutral urine pH that will not injure the kidneys or bladder.

CURRENT MEDICAL TREATMENTS

"To keep the body in good health is a duty... otherwise we shall not be able to keep the mind strong and clear."

— Gautama Buddha

I will briefly mention some current treatments for IC used in traditional allopathic medicine and do not intend to cover them thoroughly. There are numerous allopathic treatments currently for IC with most of the focus on the bladder. Since my resolution is a holistic approach, which addresses the *whole* body, I will not cover in detail current urologic interventions, but will mention them in passing.

Hydrodistension is a treatment whereby the bladder is distended under anesthesia with sterile fluid for three hours. Some patients report being symptom-free for up to 6 months after this treatment. Intavesical therapy has been one of the cornerstones of treatment.

Silver nitrate, DMSO, and Chlorpactin are drugs that have been used intravesically (instilled into the bladder) with varying satisfactory responses with follow-ups of 6 to 24 months.

Some oral medications such as the following have been prescribed: Elmiron, antihistamines, muscle relaxants, narcotic pain meds, steroids, and anti-depressants.

For further information on current allopathic medical treatments for IC, Dr. Moldwin's book, *The Interstitial Cystitis Survival Guide,* is a good reference.

Solving the Interstitial Cystitis Puzzle

FOUNDATION OF ACID-ALKALI IMBALANCE

"If I could live my life over again, I would devote it to proving that germs seek their natural habitat—diseased tissue—rather than being the cause of the diseased tissue; e.g., mosquitoes seek the stagnant water, but do not cause the pool to become stagnant."

— Dr. Rudolph Virchow, MD, founder of modern pathology

The following individuals and the research they pursued help to support my understanding of the importance of maintaining a proper acid-alkali balance in the body.

Dr. Alexia Carrel, MD

Alexia Carrel, 1912 Nobel prizewinner, surgeon, and physiologist, kept a chicken heart alive for about thirty years. He incubated a chicken egg. The heart of the developing young chick was taken out and cut in pieces. These pieces, consisting of many cells, were transferred into a saline solution that contained minerals in the same proportion as chicken blood. He changed this solution everyday, and he kept the chick's heart alive for about thirty years. When he stopped changing this solution, the heart cells died. The secret of the chick's heart surviving so many years lies in the fact that he kept the extra cellular fluids constant and that he disposed of the acidic cellular waste products every day by changing the fluid in which the chick's heart was kept. Cells will deteriorate when acid waste products accumulate.

Dr. Otto Warburg

In 1931, German biochemist, Dr. Otto Warburg, won his first Nobel Prize for work proving cancer is caused by a lack of oxygen in the cells. He states in *The Prime Cause and Prevention of Cancer* that the cause of cancer is no longer a mystery; we know it occurs whenever any cell is denied 60% of its oxygen requirements. This occurs through a buildup of pollution or acidity within and around the cell that blocks and then damages the cellular oxygen respiration mechanism. In 1944, he won a second Nobel Prize for his work linking cancer to damaged cell respiration due to a lack of oxygen at the cellular level.

In his book, *The Metabolism of Tumors*, Dr. Warburg demonstrates that the primary cause of cancer was the replacement of oxygen, an alkaline element, in the respiratory chemistry of normal cells by the fermentation of sugar, an acidic environment. The growth of cancer cells is a fermentation process that can be initiated only in the relative absence of oxygen.

Dr. Keichi Morishita, MD

According to Keichi Morishita, MD, in his *Hidden Truth of Cancer*, "if the blood develops a more acidic condition, then our body inevitably deposits these excess acidic substances in some area of the body such so that the blood will be able to maintain an alkaline condition. As this tendency continues, such areas increase in acidity and some cells die; then these dead cells themselves turn into acids. However, some other cells may adapt in that environment. In other words, instead of dying, as normal cells do in an acid environment, some cells survive by becoming abnormal cells. These abnormal cells are called malignant cells. This is cancer. In other words, a deficiency of oxygen (an alkaline element) in human cells in an acid environment is the cause of cancer growth." [1]

Pasteur, Bechamp, Enderlein: Monomorphism, Pleomorphism and the Inner Terrain

French chemist Louis Pasteur's (1822-1895) theory is described as *The Germ Theory of Disease*. Modern medicine is based on Pasteur's theory that bacteria and viruses cause infectious diseases or exogenous infections. Pasteur claimed that fixed species of microbes from an external source invade the body and are the first cause of "infectious" disease. This concept of specific unchanging types of bacteria causing specific diseases is also called monomorphism (one-formism). Current pharmaceutical and medical industries have built a trillion-dollar-a-year business around this concept.

A contemporary of Pasteur, Antoine Bechamp (1816-1908) Master of Pharmacy, and Doctor of Medicine brought his attention to tiny "molecular granulations" found in body cells, which other observers before him had noted. After ten years of observation he brought to the world in 1866 the profound revelation that these granules were living elements. He named them microzymas, meaning "small ferments." The essence of the theory is that the microzyma, an independently living element, exists within all living things, and is both the builder and recycler of organisms. It inhabits cells, the fluid between cells, the blood and the lymph. Bechamp's microzyma is capable of multiplying and it reflects either health or disease. In a state of health, the microzymas act harmoniously and beneficially. But in a condition of disease, microzymas become disturbed and change their form and function. They evolve into microscopic forms (germs) that reflect disease and produce symptoms. This transformation of the microzymas occurs due to a modification of the inner terrain or inner environment (acidity/toxicity) of the body by an inverted way of eating and living. He observed and explored the concept of pleomorphism (multi-formism) at its earliest.

Bechamp never denied that the air carried germs and could contribute to a disease state, but maintained that airborne germs were not necessary for disease to occur. Louis Pasteur himself prior to his death admitted that he was wrong and his contemporary, Antoine Bechamp, was right..."it isn't the seed, but the ground" that causes disease.

Gunther Enderlein (1872-1968), a brilliant German researcher, continued Bechamp's discoveries of the pleomorphic cycle of disease. His discovery showed that in a healthy state, the blood cells continue to do their job properly, supplying nutrients and oxygen to the tissues of the body. However, when the balance [of internal environment] is disrupted, a tiny biological unit of life which he called a "protit" begins to assume certain shapes in a degenerative 16-stage cycle (similar to the way in which the malaria parasite goes through various stages of maturation).

In more understandable terms, pleomorphism is similar to the profound changes we may observe when a caterpillar transforms into a butterfly. The stages of a butterfly start when an egg transforms into a caterpillar that hibernates in the chrysalis and leaves in the form of a butterfly. Enderlein observed these pleomorphic changes by looking at live blood under a microscope without staining or disturbing the specimen. He observed that protits remained small in response to a healthy condition. When the life units, or protits, encountered a disturbed inner condition (acidity and/or toxicity) they became enlarged and evolved into more complex forms including bacteria and fungi.

The evolvement of a protit to a more complex bacteria or fungi is actually the body's adaptive reaction to clean-up an acidic or toxic environment. To make this concept clearer, in death, the body tissues become acidic in order to aid in the process of decomposition. The acidity of body tissues creates an environment conducive to the growth of bacteria and fungi. Microorganisms aid in the breakdown of the body. If one extends this model, there would exist areas of the *living* body with an abnormally low tissue pH wherein the body would respond with the growth of bacteria or fungi because of this tissue acidiosis.

Four things determine a healthy or diseased inner terrain: its acid/ alkali balance (pH); its electric/magnetic charge (negative or positive); its level of poisoning (toxicity); and its nutritional status.

Dr. Paul W. Ewald: A New Germ Theory

A lengthy article entitled "A New Germ Theory" in the Atlantic Monthly, February 1999, centers around the brilliant evolutionary biologist, Professor Ewald at Amherst College. Professor Ewald's theory is that an organism (microorganism) evolves according to Darwinian Theory in response to its environment. The article uses an example of the recent discovery that Helicobacter pylori is found in the stomachs of a third of adults in the United States, causing inflammation of the stomach lining. In 20% of the infected people, it produces an ulcer. Nearly everyone with a duodenal ulcer is infected with these H. pylori. H. pylori infections can be readily diagnosed and cured in less than a month with antibiotics. However, a standard medical textbook from the 1970's until recently under etiology of stomach ulcers reads as follows: environmental factors, smoking, diet, ulcers caused by drugs, aspirin, psychonomic factors, and lesions caused by stress. There is no mention of infection at all. It is interesting to note that a Colorado survey found that

46% of patients seeking medical attention for stomach ulcer symptoms are never tested for H. pylori by their physicians.

Professor Ewald noted that if we looked up atherosclerosis in a textbook ten years ago, we would find similar etiologies: stress, lifestyle, lots about diet and nothing about infection. Heart disease is now being linked to Chlamydia pneumoniae, a newly discovered bacterium, that also causes pneumonia and bronchitis. Saikku and Leinonen found that 68 % of Finnish patients who had suffered heart attacks had high levels of antibodies to Chlamydia pneumoniae, in contrast to 17 percent of the healthy controls. Ewald is confident, according to this Atlantic Monthly article, that the association of Chlamydia pneumoniae and heart disease is real. Ewald's theory about evolution and infectiousness provides a framework that will provoke diverse research on the front lines of various diseases.

Dr. Stephen S. Morse, an expert in infectious diseases at Columbia University School of Public Health, states, "Helicobacter is probably the tip of the iceberg. Although science has developed tools of microbial cultivation for a hundred years, much of the microbial world is still as mysterious as an alien planet. It has been estimated that only 0.4 percent of all extant bacterial species have been identified." [2]

"Some people think that it is scary to have these time bombs in our bodies," Ewald says, "but it's also encouraging—because if it's disease organisms, then there's probably something we can do about it. The textbooks say, In 1900 most people died of infectious diseases, and today most people don't die of infectious diseases; they die of cancer, and heart disease and Alzheimer's and all these things. Well, in ten years I think the textbooks will have to be rewritten to say, 'Throughout history most people have died of infectious disease and most people continue to die of infectious disease.'" [3]

It appears if you combine the genius of Bechamp, Enderlein, and Ewald's theories they would all agree that infectious disease is a common underlying theme of human illness. It would be interesting to determine if Ewald would further agree with Bechamp and Enderlein that the imbalance of the body's inner terrain is the real breeding ground for the evolution of these microorganisms and disease. It is something to ponder regarding the etiology of interstitial cystitis as well as other illnesses with *unknown causes*.

It is interesting to note that medical texts do suggest that such factors as stress, diet, and smoking have been linked to most disease. Is this because these acid-forming factors do in fact contribute to a toxic/acidic inner terrain, which then leads to the spontaneous evolution of microorganisms and disease?

Again, recall that Enderlein's theory was that the protit (the smallest biological unit of life in the body) only evolves into more complex organisms such as bacteria, fungi, and mold under toxic conditions in order to clean up a toxic and acidic inner terrain.

Solving the Interstitial Cystitis Puzzle

It is possible that the answer to interstitial cystitis is some undiscovered antibiotic for an obscure microorganism—and in the future, this may prove valid as with H. pylori and stomach ulcers. In some cases, an association with IC and Chlamydia pneumoniae has been found. The following is an excerpt from OB-GYN.NET:

"Researchers at Vanderbilt University Medical Center, Nashville, Tennessee, have discovered a potential role of Chlamydia pneumoniae in the pathogenesis of interstitial cystitis (IC).

"The C. pneumoniae organism, first described in 1988, is an airborne organism transmitted via cough. As an obligate intracellular parasite, it is difficult to detect by routine cultures, can cause chronic infections, and may not elicit an acute inflammatory response. C. pneumoniae is commonly associated with respiratory tract infection, but has also been implicated in the development of coronary artery plaques.

"The data, using polymerase chain reaction (PCR) analysis of urine, revealed that 81% of patients with IC and 16% of controls were positive for C. pneumoniae, suggesting a potential role for this organism in the development of IC.

"Seventeen patients with IC as outlined by NIADDK criteria and six control patients underwent bladder biopsy. Selection of control patients was limited to those patients without history of irritative voiding systems, transitional cell carcinoma, or recurrent urinary tract infection. Biopsy specimens were analyzed for C. pneumoniae using standard tissue culture technique. Of those patients with IC, 82% (14/17) had tissue culture positive for C. pneumoniae. In control patients, 16% (1/6) had tissue cultures positive for C. pneumoniae.

"'We found a statistically significant correlation between IC and infection with C. pneumoniae based on tissue culture,' said Dr. Jenny J. Franke, assistant professor of Urologic Surgery at Vanderbilt. 'These results also parallel those obtained with urine PCR. The possible role of C. pneumoniae in the pathogenesis of IC remains to be determined by further analysis of tissue culture results as well as monitoring patient response to appropriate antimicrobial therapy.'

"The Vanderbilt researchers presented their data at the American Urological Association's 2001 Annual Meeting held in early June 2001.

"The study of the organism has intensified as Vanderbilt and other medical centers around the country, including Johns Hopkins and The Mayo Clinic, look at the role of Chlamydia in diseases such as multiple sclerosis, rheumatoid arthritis, pyoderma gangrenosum, coronary artery disease, and IC."[4]

Please note that the above study is *small*—only 17 IC patients. I was tested for Chlamydia pneumoniae, mycoplasma, and ureaplasma by PCR analysis of urine. All of my test results were negative.

Chlamydia pneumoniae, Interstitial Cystitis and Chronic Prostatitis

The following comments were made by Dr. Sandra Mazzoli, PhD, researcher at Sexually Transmitted Disease Centre, Florence, Italy:

"Chlamydia pneumoniae is one of the newest pathogens of the respiratory tract in humans. Every year almost 10% of communicable pneumonitis is caused by this microorganism. The seroprevalence of Chlamydia pneumoniae in normal populations is high, estimated to be 50% at the age of fifty, confirming its wide diffusion. Recently, Chlamydia pneumoniae has been connected with coronary chronic disease and myocardial infarction. Very recently, Chlamydia pneumoniae has been found in patients with interstitial cystitis, a condition related to prostatitis.

"We have analyzed for the presence of Chlamydia pneumoniae DNA, by nested PCR, prostatic biopsies, EPS, post EPS urine, total ejaculate, and first void early morning urine from patients affected by different prostatic pathologies: chronic abacterial prostatitis, benign prostatic hyper-plasia (BPH) and prostate cancer. Forty patients were included in the study and 87% resulted positive for Chlamydia pneumoniae DNA. 100% of the prostate biopsies (N. 10 patients) were positive, demonstrating the presence of the microorganism inside the prostate gland in prostatitis, BPH, and prostate cancer patients.

"Chlamydia pneumoniae, a microorganism inducing chronic body damages, has to be better studied in relation to chronic prostatic pathologies and prostate cancer. Several interrogatives remain also open: the role of macrophages and other immunologically related cells in transporting the microorganism inside the prostate gland and in modulating the infection; its persistence in relation to the various stages of prostate damage.

"Chlamydia pneumoniae positivity in this chronic prostatitis is *resistant* to several therapeutic regimens of antibiotics and is open to new pharmacological approaches. The constant presence of Chlamydia pneumoniae in all the prostate pathologies examined opens a discussion about the role of this microorganism in their development. We postulate that the three conditions—prostatitis, BPH, [and] prostate cancer—may represent different moments of the same process in which external conditions due to the host, especially immunological conditions, can induce the determinism of the one instead of the other pathology.

"We perform very long term follow up in our prostatitis patients with Chlamydial infections by DNA detection and specific Chlamydial immunological markers, and, recently, we have found intra-macrophage Chlamydial bodies after repetitive cycles of tetracycline therapy in some of our patients. So, we have evidence that Chlamydia is maintained inside immunocompetent cells in a state able to re-induce possible infection in permissive conditions. This is experimental evidence in our chronic

Chlamydial prostatitis patients. So that we have to go on with further studies. Of course, this is a very serious problem! It seems we are in front of a very 'smart' organism!"

I am questioning the possibility given Bechamp's, Enderlein's, and Ewald's theory that disease is a product of a microorganism's evolution in relationship to its environment. In the case of IC, the environment is a toxic tissue acidosis. I encourage the reader to look at the alternative of adjusting one's inner environment. If some undiscovered microorganism (i.e., antibiotic resistant microorganism such as Chlamydia pneumoniae) has evolved to gain some foothold with respect to IC, it may be eradicated by changing one's inner terrain. If Ewald's and Enderlein's theory is correct—that infectious disease is the underlying theme of human illness—, this, of course, could be true for other diseases: vulvodynia, fibromyalgia, irritable bowel, Sjogren 's syndrome, heart disease, multiple sclerosis, rheumatoid arthritis, and interstitial cystitis.

Solving the Interstitial Cystitis Puzzle

Understanding Acid-Alkali Balance and its Effect on Interstitial Cystitis

"Evident facts having an unorthodox appearance are suppressed."

— Dr. Alexis Carrel

Introduction

The majority of people in our American society today suffer from overacidity of the body's fluids that make up 70% of the body's weight. An interesting fact to note is that both our bodies and the earth are approximately 70% water. It is also known that our bodily fluids are related to the sea. The pH of seawater is approximately 7.8 while that of human blood is 7.4. This very sea inside each one of us is known as plasma, lymph, and cellular fluids that resemble the chemical composition of seawater. This "inner sea" circulates throughout our bodies and surrounds our cells, carrying life to every cell. "In Germany this extacellular space is called *Pishinger's Space* named after the German scientist who described it. This is the extracellular space that contains the fluids that bathes each and every cell. This Pishinger's Space serves as a 'pre-kidney' which stores excess acids prior to delivery to the kidneys." [1]

The maintenance of robust health comes from whole natural foods, oxygen, and pure water. One could compare our body's fluids to a fishpond. If the pH of the pond becomes out of balance either too alkaline or too acidic no fish can survive. The cells of our body are no different. The environment in which our cells survive is in a pool of water. With IC, our body's pool of water has become too acidic.

Defining pH

Briefly, we need to review some basic facts about acid-alkali balance to understand the chemical processes of the body and how our bodies develop this pH imbalance. An acidic or alkaline substance is measured with a pH scale. pH stands for "potential of hydrogen." pH measures the amount of concentration of hydrogen ions in a solution. Hydrogen ions are acids that must be maintained within strict limits in the body. A high concentration of hydrogen ions indicates a solution is acidic. A low number of hydrogen ions indicates the solution is alkaline. The pH scale is logarithmic, which means a difference of one pH unit represents a ten-fold increase or decrease in the concentration of hydrogen ions.

The pH scale, which determines whether something is acidic or alkaline, is numbered from 0 to 14. The pH of a solution is a measure of the number of hydrogen ions. A neutral solution has a pH of 7. That is, there are an equal number of hydrogen ions (H+) and hydroxide ions (OH-). Solutions less than 7 are considered acidic and have a greater concentration of H+.

Table 1: pH Values for Common Substances

Substance	pH Value	State
Hydrochloric Acid, (Drain Cleaner)	1.0	Acid
Sulfuric Acid (Battery Acid)	1.0	
Cola	2.5	
Vinegar (5% Acetic Acid)	2.8	
Wine	2.8 - 3.8	
Lemon Juice (Citric Acid)	3.0	
Orange Juice	3.0	
Apples	3.0	
Tomato Juice	4.0	
Black Coffee	5.0	
Detergent	6.5	
Milk	6.8	
Distilled Water	**7.0**	**Neutral**
Seawater	7.8	Alkali
Baking Soda	8.3	
Milk of Magnesia	10.7	
Household Bleach	11.0	
Household Ammonia	11.0	
Caustic Soda (Drain Cleaner)	14.0	

Solutions with a pH greater than 7 are basic or alkaline and have a greater concentration of OH-.

Some examples of acid solutions are vinegar with a pH of 2.8 and cola with a pH of 2.5. Some cite that it takes 32 glasses of alkaline water to

Solving the Interstitial Cystitis Puzzle

Table 2: pH Values for Bodily Substances

Substance	pH Value
Stomach Acid	1.0
Vagina	4.0
Skin	4.5 - 6.0
Urine	4.6 - 8.0
Saliva	5.0 - 7.5
Breast Milk	6.6 - 6.9
Perspiration	7.0 - 8.0
Tears	7.2
Arterial Blood	7.4
Semen	7.5
Small Intestines	7.7
Liver Bile	8.0
Pancreatic Fluid	8.8

neutralize one cola drink. Arterial blood with a pH of 7.35 to 7.45 is alkaline. Blood needs to be slightly alkaline. A variation of 0.4 in either direction in the pH of the blood can be fatal. A pH less than 7.35 indicates a state of acidosis. A pH greater than 7.45 indicates a state of alkalosis.

A pH of 7 means the solution is neutral; it is a combination of acid and alkali together to create a neutral solution. Pure distilled water has a pH of 7. Pure distilled water is not acidic or alkaline; it is considered neutral. Baking soda, the household name for sodium bicarbonate, is an alkaline substance with a pH value of 8.3. Household ammonia is a strong alkali with a pH of 11.

There are a number of body systems that have their preferred pH, as presented in Table 2. Examples are stomach acid with a pH of 1.0 or pancreatic fluids with a pH of 8.8. Urine pH range is 4.6 to 8.0. Arterial blood has a pH of 7.4. Overall, the body's internal chemistry changes from a weak acid to a weak alkali within a 24-hour period, usually more acidic at dawn and more alkaline at sunset.

When the urine pH is in its normal range of 6.8 to 7.5, the blood pH is normal. A urine pH less than 6.0 is unhealthy (too acidic) and a urine pH greater than 8 is unhealthy (too alkaline). When urine pH is 6.0 and below it indicates the body is ridding itself of excess H+ ions or acid, and it indicates the body is in an acidic state. In my case, my urine pH was very acidic around 4.6 because of my high acid-forming diet.

Acid and Alkali Regulation and Buffer Systems

We need to understand that in the process of daily activities as well as digesting our food, our bodies produce acids. Our bodies' movements and exercise produce acids such as lactic acid and carbon dioxide. Phosphoric and sulfuric acids are produced from the metabolism of proteins, legumes, most nuts, seeds, and grains. These acids must be buffered and eliminated from the body. The body buffers and eliminates acids to maintain its acid-alkali balance. The blood pH is the most critical to maintain at a pH between 7.35 and 7.45.

The pH regulating system of the body includes:

- Alkaline minerals inside and outside our cells
- Alkaline mineral reserves in our bones
- Three main buffering systems in the blood
- Lungs
- Kidneys

The main alkaline minerals found inside and outside our cells and in our bones are sodium, potassium, magnesium, and calcium.

The three main blood-buffering systems are the bicarbonate/carbonic acid system, the phosphates, and protein/ hemoglobin buffer systems. The bicarbonate/carbonic acid system is the most important. Sodium bicarbonate and carbonic acid are the two buffers in this system and work together to neutralize acids or alkalis released in the bloodstream. The bicarbonate/carbonic acid buffer system is immediate and can respond in fractions of a *second*.

The lungs exhale CO_2 or carbon dioxide—an acid waste from metabolism—and inhale O_2 or oxygen—an alkaline element that is diffused into the blood stream. The lungs can help correct pH imbalances in a matter of *minutes*.

The kidneys can generate, retain, or excrete bicarbonate ions (alkali) or hydrogen ions (acid) thereby increasing or decreasing the body's pH. The kidneys can help correct pH disturbances but this can take several *hours* to several *days*. The kidneys can normally handle a significant amount of acid or alkaline waste products, but the production or ingestion of too much acid or alkaline substance can eventually overburden the kidneys to regulate the pH.

All these systems keep the blood and the body from becoming too acidic or too alkaline. If for some reason these organ-buffering systems weaken, the body's pH balance will be upset. Either too much or too little acid will be neutralized. As we age, these organ-buffering systems weaken and our alkaline reserves diminish.

Weak Acids

"Your body is alkaline by design and acid by function. Although your cells live in an alkaline environment, they produce acids as they function. Acid must be neutralized or eliminated from the body. Acid produced by the cells in cellular metabolism is 'natural' and self-made acid easily eliminated through the lungs, the urine and feces..." [2]

Normal cellular metabolism creates carbonic acid, a weak acid. This carbonic acid (H_2CO_3) can be readily converted to a gas, carbon dioxide (CO_2) and water and vice versa. Carbon dioxide is exhaled through the lungs, and the water is excreted by the kidneys. Carbonic acid is easy for the body to deal with.

$$\text{Carbonic acid} <\longrightarrow \text{Carbon dioxide and water}$$
$$H_2CO_3 <\longrightarrow CO_2 + H_2O$$

Generally, when persons with IC are fasting, they state they have decreased IC symptoms. There are several reasons for this:

1. The acid load of the body is reduced.
2. No demands are made on the liver or pancreas to produce alkaline fluids for digesting food.
3. Food allergens or food sensitivities do not trigger a histamine reaction or aggravate a leaky gut.

It is this writer's opinion that IC is a whole body condition and needs to be addressed as such to heal. The involvement of different body systems, of course, is what makes the etiology of IC difficult to pinpoint.

Strong Acids

"The body can handle reasonable quantities of dietary acid. However too much acid-producing food overloads neutralizing mechanisms; the environment of your cells deteriorates; and your body becomes acid-it becomes toxic. Too much acid is termed acidosis. ACIDOSIS=TOXICITY." [3]

Examples of strong acids are sulfuric acid, nitric acid, and phosphoric acid. These acids form when we eat too much acid-forming foods such as sugar, grains, legumes, nuts, seeds, and all animal protein. When we eat these acid-forming foods, they are metabolized into strong acids. *Lactic acid is another acid that is created when we exercise.* These must be neutralized and they are neutralized by combining with an alkali or a base such as organic sodium, potassium, calcium, and magnesium. An acid combined with a base or alkali will form a salt that has a neutral charge. This salt will be excreted through the kidneys or bowel and will not burn or injure these organs. If we consume too many acid-forming foods and do not eat enough alkali or base foods (fruits and vegetables), the body will *rob* alkali or base elements from our own body reserves. The body must do this in order to maintain the critical blood pH between 7.35 and 7.45.

The body's alkaline reserves help to buffer and neutralize strong acids. Where are these so-called reserves in our body? Ninety-eight percent of the body's alkaline reserve element *potassium (K)* is found inside our cells. Ninety-nine percent of the body's alkaline reserve element *calcium (Ca)* is found in bones and teeth, while seventy percent of the body's alkaline reserve element *magnesium (Mg)* is found in the bones and muscles. Forty percent of the body's alkaline reserve element *sodium (Na)* is found in bone and fifty percent is found in the extracellular fluid. The major proportion of another alkalizing mineral, *iron (Fe)*, is found in the blood in the form of hemoglobin.

We can see how consuming an acid-forming diet and being alkali or base deficient will eventually deplete our body's alkaline reserves, producing latent tissue acidosis. This creates a host of body symptoms. The body will maintain the proper blood pH in order to survive even if that means "robbing" our alkaline reserves and storing acids and toxins. This process will create imbalance and dis-ease in all parts of our bodies.

When buffering the body's acids in the bloodstream the following events occur: "The families of mineral compounds which neutralize acids are the carbonic salts, symbolized as $BaCO_3$ where the *Ba* stands for any one of the four base or alkaline elements. Na, Ca, K, Mg (sodium, calcium, potassium, magnesium). When carbonic salts meet with strong acids such as sulfuric acid, phosphoric acid, acetic acid, and lactic acid, the alkaline minerals making up the carbonic salt leave the salt and combine with the acids to make new salts.

For example:

$$BaCO_3 + H_2SO_4 = BaSO_4 + H_2O + CO_2$$

Carbonic Salt + Sulfuric Acid = Sulfuric Salt + Water + Carbon Dioxide

"In the result, carbonic salt changes sulfuric acid, which is a strong acid, to sulfuric salt, which can be eliminated through the kidneys without any harm. In the same way, some other acid may be changed to another salt and be eliminated through the wall of the large intestine. In short, the acids, which are the product of metabolism, can be eliminated only after they are changed to neutral salts. Then they are no longer harmful to the kidneys and to the wall of the intestine.

Solving the Interstitial Cystitis Puzzle

"The result of this change, that is to say, from acid to neutral salt is to reduce the concentration of alkaline elements such as Na, Ca, Mg, and K in the blood and then in the extracellular fluid. It is the lowered concentration of alkaline elements, which is referred to as the acidic condition of the body fluid. Since in order for us to be healthy our body fluid must be kept at an alkaline level (pH of 7.4) we must re-supply the lost alkaline elements through the foods we eat."[4]

What Medical Doctors Have to Say about pH Factor and Health

Dr. Shaun Kerry, MD, says, "One school of thought says…disease is caused by germs or some form of static disease-causing microbe (the germ theory)… Kill whatever is making you sick. Treat the disease with drugs, antibiotics, chemotherapy, radiation, or surgery.

"The other school of thought says most disease is caused by some imbalance in the body brought about by some nutritional, electrical, structural, toxicological, or biological equation. In order to get well, you need to re-establish balance in your body. Embracing the biological view gives new insights to the disease process and is truly another paradigm for understanding health.

"Acids are a normal by-product of metabolism. The body has the mechanisms in place to eliminate these acids. But poor dietary habits, prolonged stress, lack of exercise, and toxicity exposures can lead to liver and kidney malfunction, and the acids in the body do not always get eliminated as they should.

"When the body has an excess of acid it can't get rid of, it gets stored for later removal. Where is this acid stored? In the interstitial spaces, also called the extracellular matrix—the spaces around the cells; the mesenchyme. When the body stores the acid in the extracellular matrix, it believes that one day the acid is going to be removed. Therefore, in order to be in balance, it knows that for every molecule of acid that gets stored in the tissues, an equal molecule of bicarb or base needs to be put into the blood because one day it will need to escort the acid out of the body. If the body has an acid overload, it stores the acid in the tissues (the tissue pH decreases) and the blood compensates and becomes alkaline (the blood pH increases).

"The total healing of chronic illness only takes place when and if the blood is restored to a slightly alkaline pH. Normally, human blood stays in a very narrow pH range…around 7.3. Below or above this range means symptoms and disease.

"When pH is too high or low, microorganisms in the blood can change shape, mutate, become pathogenic, and thrive. When there is a pH imbalance…enzymes that are constructive can become destructive, and oxygen delivery to cells suffers.

"Minerals have different pH levels at which they can be assimilated into the body. Minerals on the lower end of the atomic scale can be assimilated in a wider pH range, and minerals higher up on the scale require a narrower and narrower pH range in order to be assimilated by the body. For example, as more acid accumulates in our body, it gets stored and pushed further, and ultimately it gets pushed into the cell. When it gets pushed into the cell, the first thing it does is displace potassium and then magnesium and then sodium.

"Those are three critical minerals in our body. The potassium and magnesium will leave the body, but as a preservation mechanism, the sodium will be retained. Remember, the body knows it must place an alkaline molecule in the blood to escort out this increasing acid that is being stored in the tissues and cells. What it will often do (when mineral reserves are low which is often the case when eating a modern American diet) is draw calcium the most alkaline mineral known from the bones and put it into the blood. This leads to something called free calcium excess.

"This is something you don't want and it is what's behind osteoporosis, arthritic pain, etc. It is brought about by the body compensating for an ever-increasing tissue acidosis somewhere in the body. What you don't want to do in this case is take more calcium supplements. With that said, you can now understand why calcium is one of the most over-prescribed supplements. In these situations what the body really needs is more potassium, and magnesium, perhaps organic sodium, and possibly zinc which lends help to the whole proper acid breakdown process."[5]

Dr. Dennis Myers, MD, in his book, *The New Biology*, states that because of our acid-forming diet and lifestyle choices we develop what he describes as a latent acidosis. He actually describes this latent acidosis as becoming base or alkali deficient.

Dr. W. Lee Cowden, MD, clinical researcher and professor of alternative medicine at the Conservative Medicine Institute in Richardson, Texas, has this to comment on the pH factor and health:

"First it is absolutely true that we live and die at the cellular level.

"All the cells (billions of them) that make up the human body are slightly alkaline, and must maintain alkalinity in order to function and remain healthy and alive.

"However, their cellular activity creates acid and this acid is what gives the cell energy and function. As each alkaline cell performs its task of respiration, it secretes metabolic wastes, and these end products of cellular metabolism are acid in nature.

"Although these wastes are used for energy and function, they must not be allowed to build up. One example of this is the often-painful lactic acid, which is created through exercise. The body will go to great lengths to neutralize and detoxify these acids before they act as poisons in and around the cell, ultimately changing the environment (Pasteur called it 'the Terrain') of the cell.

"Most people and clinical practitioners believe the immune system is the body's first line of defense, but in actuality, it is not. It is very important, but more like a very sophisticated cleanup service. We must instead look at the importance of pH balance as the first and major line of defense against sickness and disease and for health and vitality.

"If we were to ask, 'What is killing us?' The answer might be 'ACIDOSIS'! It has been demonstrated that an acidic, anaerobic (lacking oxygen) body environment encourages the breeding of fungus, mold, bacteria, and viruses. It is said that cancer cells cannot grow in a well-oxygenated environment.

"Let's look at an example. If we were to seal the door to our freezer and then unplug it, come back and open the door in two weeks, what would we find? We would find mold, bacteria, and microscopic bugs. Things will be growing and multiplying. Where did they all come from? They did not sneak in - remember the door was sealed. The answer is...'they were always there'. It is simply that the environment changed to a more inviting and healthy one for the 'critters' to live in. This can be likened to a shift in our biological terrain from a healthy oxygenated, alkaline environment to an unhealthy anaerobic acidic environment. You see what is healthy for us is unhealthy for the body attackers and what is healthy for them is what is unhealthy for our body."

Dr. Susan Lark, MD, states, "As we age, our ability to maintain a slightly alkaline balance in our cells and tissues diminishes. All too many factors in modern life, including the standard American diet, also affect acid alkali balance in the body. Our diet is high in acidic and acid-creating foods, and the fast pace of life today increases acidity." [6]

"Maintaining the cells and tissues of the body in their healthy, slightly alkaline state helps to prevent inflammation. In contrast, over acidity promotes the onset of painful and disabling inflammatory conditions as diverse as colds, sinusitis, rheumatoid arthritis, and *interstitial cystitis*." [7]

When our diets are deficient in the alkaline elements (Na, Ca, K, Mg, Fe), the body will strip calcium (Ca) from bone or arterial walls in order to render phosphoric acid harmless by converting it into a salt. This is the cause of such diseases as osteoporosis and the so-called "hardening of the arteries." If the body sees a need for magnesium (Mg) and the person's diet is deficient in magnesium, the body may extract magnesium from the muscles (fibromyalgia). Obviously if the body deficits of magnesium and potassium affect the muscles of the heart, one can see disastrous results with this scenario: cardiac arrhythmias and heart attacks. One's blood lab results may look "normal," but this does not reflect the condition of the tissues or cells of the body.

How Latent Acidosis or Tissue Acidosis Manifests

Again, the blood stream is the most critically buffered system of the entire body. In hospital medicine, doctors are usually only concerned with a critical acidosis of arterial blood pH in an emergency.

Arterial and venous blood must maintain a slightly alkaline pH: arterial blood pH is 7.4, but venous blood is 7.36 due to a higher level of carbonic acid. The pH of interstitial fluids and connective tissue—body tissues, organs, and joints—is 7.34 to 7.36, a slightly more acidic profile, because cells dump acids into these areas to buffer the blood.

The blood pH is maintained slightly alkaline at the expense of the tissues, organs, and joints by dumping excess acids into the cells and extracellular space (Pishinger's Space) when the alkaline buffer system becomes critically low. pH measurements in the extracellular spaces can drop dangerously to concentrations of pH equal to 5.0.

Medical doctors are familiar with the medical condition called gout. The reader may be familiar with this too. Gout is a disease where uric acids are deposited into joints. Gout develops when a high protein diet is converted to uric acid in the body. These uric acid deposits settle in different joints, and gout is exacerbated by alcohol and a high protein diet, which are acidifying.

In tissue acidosis, where there is an alkali deficit and acids are stored in different parts of the body, one can see a multitude of diseases. In conditions of chronic pain, the complaint is one of aches, pains and burning; certainly stored acids and toxins will not feel good. In fibromyalgia, it affects the muscles, in vulvodynia, the tissues, and in interstitial cystitis, the bladder.

Latent Acidosis and Decreased Blood Circulation

In tissue acidosis overly acidic cells lose their flexibility. In the case of red blood cells, for example, the loss of flexibility inhibits the elasticity and adaptability of the cells, thus impeding blood flow.

Dr. Kern, a German heart specialist, discovered that one cause of heart infarct is overacidity. His research revealed that blood that flows through acid tissue itself becomes acidic. When the pH of the heart is at or below 6.4, the red blood cells become inflexible and unable to deform sufficiently to pass through the narrow capillaries. Once the red blood cells are attached against the capillary walls, they cause a blockage.

Dr. Moldwin in his book *The Interstitial Cystitis Survival Guide* reports, "Dr. Irwin and Galloway (1993) were the first to report a relative lack of blood flow in the bladders of IC patients when compared to non-IC patients during bladder filling." [8]

"As the pH of the blood goes more acid, fatty acids which are normally electro-magnetically charged on the negative side switch to positive and automatically are attracted to and begin to stick to the walls of arteries

Solving the Interstitial Cystitis Puzzle

which are electro-magnetically charged on the negative side. (And as science states, opposites attract.) It should start to make sense that a society which over-emphasizes food that could push blood more acid will have a high rate of heart disease." [9]

The lack of blood flow in the IC bladder might be related to tissue acidosis that leads to red blood cell deformation. When the tissue pH is acidic, deformed red blood cells obstruct the capillaries, and this would cause a decrease of blood flow to the bladder. Decreased circulation to the bladder will cause pain. The GAG layer will also be diminished related to decreased oxygen and nutrients. By taking a dose of sodium bicarbonate, one can quickly eliminate IC symptoms, at least temporarily. By raising the pH of the blood you increase circulation to the bladder.

Latent Acidosis and Mast Cell Breakdown in IC

Mast cell secretion of histamines plays a large part in the painful symptoms of IC. According to Dr. Theoharides, mast cell secretion of histamines is triggered by the following factors: stress, bacteria, chemicals, drugs, free radicals, certain hormones (estradiol/neural activation of mast cells is augmented by estrogens), IgE and antigen (allergies), viruses, toxins, radiation, and exercise. These triggers of mast cell secretion of histamines are acid-forming.

Dr. Lark states the severity of allergic reactions depends on the degree of acidity of the internal environment of the body. "When the body is overly acidic, and mast cells are activated by an allergen, they will tend to break down more quickly and are more likely to generate histamines and other inflammatory chemicals. Chronic inflammation can, in turn, damage cells and tissues, causing them to become more acidic thereby sending the body into a destructive downward spiral.

"Overacidity can both trigger the symptoms of and lengthen the period of convalescence in allergic individuals. Unfortunately, the underlying cause is often over-acidity, which is rarely treated. Obviously, environmental and food allergens and sensitizing agents should be avoided as much as possible. However, when a person is exposed to these substances, they should begin an aggressive alkalinizing program. Allergic or sensitivity reactions can often be contained very quickly. Many people are unaware of the role that overacidity plays in the reactivity to allergens." [10]

Exogenous Conditions Contributing to Latent Acidosis

Latent acidosis can be aggravated by conditions coming from *outside* the body.

Lifestyle

- Diet with excess of foods such as proteins and animal products, grains, legumes, nuts, seeds, sugar, table salt, sodas and carbonated beverages, caffeine, alcohol, smoking, and refined and processed foods deplete alkaline reserves

- Drinking acidic water (pH < 7)

- Inhaling polluted acidic air (sulfuric, carbonic, nitric acids)

- Diet deficient of the foods that help neutralize acid such as fresh fruits, vegetables, and sprouts

- Sedentary life styles

- External stress (new job, divorce, death of a loved one, illness)

- Exposure to toxic chemicals in our environment and personal care items

- Consuming foods grown in mineral and nutrient depleted topsoil

- Shallow breathing, limiting our inhalation of alkalizing oxygen and retaining acidic carbon dioxide

- Eating on the go, neglecting to relax and chew adequately. This does not allow the alkaline fluids from the salivary glands in the mouth to start digestion.

- Over-exercising increases the acid load by producing lactic acid

- Swimming in chlorinated pools or jacuzzis. Showering and bathing in chlorinated water. Chlorine gas is inhaled and chlorine is absorbed through the skin while swimming and bathing. Inside the body, the chlorine combines with water to form HCl (hydrochloric acid) and HOCl (hypochlorous acid). This leads to an increase in acid load. Choose instead to swim in clean lakes, ponds, rivers and the ocean or in pools treated with ozone or salt. Using a filter to eliminate chlorine while showering and bathing might be necessary.

- Drugs: "As far as acids are concerned, the only things more acid than protein are drugs, all of them. Most drugs are alkaloids that, as with protein, contain nitrogen. These drugs have to be converted first to their corresponding strong acid, nitric acid in this case, and then to the mineral salt, sodium, potassium, or calcium nitrate... Coffee is a drug, herbal medicines are drugs. All things like these have alkaloids as their active ingredients and are drugs." [11]

Solving the Interstitial Cystitis Puzzle

Endogenous Conditions Contributing to Latent Acidosis

Latent acidosis can be aggravated by conditions coming from *inside* the body.

⚘ Dysbiosis or intestinal fermentation is where *"bad"* bacteria live in the intestines, i.e., parasites and yeast. By-products of unwanted parasites and yeast create fermentation and acids.

⚘ Malfunctioning of *any* organ inside the body will increase the acid load such as the intestines, liver, adrenal glands, thyroid, kidneys, lungs, heart etc. Base or alkali *undernourishment* is a contributing factor that leads to the malfunctioning of organs.

⚘ Allergic conditions lead to inflammation and acid production

⚘ Psychosomatic stress increases acid load

⚘ Inflammatory conditions in the body generate acid

⚘ An infection of any sort—bacterial, viral, or yeast—generates acids

Cover Cells of the Stomach

Acid production (HCl or hydrochloric acid) by the cover cells of the stomach is matched by the production of an equivalent amount of sodium bicarbonate or potassium bicarbonate. As we age, the stomach produces less acid and hence less sodium/potassium bicarbonate. Sodium bicarbonate or potassium bicarbonate produced by the cover cells of the stomach is circulated to the blood stream and is supposed to be picked up by the liver and pancreas to make their alkaline fluids. However, due to latent tissue acidosis, sodium bicarbonate or potassium bicarbonate gets "used up" attempting to neutralize acid residues stored in the Pichinger's Space.

Many people with IC complain of too much stomach acid (GERD or Gastroesophageal Reflux Disease); GERD is a often a *compensatory* factor as the body is actually attempting to produce more sodium bicarbonate ($NaHCO_3$) or potassium bicarbonate ($KHCO_3$) in order to neutralize tissue acidosis.

Again, for every hydrochloric acid molecule the stomach makes, it also creates an alkalizing sodium bicarbonate molecule or potassium bicarbonate molecule.

The "ingredients" in the stomach's cover cells needed to make hydrochloric acid (HCl) are carbon dioxide (CO_2), water (H_2O), and sodium chloride (NaCl) or potassium chloride (KCl).

$$NaCl + H_2O + CO_2 = HCl + NaHCO_3$$

$$KCl + H_2O + CO_2 = HCl + KHCO_3$$

Allergies and Acidity

One of the factors in the etiology of allergies is that there is a latent tissue acidosis. With allergies, there is inflammation and cell destruction related to the inflammation. This contributes to an acidic state and thus creates a vicious cycle. Dr. Lark states the severity of allergic reactions depends on the degree of acidity of the internal environment of the body.

"When the body is overly acidic, and mast cells are activated by an allergen, they will tend to break down more quickly and are more likely to generate histamines and other inflammatory chemicals. Overacidity can both trigger the symptoms of and lengthen the period of convalescence in allergic individuals. Unfortunately, the underlying cause is often over-acidity, which is rarely treated. Many people are unaware of the role that overacidity plays in the reactivity to allergens."[12]

The Aging Process and Acidity

The organs in the body diminish in function by approximately one percent per year after the age of forty and faster in some cases depending on the person's diet, stress level, exposure to pollutants, and general life style. As we age, the slightly alkaline balance in our cells and tissues is reduced. As our cells and tissues, become more acidic over time, the ability to deliver nutrients and oxygen to the cells declines. An example of acid buildup and decreased blood flow is when your leg "falls asleep." Blood flow is decreased allowing acid buildup. The leg has a painful "pins and needles" feeling most of us have experienced. Upon standing, blood flow is restored. The tingly pins and needles sensation subsides.

Standard American Diet (SAD)

Most Americans are eating an inverted diet of 80% *acid-forming* foods and only 20% *alkalizing* foods. Acid-forming foods are high in sulfur, phosphorus, nitrogen, and chlorine. These foods include high protein foods: animal products, grains, legumes, nuts, seeds, acidic water, and soft drinks or carbonated drinks. Additionally, coffee, alcoholic drinks, sugar, and table salt are all acid-forming.

Alkalizing foods are rich in potassium, calcium, magnesium, iron, and organic sodium. These alkalizing foods include especially fruits and vegetables.

"In fruit and most vegetables, the organic acid (such as the acidity of an orange which you can taste) contains many elements such as potassium, calcium, and magnesium. Organic acids, when oxidized, become carbon dioxide and water; the alkaline elements (K, Na, Ca, and Mg) remain and neutralize body acid. In other words, strangely enough, acid foods reduce body acids. This is the reason that fruits and most vegetables are considered alkaline forming foods. Conversely, high protein foods and most grains, when metabolized, produce acid that must be neutralized; therefore they are generally acid forming foods."[13]

Alkalinity and Mental Health

It is a known fact that persons with IC suffer from depression. Although having a condition of chronic pain and discomfort can contribute to a state of depression, the following information may shed some more light on this connection between overacidity and depression. "The effect of pH on mental health is well demonstrated in the work of Dr. William H. Philpott, MD, an environmental psychiatrist who spent many years researching the links between food allergies, overacidity, and mood. In treating mental illness over a twenty-five year period, he frequently observed that these conditions were often not emotional in origin but rather were due to chemical imbalances." [14]

"One physiological reason for the link between alkalinity and optimism is that over acidity acts as a depressant to the central nervous system, whereas alkalinity acts as a natural mood elevator. When acids accumulate in tissues throughout the body, they can directly affect the mental energy underlying our ability to create and maintain a positive outlook..." [15]

"An acidic condition inhibits nerve action and an alkaline condition stimulates nerve action. One who has an alkaline blood condition can think and act (decide) well...Therefore, it is very important to maintain an alkaline blood condition all the time—not only for physical health but also for mental awareness." [16]

Autonomic Nervous System, Immunity and pH Balance

The Autonomic Nervous System includes the Sympathetic Nervous System (Fight or Flight Response) and the Parasympathetic Nervous System (Relaxation Response).

Acidity stimulates the Sympathetic Nervous System, making us feel energized initially, then nervous, jumpy, and irritable. In addition, chronic acid-forming stress leads to over stimulating the Sympathetic Nervous System. Over-stimulation of the Sympathetic Nervous System leads to a decreased immune response, which we see in the form of colds and flu when we are under stress. However, long-term chronic stress leads to chronic over stimulation of the Sympathetic Nervous System, which eventually puts our immune system into overdrive. The Sympathetic Nervous System in chronic overdrive is linked to all types of autoimmune diseases. Some examples are rheumatoid arthritis, multiple sclerosis, and Grave's disease, an attack on the thyroid. It has been theorized that IC might be an autoimmune disease.

Alkalinity stimulates the Parasympathetic Nervous System, which controls our digestion and rest. The Parasympathetic Nervous System allows the body to conserve and restore energy and helps to balance the immune system response. Alkalizing and finding ways to reduce acid-forming stress is mandatory to support a healthy immune system, one that is not under or overactive.

Early, Intermediate and Late Signs and Symptoms of Tissue Acidosis [17]

Early Symptoms

- Acne
- Agitation
- Muscular pain
- Cold hands and feet
- Dizziness
- Low energy
- Joint pains
- Food allergies
- Chemical sensitivities
- Hyperactivity
- Panic attacks
- Pre-menstrual and menstrual cramping
- Pre-menstrual anxiety and depression
- Lack of sex drive
- Bloating
- Heartburn (acid reflux)
- Diarrhea
- Constipation
- Strong smelling urine
- Mild headaches
- Rapid heartbeat
- Irregular heartbeat
- Hard to get up in the morning
- Excess head mucous (nasal stuffiness)
- Metallic taste in the mouth

Intermediate Symptoms

- Cold sores (Herpes I and II)
- Depression
- Loss of memory
- Loss of concentration
- Migraine headaches
- Insomnia

- Disturbance in smell, taste, vision, hearing
- Asthma
- Bronchitis
- Hay fever
- Earaches
- Hives
- Swelling
- Viral infections (cold, flu)
- Bacterial infections (staph, strep)
- Fungal infections (Candida albicans)
- Impotence
- Urethritis
- Cystitis
- Urinary infection
- Gastritis
- Colitis
- Excessive falling hair
- Psoriasis
- Endometriosis
- Stuttering
- Numbness and tingling

Advanced Symptoms
- Chron's disease
- Schizophrenia
- Hodgkin's Disease
- Systemic Lupus Erythematosis
- Multiple Sclerosis
- Sarcoidosis
- Rheumatoid arthritis
- Myasthenia gravis
- Scleroderma
- Leukemia
- Tuberculosis
- All other forms of cancer

Summary

To summarize, what has been explained thus far is that as one ages an acid-alkali imbalance develops and we live in a state of over acidity of the body's cells, tissues, and extracellular fluids (Pishinger's Space). The causes of this latent acidosis can be attributed to many factors: the aging process and decreased function of the organs, a highly acid-forming diet, stressful life style, medications, breathing polluted air, exposure to toxins, allergies, poor intake of alkalizing foods like fruits and vegetables, consuming acidic water, colas, coffee, or alcohol, over-exercising, under-exercising, and shallow breathing.

Our body needs to maintain a critical blood pH of 7.35 to 7.45 and needs to neutralize and eliminate acids at all costs, even if that means discarding acids inside and around our cells, tissues and organs. In the case of IC, when our alkaline reserves are critically low these acids are disposed into the extracellular spaces. Acid wastes cause an inflexibility and deformity of the red blood cells flowing through the capillaries of acid tissues. These red blood cells deform and occlude the capillary flow of blood to the tissues. The lack of blood flow causes a decrease of nutrients and oxygen to the bladder and nerves. In addition, when the pH is too low, the oxygen delivery to our cells suffers. With decreased oxygen and decreased blood flow, you experience pain. Decreased blood circulation to the bladder would play a part in the reduction of the GAG layer as well. This same mechanism of tissue acidosis leading to mineral deficits, acid dumping, and compromised circulation would play a significant part in vulvodynia, fibromyalgia, irritable bowel, etc. These are all common conditions with IC.

With IC, acids are discarded into Pishinger's Space (extracellular spaces). There is an alkali or base deficit when adequate minerals are not consumed through diet. Minerals are stripped from bones, muscles, tissues, and cells in order to maintain a proper blood pH. This state of tissue depletion and toxicity will cause symptoms of pain and inflammation.

A prevalent etiologic theory of IC is the patho-physiologic role of the mast cell. Mast cell secretion of histamines in the bladder leads to the chronic break down of the GAG layer. Histamines will cause inflammation, swelling, and the pain response seen in interstitial cystitis. We have seen that mast cell secretion triggers are acid-forming conditions such as exercise, stress, bacteria, viruses, chemicals, drugs, free radicals, antigens or allergies, radiation and toxins.

Essentially, what is happening in the body can be explained using simple chemistry. Life and the process of metabolism create an acid load in the body that must be neutralized or buffered by an intake of alkaline food and drink. In other words, we are attempting to combine an acid (body metabolism) and an alkali (alkalizing diet/lifestyle) in approximately equal amounts in order to maintain a neutral or balanced state in our bodies. By working to establish this balanced state, we will maintain our blood, tissues, organs, cells, and Pishinger's Space (extracellular fluids) in a slightly alkaline condition, which will provide the healthy environment we need to heal. Neutrality is an ideal condition in which the amount of acid and alkali is equal. It is an ideal condition and not realistic. However, in reality, our diet and lifestyle choices are typically more acidic or alkaline.

How to Measure your Body's pH

"Unless the doctors of today become the dietitians of tomorrow, the dietitians of today will become the doctors of tomorrow."

— Dr. Alexis Carrel, *Man the Unknown* (1935)

Urine pH

Normally, urine is slightly acidic in the morning because the body produces acids in the metabolic processes that occur continuously. In a *healthy pH-balanced* body, urine is slightly acidic in the morning (pH is 6.8 to 7.0) generally becoming more alkaline (pH is 7.5 to 8.0) by evening as the body digests food and releases alkali elements. Urine pH fluctuates throughout the day depending on diet, illness, stress, and activity level. Stress, infections, fasting, allergies, and vigorous exercise will lower your pH readings. Most medications (over the counter or prescribed) are acid-forming.

According to Dr. Dennis Myers, MD, healthy urine pH readings throughout the day would be the following:

The urine is most acid at 2 A.M. with a pH reading of 5 to 6.8. This is because at night while the body is fasting it attempts to remove accumulated acids from the Pishinger's Space (the extra cellular space). The *second* urine voiding first thing in the morning would be 6.8. Between breakfast and lunch and between lunch and dinner a healthy urine pH would be 7 to 8.

Two times a day the urine should be the most alkaline at 10 A.M. and 2 P.M. (7 to 8.5) because of the *alkaline tide* after meals. These are optimal urine pH readings. My urine pH was consistently below 6 during my assessment process, indicating my body was excreting excess acid.

A person consuming an acid-forming diet will generally have a urine

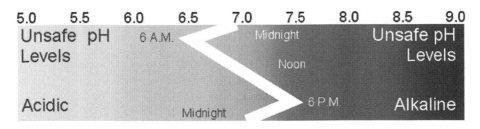

pH below 6 indicating the body is attempting to eliminate excess acids.

In order to accurately assess urine and saliva pH purchase *Hydrion* pH paper usually sold at pharmacies or health food stores. You may also purchase Hydrion pH paper over the internet. There is a color chart included with the roll of pH paper. Yellow indicates acid; green is weakly acidic and blue, alkali.

When checking your urine, you simply tear off a strip of pH paper, dip it into the urine stream, and read the results. Hold the strip and compare the strip to the corresponding color chart. Hold the strip close to the color blocks and match carefully. The pH may be read up to one minute after dipping.

Urine pH ranges from 4.6 to 8.0 however; urine pH below 6 usually indicates an overly acidic state in the body. A healthy alkalized person will have a urine pH range of 6.8 to 7.5.

Acidity and Alkaline Urine pH Readings

As noted before, some individuals may be consuming an acid-forming diet and still produce alkaline urine. Dr. Gillespie and Dr. Lark feel the reason for this is because the bladder cells are injured, thereby releasing alkaline minerals into the urine, which raises the pH of the urine.

Dr. Gillespie has reported the urine pH in the bladder of certain persons with IC to be on the alkaline side. However, she also reports the urine samples of these IC patients taken with a catheter from their kidneys were acidic.

The following excerpt from Dr. Lark reads as follows regarding the urine pH of persons with IC.

"To test for interstitial cystitis, a urine sample is normally analyzed for the presence of bacteria. The urine should show no sign of bacterial infection and often has an alkaline pH. As mentioned above, when bladder cells are damaged, they become more acidic. They leak their contents into the urine, losing their alkaline minerals while, at the same time, gaining acidic hydrogen ions from the surrounding environment. Thus, the cells become more acidic while the urine pH begins to rise. The overacidity of the cells makes it more difficult for the bladder tissue to repair itself."[1]

Dr. Ted Morter has a different theory about how we may have an alkaline urine reading when we have a tissue acidosis. Dr. Morter has been working with patients and using an alkalizing program for over thirty years to help heal disease. He has determined that after many years of putting a strain on the bodies' alkaline reserves to neutralize acids, these reserves begin to run critically low. He believes the body begins using an "emergency back-up system" of neutralizing highly acidic urine with ammonia.

The pH of ammonia is alkaline (pH 11). One way this ammonia is produced is to break down muscle tissues that is made of protein and can be used to produce ammonia. Thus, ammonia is produced from muscle breakdown to help neutralize a chronic acid state. Hence, you might see alkaline urine even though you are consuming a highly acid-forming diet. The smell of ammonia is a strong smell. I know many persons with IC have written to me complaining about the strong and unpleasant odor of their urine.

Solving the Interstitial Cystitis Puzzle

Dr. Myers agrees with Dr. Morter and describes alkaline urine findings with the depletion of the alkaline reserves. Dr. Myers indicates that nitrogen is eliminated as ammonia to neutralize metabolic acidosis. Calcium from bones is used as a secondary buffer as well as bicarbonate that will present an alkaline urine reading even though one is leading an acid-forming lifestyle.

Dr. Kerry has this to say about biological terrain: "As acids accumulate in our body, they get stored and pushed into the tissues. Where they get pushed, on a local level, is going to be in large measure where in your body or with what organ you experience problems. When the body stores this excess acid, it will compensate and place an alkaline atom/molecule in the blood, and the blood will therefore become increasingly alkaline." [2]

Saliva pH

To check the saliva, wait at least 2 hours after eating or drinking, fill your mouth with saliva, and then swallow it. Do this again to help ensure that the saliva is clean. On the third time, put some saliva onto pH paper.

The pH paper should turn blue. This indicates that your saliva is slightly alkaline at a healthy pH of 7.4. If it is not blue, compare the color with the chart that comes with the pH paper. Saliva pH ranges from 6 to 7.4. A healthy saliva pH range for someone working on alkalizing is 6.8 to 7.4.

"When healthy, the pH of blood is 7.4, the pH of spinal fluid is 7.4, and the pH of saliva is 7.4. Thus the pH of saliva parallels the extra cellular fluid...The pH of the non-deficient and healthy person is in the 7.5 (dark blue) to 7.1 (blue) slightly alkaline range. The range from 6.5 (blue-green) which is weakly acidic to 4.5 (light yellow) which is strongly acidic represents states from mildly deficient to strongly deficient, respectively. Most children are dark blue, a pH of 7.5. Over half of adults are green-yellow, a pH of 6.5 or lower, ...cancer patients are usually a bright yellow, a pH of 4.5, especially when terminal." [3]

According to Dr. Morter lower saliva pH readings indicate that too much emotional stress is taking its toll on your mineral reserves. In addition, low saliva pH readings can be indicative of low liver and pancreatic enzymes. Testing your urine pH readings a few times a day over a long period of time will give you a better indication of how well you are doing with your alkalizing program.

One should check the urine pH the same time each day over a period of weeks or months to determine the *trend* of the body's pH. We are measuring the effect of diet and lifestyle changes on the pH of our bodies. Maintaining your urine between 6.8 and 7.5 should be a realistic healthy goal on this alkalizing program.

Some individuals have mentioned since the first edition that even though their urine pH was more alkaline they still have IC symptoms. This is due to the fact that irritants such as histamines, toxins, and allergens still play a part in IC symptoms. We are working to alkalize the entire body not just the urine. Alkalizing helps to decrease inflammation and will gently detox the body which contributes to long-term healing. Keeping the urine pH on the alkaline side will help the bladder to repair. Long term acidic urine will damage the urinary system.

Over time, alkalizing will allow *all* our body systems to function properly (kidneys and bladder, liver, adrenals, GI tract, nervous system, muscles, etc). A healthy proper alkaline state for all the cells of the body is what we are aiming for, and we must maintain this approach to guarantee long term health and recovery from all disease not just IC. The body will use a "triage system." When you replace lost alkaline elements with diet and supplements, you have no control over where the body "chooses" to use them.

For example, if organic sodium from the vegetables you eat is needed to repair the liver and pancreas, the body may decide this is where the repair work will begin. You might like the body to "fix" the bladder first, but the body has other priorities. At least when you stay on an alkalizing program and you see that your urine pH readings are more alkaline, you know that every day you are adding to your alkaline reserves not subtracting from them. You are rebuilding your health each day.

Solving the Interstitial Cystitis Puzzle

Solving the Interstitial Cystitis Puzzle

LEAKY GUT SYNDROME

"If we could give every individual the right amount of nourishment and exercise, not too little and not too much, we would have found the safest way to health."

— Hippocrates c. 460 - 377 BC

Dr. Beiler, MD, author of *Food is Your Best Medicine,* states that the gastrointestinal (GI) system is the *first line of defense against disease.* First, let use briefly describe the GI tract. It is about 28 feet long. The digestive tract consists of the mouth and salivary glands, the esophagus, stomach, liver, gallbladder, pancreas, small and large intestines, the rectum, and anus. In the small intestine there are microscopic finger-like projections called villi that absorb the food we eat. It is estimated that the micro-villi absorption capacity, if it were laid out over a flat area, would approach the *size of a tennis court or almost 2,700 square feet!*

The purpose of the gastrointestinal tract is multifold:

- Digests foods
- Absorbs food particles to be converted into energy
- Carries nutrients like vitamins and minerals attached to carrier proteins across the gut lining into the bloodstream
- Contains immunoglobulins or antibodies that act as the first line of defense against infection
- Beneficial bacteria also metabolize hormones (e.g. estrogen) discharged from the liver into the small intestine.
- Certain B vitamins are manufactured in the large intestines.

What is LGS?

What is leaky gut syndrome (LGS)? LGS represents a hyperpermeable intestinal lining. In other words, large spaces develop between the cells of the gut wall, and antigens leak through into the blood stream. An official definition of LGS is *an increase in permeability of the intestinal mucosa to luminal macromolecules, antigens, and toxins associated with inflammatory degenerative and / or atrophic mucosal damage.*

Antigens and Antibodies

An *antigen* is a substance that induces the formation of antibodies because an antigen is recognized by the immune system as a *threat.* An *exogenous antigen* may be a substance from the environment such as food, inhalants, bacteria, yeast, chemicals, or toxins. An *endogenous antigen* could be a toxin such as a waste product from bacteria or virus. An *antibody* is a protein produced by the immune system in response to the presence of an antigen. Antibodies defend the body against substances identified by the immune system as potentially harmful.

A Guide to Natural Healing   75

Effects of LGS

Allergies

There is only a thin lining of mucous in the GI tract that prevents antigens from entering your bloodstream. With LGS, this mucous membrane is worn away, and there are leaks in the intestinal tissues. With LGS, large food particles leak into the bloodstream and create IgG allergic reactions (histamine release and inflammation) that target organs creating arthritis, fibromyalgia, interstitial cystitis, et cetera.

Autoimmune Diseases

With intestinal leakage and inflammation, bacteria, and other harmful microbes are able to translocate. This means that they are able to pass from the gut lumen into the bloodstream and set up infection anywhere else in the body.

For example, some genetically predisposed persons with arthritis who have leaky gut might harbor a species of bacteria called proteus in the intestine. With LGS, this bacteria leaks into the blood stream. Proteus shares a structural similarity with antigens on the surface of joints. When these antigens (proteus) are abnormally "leaked" into the circulation because of a breakdown of the normal barrier function of the gastrointestinal tract, the immune system may be activated to attack the joints, resulting in an autoimmune process.

Consequently, when an antibody is made to attack proteus, this antibody also attacks the tissues. This is probably how autoimmune diseases such as rheumatoid arthritis, lupus, multiple sclerosis, thyroiditis and many other members of the ever-growing category of "incurable" diseases start.

Immune System Stressed and Depressed

The immune system is highly stressed with LGS. As toxins, allergens, and harmful parasites contact the damaged mucosa, the immune system is activated to neutralize them from entering the body. Normally, when the gut lining is intact and healthy beneficial bacteria are present, this will maintain immunity. With LGS, antigens contact the mucosa where they will be tagged with secretory IgA (SIgA), which attracts macrophages and other white blood cells to neutralize them. When the gut lining is inflamed, the protective coating of IgA (immunoglobulin A) is overwhelmed, and the body is not able to ward off protozoa, bacteria, viruses, and candida. Of course, if there are too many toxins or undigested food particles, the immune response is overwhelmed, and not only do some toxins and allergens enter the body but the immune system becomes depleted.

LGS and Liver Stress

In LGS, the leakage of toxins and large food particles overburdens the liver so the body is less able to handle everyday chemicals.

Solving the Interstitial Cystitis Puzzle

LGS and Adrenal Exhaustion

Since the small intestines are inflamed and the area of the small intestines is so large, the adrenal glands are provoked to produce huge quantities of cortisol to attempt to suppress this inflammation. LGS slowly diminishes adrenal function. In the early and middle stages of LGS, there is actually an adrenal excess, as measured by excess cortisol output. Eventually, cortisol levels drop, and exhaustion develops. (Note: With adrenal exhaustion, the body "borrows" progesterone in order to maintain the high level of cortisol needed to suppress LGS inflammation. This sets us up for estrogen dominance, since adequate progesterone is not present to help balance estrogen.)

Dysbiosis

"First, IBS and IC are related, and most of these women have what is known as dysbiosis, which is an imbalance in the bacteria and the yeast that are normally in the bowel. Those bacteria and yeast, if they get out of equilibrium, can result in an imbalance in the gut flora, which we call 'leaky gut syndrome.' This allows foods that we would normally eat to be exposed to the immune system, which results in the development of food allergies. Diagnosing dysbiosis involves doing a specialized stool culture. Treating dysbiosis involves a low glycemic diet, acidophilus, and antifungal medications..."[1]

Eubiosis

Eubiosis, the balanced condition we are working toward, is the state of having a healthy population of bacteria in your intestines. It is the opposite of dysbiosis.

What Causes LGS?

§ *Disbiosis* is an imbalance of bacteria. Antibiotics wipe out "friendly" bacteria in the intestinal tract and allow yeast and disease-causing bacteria to flourish. Harmful parasites increase damage to the gut lining and can enter the blood stream causing disease in other parts of the body.

§ *Nonsteroidal anti-inflammatory drugs* (NSAIDS) like aspirin and Ibuprofen (Motrin, Advil) can irritate and damage the gut wall.

§ *Gut Irritants*: alcohol and caffeine are strong gut irritants.

§ *Stress* (having a chronic condition like IC is a big stressor). When we are in a "fight or flight" mode, there is *decreased* blood circulation to the gastrointestinal tract. If you have been storing up stress responses for a long time, your intestinal tract will be *chronically* "starved" for blood, and your intestinal tract will start to function imperfectly.

§ *Gluten intolerance and food allergies*. True food allergies (IgE) provoke intestinal inflammation and contribute to LGS. With LGS, large food particles are absorbed before they are fully digested into the bloodstream. This provokes an immune response creating an IgG food allergy. Every time a particular food allergen (IgE or IgG) contacts the lining of the intestines, an inflammatory immune response is mounted that further damages the epithelial lining of the intestines.

🔸 *Poor food combining* which leads to gut fermentation and acid production which increases intestinal inflammation

🔸 *Pancreatic enzymes:* low production levels

🔸 *Hydrochloric acid:* low production levels

🔸 *Bile production:* low levels or toxic bile production.

Healing LGS—"Weed, Seed, and Feed the GI Tract"
1. The Intestinal Permeability Assessment
The Intestinal Permeability Assessment from Great Smokies Labs directly measures the ability of two nonmetabolized sugar molecules—mannitol and lactulose—to permeate the intestinal mucosa. Mannitol is easily absorbed and serves as a marker of transcellular uptake, while lactulose is only slightly absorbed and serves as a marker for mucosal integrity. To perform the test, one mixes premeasured amounts of lactulose and mannitol and drinks the challenge substance. The test measures the amount of lactulose and mannitol recovered in a urine sample over the next 6 hours. *Increased* lactulose recovery has been associated with food allergy, leaky gut syndrome, and other inflammatory conditions. The *reduced* mannitol recovery indicates malabsorption as well as a decreased permeability to small molecules through the intestinal mucosal cells. Low mannitol recovery has been associated with gluten enteropathy, malabsorption and failure to thrive in children, typically a result of damage to the intestinal micro-villi.

2. Food Allergy Testing
Initially I used MRT testing with my chiropractor. Later I used York Labs and Immuno Labs to test for IgG and IgE allergies. The tests from the MRT and the labs did vary some, but the results did help me to eliminate food triggers. I also encourage an allergy elimination diet and food challenges. Once you have a list of your food allergens, eliminate them from your diet for at least three to six months. You may carefully rotate one IgG food allergen back one at a time after three to six months to see how you tolerate it. Test each new food for three days. If you do tolerate the food, then rotate your food selections. You *must* always avoid IgE food allergies, as these are permanent. See appendix D for information on labs.

3. Parasite Testing and Treatment
I recommend doing a stool test for parasites. I use Diagnos-Techs, as they are excellent. Diagnos-Techs will test stool for 19 different parasites through stool and saliva sampling that you do in the convenience of your

home. They offer a GI-1 panel that tests for parasites and gluten allergy. GI-2 panel tests for parasites as well as gluten, dairy, egg and soy allergies. After detecting allergens eliminate them. After detecting your parasites, treat them. I suggest using Clark Pharmacy and take a compounded antimicrobial to "**weed**" out harmful parasites in the GI tract. You will need an MD to prescribe antimicrobials if certain parasites are detected.

4. Probiotics and Prebiotics

In addition to a good intestinal cleanse to help repair leaky gut, probiotics are critical. *Lactobacillus acidophilus and lactobacillus casei are the primary probiotics found in the small intestines. Bifidobacterium bifidum is the predominant beneficial bacteria found in the large intestine.* It is *vital* to "seed" with beneficial bacteria that have been destroyed with the use of antibiotics. Probiotics also help by killing hostile bacteria and yeast in the intestinal tract. The following are some protective and therapeutic roles probiotics perform in the intestinal tract:

- Kill and deactivate hostile and disease causing bacteria and yeast
- Detoxify pollutants and carcinogens
- Improve the efficiency of the digestive tract
- Eliminate constipation, diarrhea
- Manufacture certain B vitamins
- Breakdown hormones such as estrogen

Prebiotics are foods or nutrients that are used by specific bacteria that can be added to the diet to increase the chances of probiotics to grow and thrive in the intestine.

Fructooligosaccharides (FOS) are known as prebiotics. FOS are compounds made up of fructose sugar molecules linked together in long chains. They can be found naturally in such foods as Jerusalem artichoke, tubers, onions, leeks, some grains, and honey. Some probiotics contain prebiotics in them.

Generally, probiotics should not be taken with food to avoid extreme acidity during mealtimes, but follow the directions on the probiotic product that you purchase. Good products should carry a guarantee of viable colonizing bacteria up to a specific date. Probiotics should be used

- During and after antibiotic therapy
- By peri- and post-menopausal women to reduce chances of osteoporosis
- By anyone having recurrent bladder and vaginal infections
- By anyone with chronic health problems
- During and after an intestinal parasite cleanse

Tip: Open a capsule of your probiotic and pour the contents of the capsule into your mouth so it dissolves and coats the mouth and esophagus. This helps to rebalance the flora in the mouth and the esophagus. Wait thirty minutes before eating or drinking.

I have discovered probiotics by Pharmax called HLC Intensive and HLC High Potency capsules. Here is the summary by Pharmax on their probiotic: The HLC (*Human Lactic Commensals—Human strains*) range of probiotics have been developed by Pharmax and have been proven in both human clinical trials and by practitioner usage for over 10 years in Europe. In many countries in Europe, they are the market leading probiotic nutraceutical used by professional healthcare providers.

HLC (*Human strain probiotic*)—**Summary**

Tailored to address specific health/disease presentations:

🍥 Dysbiosis and overgrowth

🍥 Neonate immune system development

🍥 Chronic inflammatory conditions

🍥 Gastrointestinal (GI) tract syndromes

🍥 Stressful lifestyle

🍥 Immune maintenance with age

🍥 High potency

🍥 Guaranteed quality by independent potency analysis with each delivery

🍥 Unique and proven synergistic interactions with other nutritionals.

I am excited about HLC probiotics as they are a human strain of probiotic not bovine (cow) or soil based. It makes sense to use a probiotic that comes from a *human* source to colonize the *human* intestinal tract. I feel HLC is a powerful tool to help heal LGS. The directions are to take the Pharmax HLC Intensive, which are 7 individual packets of probiotics. Take one packet a day with a meal for 7 days in a row to help "load" the intestinal tract. Some individuals take one half packet twice a day with a meal when doing their loading doses. Follow up with two HLC High Potency capsules a day taken with food for one month. Maintain by taking one HLC High Potency capsule a day with food. Pharmax HLC probiotics are a bit costly, but I feel they are well worth the value. Refrigerate the product immediately upon delivery. You can purchase Pharmax HLC probiotics from Clark Pharmacy. See Resources in appendix D.

5. Perm A Vite

Perma A Vite is a hypoallergenic powder supplement made by Allergy Research Group used to help heal and **"feed"** LGS. It is to be taken one hour before a meal. See appendix E for more information on product.

6. L-glutamine

If you do not tolerate Perm A Vite, consider L-glutamine. It is an amino acid used to help heal and **"feed"** LGS and ulcers. L-glutamine *directly feeds* the tissue of the small intestine enabling the villi to grow and improve absorption of nutrients across the cell membrane. L-glutamine also works inside the liver to produce the super powerful amino acid glutathione, which is one of the main free radical fighters within the body.

Dosage of L-glutamine for healing LGS: start slowly with 500mg at bedtime on an empty stomach. You may increase the dose to 500 mg three times a day; take this on an empty stomach, with your last dose at bedtime. To help heal LGS, take this dose for at least three to six months. (Dosages of 500 mg to 40 grams have been recommended for LGS). Normal dosage is 1,500 to 2,000mg per day in divided doses. See a health care professional for doses larger than 2,000 mg a day.) Allergy Research Group makes a hypoallergenic powder L-glutamine.

7. Aloe Vera

The aloe plant is a natural anti-inflammatory, antibiotic, and antifungal agent but only when used in its whole-leaf form. Aloe vera is high in muccopolysaccarides and has been shown to have healing properties for the gastrointestinal tract and benefits the immune system. Persons with interstitial cystitis should be cautious about using liquid aloe vera since it must be preserved with citric acid, which might be irritating to the bladder. Freeze-dried aloe vera from the whole plant—with no additives, no fillers, and no heat treatment—has been proven to be the most effective type of aloe for helping to heal LGS and interstitial cystitis. Three capsules two to three times a day is recommended. Take aloe vera with or without food. I use and recommend Aloe Vera with Coral Calcium by Healthy Life Harvest.

8. Pancreatic Enzymes

Diagnos-Techs GI panel testing will report your status of the production of pancreatic enzymes. Plantizyme, by Thorne, contains plant enzymes for those wanting a vegetarian-source digestive enzyme formulation. Every IC client who was tested with the GI panel at Diagnos-Techs has shown extremely *low* pancreatic enzyme output. I like Thorne products as they are pure and hypoallergenic. See appendix E for contents and dosages. See appendix D for resources for Thorne information.

9. HCl and Pepsin

Betaine HCl and pepsin might help when digestive complaints are caused by underproduction of stomach acid. Contrary to popular opinion, this is a common condition exhibiting the same symptoms as acid overproduction. Common symptoms of unsufficient stomach acid production (hypochlorhydria) are: GI burning, indigestion, reflux, gas, bloating and fatigue after eating. Consult with your health care provider before adding this supplement. I recommend Thorne Betaine HCl & Pepsin.

10. Gluten Intolerance

Gluten intolerance can cause chronic intestinal inflammation and aggravate leaky gut. Your doctor can test you for gluten intolerance. Diagnos-Tech labs also tests for gluten intolerance. For now, avoid the following foods that contain gluten: wheat (durum, semolina), rye, oats, barley, spelt, triticale, kamut, and farina. *Read your labels.* Most baked goods, cereals, pastas, and crackers contain wheat which contains gluten. It can be listed as durum, enriched white flour, semolina, wheat, wheat bran, wheat germ, bulgar, couscous, triticale, wheat starch, orzo, vegetable gum, vegetable starch, modified food starch, wheat malt, or cracker meal.

Non-Gluten Grains and Starches

The following non-gluten grains & starches are allowed: buckwheat, rice, corn, potato, tapioca, bean, sorghum, soy, arrowroot, amaranth, quinoa, millet, teff, and nut flours. Some sources say oats may be used sparingly while others sources say to avoid oats.

Foods that Encourage Gut Fermentation—Bad

Sugar, cookies, cakes, soda, sweetened fruit juice, refined carbohydrates such as refined wheat, white bread, pasta, pizza, sweet rolls, muffins, cookies, sweet fruits, egg, and too much meat.

Foods that Discourage Gut Fermentation—Good

The following foods are helpful when one has a fermentation problem: Complex carbohydrates (e.g., brown rice, buckwheat, popcorn, rice cakes), vegetables, strawberries, and blueberries (non-sweet fruit), soy milk, aloe vera juice, unsweetened yogurt, goat yogurt, Kefir milk, tomatoes, sesame-seed paste, hominy grits (white corn grits), squashes, olives (black and green, not from metal can, without sulfite preservative), goat feta cheese (not cow feta), potatoes in small quantities, millet is OK most of the time, small amounts of turkey, fish, flax oil, olive oil, and rutabagas. One can use Stevia for sweetener.

Improper Food Combining

Proper food combining helps to decrease fermentation and leaky gut problems.

1. Don't mix fruits with any other foods.
2. If you have yeast problems, don't eat fruits, dried fruits, or fruit juices while working on an anti-yeast program.
3. If you use dried fruits, choose organic and unsulfured, and don't combine dried fruits with other foods. Eat small amounts.
4. Don't mix high starches with high proteins. (No meat and potatoes)
5. High starch foods and high water content vegetables are OK.
6. High protein foods and high water content vegetables are OK.

Solving the Interstitial Cystitis Puzzle

High Carbohydrates (High Starch)

avocado	beet	carrots	corn
eggplant	grains	parsnip	pastas
potato	rice	squash	turnip

High Water Content Vegetables

artichokes	aspargus	broccoli	Brussels sprouts
cabbage	cauliflower	celery	chives
cucumber	dandelion greens		endive
green beans	kale	kohlrabi	leafy greens
leeks	okra	onions	parsley
peppers (all)	radishes	sea vegetables	Swiss chard
watercress	zucchini		

High Protein Foods

dairy products	eggs	fish	legumes
meat (all)	nuts	poultry	seafood
seeds	wild game		

Fruits

apple	apricot	banana	berries
cherry	date	fig	grapefruit
lemon	mango	melons (all)	nectarine
orange	papaya	peach	pear
pineapple	plum	tomato	

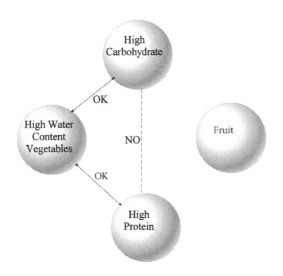

ALLERGIES

"One Man's Meat is Another Man's Poison"

—Lucretius

A person can be allergic to anything: food or beverages, chemicals, pollen and natural environmental allergens, animals, latex, et cetera. According to Dr. Moldwin, 40.6% of persons with IC also have allergies to something. [1] I suspect this percentage to be much higher.

Dr. Nambudripad, author of *Say Goodbye to Illness* states, "An allergy is an adverse physical, physiological, and/or psychological response of an individual towards one or more substances also known as allergens." [2]

The literal meaning of allergy comes from the Greek word *allos* or "altered action." A person has a biological hypersensitivity to certain substances. Traditional allergists describe an allergy as an attack of a person's own body when it is exposed to an allergen and reacts adversely even though that substance may actually be harmless to the body.

The reaction of the person's immune system towards the allergen produces IgE antibodies (immediate allergies) and IgG antibodies (delayed allergies) that release histamines. Histamines produce the different allergic reactions such as sneezing, coughing, itchy and watery eyes, sinusitis, headaches, anxiety, hyperactivity especially in children (ADHD), all kinds of inflammatory conditions.

In the case of IC, inflammation and burning of the bladder tissue when exposed to the allergen is caused by the release of histamines. The most common sites that are affected by allergic reactions are skin, eye, nose, throat, mouth, rectum, and vaginal mucosa (vulvodynia). A history of antibiotics predisposes one to LGS and its related allergies. Most persons with IC have a long history of antibiotic use.

Leaky Gut, Dysbiosis, Allergies, and IC

"First, IBS and IC are related, and most of these women have what is known as dysbiosis, which is an imbalance in the bacteria and the yeast that are normally in the bowel. Those bacteria and yeast, if they get out of equilibrium, can result in an imbalance in the gut flora, which we call 'leaky gut syndrome.' This allows foods that we would normally eat to be exposed to the immune system that results in the development of food allergies. Diagnosing dysbiosis involves doing a specialized stool culture. Treating dysbiosis involves a low glycemic diet, acidophilus, and antifungal medications..." [3]

According to Dr. Metzger, there are two types of food allergies, immediate and delayed. The immediate reaction results in an anaphylactic reaction, and there is a definite cause and effect relationship between the food eaten and the reaction. Delayed food allergies are more common, where symptoms do not develop for 12 to 72 hours after eating the food.

Food allergies can be detected by blood testing for IgE and IgG. Many allergists don't believe in IgG type of allergies. IgE allergies are considered permanent while IgG allergies are considered to be delayed food sensitivities that have developed with exposure. IgE allergies must always be avoided. To treat food allergies, start by eliminating all allergenic food for 3 months, and then gradually reintroduce small amounts of the IgG food allergens one at a time. If there is no reaction after 72 hours, add that food to your food plan.

Some persons with food allergies have fibromyalgia symptoms. The target organs for their immune complexes are the muscles. Some may get asthma, and finally others can have their bladder as their target organ. This is where one sees interstitial cystitis.

Allergists and medical doctors may order blood tests. Other non-medical health professionals can order blood tests through the mail. If you wish to save money, do self-care and go on an elimination diet. When your bladder is under good control, begin to introduce one new food every 3 days. If the bladder stays quiet, then those foods can be included in the diet. If the bladder acts up, then that food needs to be eliminated much longer. Food allergies are quite often a person's favorite foods, ones that are consumed everyday.

Leaky Gut Protocol

See the chapter on Leaky Gut Syndrome (LGS).

Vulvodynia

Pain in the vulva or vulvodynia is seen in approximately 10% of persons with IC and may be explained by a few conditions once infection or skin diseases have been ruled out:

1. A manifestation of an allergic reaction(s)
2. A consequence of decreased circulation of oxygen and nutrients related to a tissue acidosis and toxicity
3. An imbalance of essential fatty acids with a dominance of omega-6 fatty acids (See the chapter on Essential Fatty Acids.)
4. Hormone imbalances probably contribute to pain and inflammation (i.e., usually estrogen dominance with low progesterone levels).
5. Chronic yeast infection

Overacidity and Allergies

Dr. Lark states the severity of allergic reactions depends on the degree of acidity of the internal environment of the body. "When the body is overly acidic, and mast cells are activated by an allergen, they will tend to break down more quickly and are more likely to generate histamines and other inflammatory chemicals. Overacidity can both trigger the symptoms of and lengthen the period of convalescence in allergic individuals. Unfortunately, the underlying cause is often over-acidity, which is rarely treated. Many people are unaware of the role that overacidity plays in the reactivity to allergens."[4] Of course, one should avoid the offending allergens, but the key is to start an alkalizing program.

The most common food allergies are dairy, eggs, gluten grains (wheat durum, semolina, rye, oats, barley, spelt, triticale, kamut, and farina), legumes (especially soy and peanuts), nuts, corn, chocolate, fish, and shellfish. However, you can be allergic or have food intolerances to anything. I recommend getting tested initially with a blood test if possible. It is best to get an allergy test that looks for immediate food reactions (IgE) and delayed food reactions (IgG). I recommend Immuno Labs to test for IgE and IgG. (See the Resources appendix D.) Once you have a list of your food allergies, eliminate these foods immediately from your diet.

The elimination diet was developed by Dr. Albert H. Rowe and must be followed for a period of time to determine which foods are responsible for the allergic symptoms. For IC, I have discovered a group of foods that are usually well tolerated or "safe," and I suggest that you add one new food every three days to this diet to see how you react.

Some "safe" or commonly hypoallergenic foods for persons with IC to start an alkalizing program with are celery, cucumber, lettuce, yellow or green zucchini, cauliflower, cabbage, canola oil, apple, blueberries, snow peas, Chinese cabbage, jicama, Bok Choy, Chinese cabbage, avocado, rice, trout, salmon, lean turkey, or chicken. (See Getting Started chapter.)

I have found that following a "safe" alkalizing food list and then testing specific foods every three days helps one determine food intolerances. It is time consuming, but it saves you the cost of an allergy blood test. The persons I work with who do the best follow this method. After alkalizing for about a year while working on an elimination diet with food testing most of my clients' diets are quite broad, and they have no IC symptoms, vulvodynia, irritable bowel, or fibromyalgia or have very minimal symptoms. We also work on detoxing, healing the gastrointestinal tract, liver and gallbladder, adrenals, and kidneys.

Dr. Crook: Allergies and Interstitial Cystitis

"You'll probably be surprised to know that food allergies can play an important role in causing diseases and disorders in kidneys, bladder, and other parts of the urinary tract. Yet, such a relationship has been described by many observers during the past fifty years. For example, Bray in England over fifty years ago noted that bed-wetting in children was often related to food allergies. Subsequently, this same relationship has been noted by other observers including Breneman and Gerrard.

"Here's what seems to happen: When a person eats a food he's allergic to, the muscular coat around the bladder contracts. This makes the bladder smaller and keeps it from holding a normal amount of urine. As a result, the child will urinate more often during the daytime and may wet the bed at night. Although adults rarely wet the bed, a similar mechanism can make you urinate more often during the daytime and get up to go to the bathroom at night."

"Allergy may also play an important part in causing other disturbances of the urinary tract including recurrent urinary tract infections. Here is a possible mechanism. Allergic spasm of the sphincter muscle may keep you from emptying your bladder completely, which may, in turn, make you more prone to urinary tract infection. Moreover, Tatsuo Matsumura, a Japanese allergist, has carried out scientific studies which show that albumin in the urine may be related to food allergies, and Douglas Sandburg, of the University of Miami, has described other urological problems which are related to food allergies."

"Allergy can cause still other genito-urinary symptoms. The cause of such symptoms includes foods and food coloring and additives. A final note: Recently I saw a patient with extreme urinary frequency that had been diagnosed as interstitial cystitis. Following an elimination diet and challenge, her symptoms were markedly improved. Then when she added wheat and corn, her symptoms flared up." [5]

Here are some signs and symptoms of allergies:

❦ Pallor and Allergic Shiners (dark circles under the eyes)

❦ Irritable Bowel

❦ Muscle and Joint Aches

❦ Sneezing

❦ Nasal Itching

❦ Persistent Night Cough

❦ Asthma

❦ Bronchitis

❦ Headaches

❦ Irritability and Nervousness

❦ Hyperactivity (especially in children)

❦ Fatigue

❦ Urinary Problems

If you are interested in testing yourself at home, inexpensively, there is a simple, pain-free procedure called Muscle Response Testing (MRT). Biokinesiology (MRT) was discovered by a chiropractor, Dr. George

Goodheart, in the 1960s. He found that certain muscles were weak or strong muscles became weak when he touched certain acupuncture points on the body. He was able to determine organic imbalances in the person. Later he related the differences to foods and food supplements that would strengthen weak muscles and tonify the individual.

In her book, Dr. Nambudripad describes the MRT procedure: "Muscle Response Testing is the body's communication pathway with the brain. Through MRT, the patient can be tested for various allergens. MRT is a standard test used in applied kinesiology to compare the strength of a predetermined test muscle in the presence and absence of a suspected allergen. If the particular muscle (test muscle) weakens in the presence of an item, it signifies that the item is an allergen. If the muscle remains strong, the substance is not an allergen." [6]

In a pilot study attempted to determine the efficiency of MRT in detecting food allergies, the serum test for IgE and IgG confirmed 19 of 21 food allergies that tested positive (muscle weakening or inhibition) with MRT having a screening efficiency rate of 90.5%.

Regarding MRT, simply stated, the human body is generally an efficient electrical current and when it is exposed to an allergen, this allergen "short-circuits" our system and causes a weakness in the current (muscle weakness when tested with MRT).

MRT Technique: There is an examiner and an examinee (the one being tested). Stand about two feet apart facing each other. Face each others left or right shoulder. Take care that you do not stand right in front of each other. You can choose either arm to start, and you can alternate them when one arm tires.

Let us say we will start with testing the examinee's left arm strength. You are about two feet apart from each other and you, the examiner, are looking at the examinee's left shoulder. Next, place your left palm firmly on the examinee's right shoulder to begin a circuit of energy flow. The examinee's arms are hanging loose at her sides, and the examinee is looking straight ahead. Now have the examinee raise her left arm straight out approximately 90 degrees (it does not have to be exactly 90 degrees) in front or off to the side with the left hand hanging loose, slightly flexed downwardly. The examiner will press down with the right hand on the examinee's left wrist joint (examiner's skin touching the examinee's wrist). You only need a gentle exertion of about 5 to 7 pounds of pressure. Both examiner and examinee need to keep their hands open and relaxed. Next, you need to press gently on the examinee's wrist while the examinee resists.

You are not trying to overpower the examinee; you are determining, as examiner and examinee, the relative strength of the indicator muscle of the examinee. The examiner will press downward for a second or two to determine the indicator muscle strength or resistance of the examinee. The

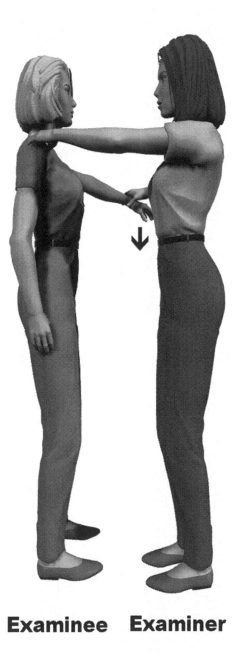

Examinee Examiner

examiner needs to press with the same pressure each time, and the examiner needs to resist with the same effort each time. If you or the examinee begins to tire, switch to the other arm, or take a break.

Now that you have determined the relative strength of the indicator muscle of the examinee's left arm place the allergen in the examinee's right hand that is hanging loosely at her side and muscle test again for any signs of weakening of the indicator muscle of the examinee's left arm when the allergen is introduced. If you find that the examinee's baseline indicator muscle strength is weak initially, you can gently massage the examinee's acupuncture point an inch under the navel for 30 seconds to help rebalance energy, and try retesting the muscle strength again before testing with an allergen.

Oval Ring Test: You can also perform MRT with an oval ring test. The examinee sits in a comfortable chair while pressing the ring finger and thumb together firmly while the examiner applies a gentle pressure to pull the fingers apart.

You can determine the indicator muscle strength of the examinee's finger grip and then introduce an allergen and test for any weakening. When the indicator ring finger gets tired, you can use the index and thumb or the middle finger and thumb then switch hands when the examinee gets tired. I prefer the oval ring test myself.

It will take some practice to determine the baseline strength of the muscles or grip being tested, but with practice, you can become very proficient with MRT.

If you wish to test a surrogate such as a pet, infant or child, or invalid have the examinee hold the pet or infant/child. The child or invalid can touch the skin of the examinee while the examinee holds the allergen. You must maintain skin to skin contact of the examinee and surrogate otherwise the surrogate will not receive the results of the testing. The examiner's hand needs to touch the skin of the examinee respectively.

Conclusion

If the examinee is allergic to an allergen, the indicator muscle will weaken. If the examinee is not allergic to the allergen, the muscle will remain strong. If the surrogate is allergic to an allergen, the indicator muscle of the examinee will weaken. If the surrogate is not allergic to the allergen, the indicator muscle of the examinee will remain strong.

Rules to Follow While Doing MRT
- Avoid fluorescent lighting
- Remove jewelry
- No music or noise while testing
- No eating, drinking, smoking or chewing gum
- Examiner and examinee look straight ahead and try to relax

Oval Ring Test

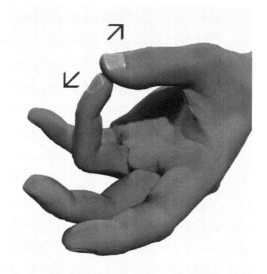

- Do not cross hands, arms, legs, or feet
- If the arm being tested weakens when testing an allergen, push the arm all the way down with a full swing to the examinee's side
- Examiner always tests with the same pressure
- Examinee always resists with the same pressure
- Be patient, and practice the MRT technique for best results

Finally, for those of you who are open-minded, curious, and wish to eliminate all of your allergies, Dr. Nambudripad, has written a book *Say Goodbye to Illness*. In her book, she discusses allergies and related health disorders and has established NAET (Nambudripad's Allergy Elimination Techniques) where she claims to combine allopathy, acupuncture, chiropractic, kinesiology, and nutrition to create a unique healing technique to permanently eliminate allergies. She states that over 2,500 licensed medical practitioners have been trained in NAET worldwide.

Personally, I have not found NAET to be effective, but several members of the IC Puzzle group have reported positive results.

Tips for Living with Allergies
- Stay inside in an air-conditioned building or car and keep the windows closed when pollen counts are high.
- Shower and change clothes after spending time outdoors.
- Don't hang clothes out to dry.

- Sleep on a hypoallergenic mattress and pillow. (No feathers or down)
- Have someone else do yard work.
- Use unscented soap, shampoo, and laundry detergent.
- Use environmentally sensitive cleaning supplies such as tea tree oil, baking soda, and vinegar.
- Eliminate mucous-forming foods, such as sugar, wheat, dairy products.
- Eat fruits and vegetables rich in the bioflavonoids, including quercetin, which is found in apples, onions, green tea, black tea, green leafy vegetables, and beans.
- Request that people you work with refrain from wearing perfume or cologne.

Solving the Interstitial Cystitis Puzzle

THE LIVER

"Life loves the liver of it."

— Maya Angelou

The liver is miraculous because of its diversity of life-sustaining functions. If we had to list the functions of the liver in the body, we would list over five hundred functions. The average healthy liver produces over 2,000 recognized enzymes and 2,000 unrecognized enzymes. It filters a liter (one quart) of blood every minute and produces one to one and a half quarts of bile each day. It is the central chemical laboratory in the body as well as the body's most important detoxifier. It is so important that man can only live a few hours without liver function. The liver is the body's primary "anti-pollution" organ. It is in charge of removing potential toxins from the blood stream. The liver detoxifies and excretes into the bile drugs, pesticides, and hormones such as estrogen and chemicals such as histamines. Through the bile, the liver is able to remove certain drugs and heavy metals such as mercury. It is responsible for destroying and removing red blood cells that have out lived their effectiveness. It is also responsible for the formation of most of the blood's clotting agents. It cleanses poisons, toxins, and excessive build up of wastes. The liver aids in the metabolism of carbohydrates, fat, protein, and the storage of vitamins and minerals. Other functions include regulating blood sugar levels and balancing hormone levels by breaking down estrogen to a weaker form of estriol.

The liver has almost detergent like abilities to break up saturated fats and oils making it possible to eliminate them. It breaks down poisons from alcohol, soda, hair sprays, deodorants, *et cetera*. In a healthy detoxified liver, the left lobe is the area that produces the anti-allergens and antihistamines which control hay fever, allergies, and sensitivities

Most of us eat the wrong things and pass up what would nourish the liver and other organ systems. Stressful lifestyles, high fat, high sugar, high protein diets stress the liver. We are routinely exposed to nicotine, toxins of various kinds, and a whole host of synthetic drugs from Ibuprofen to steroids. Overeating especially overcooked, fatty foods puts added strain on the liver. With interstitial cystitis, LGS puts another stress on the liver. The liver is responsible for detoxifying *everything* that enters the body. Everything that enters the liver through the portal vein from the digestive system must be detoxified and neutralized. Everything we eat or drink, breathe, and absorb through our skin must be detoxified by the liver.

Some of the more detrimental compounds we ingest that increase the liver's workload include

§ High protein diets

§ Alcohol

- Caffeine
- Nicotine
- Pesticides and herbicides
- Saturated fats
- Heavy metals

The American Liver Foundation reports that more than 25 million people are afflicted with liver and gallbladder disease each year. Over 27,000 Americans die from cirrhosis annually, making it the country's third leading cause of death for people between the ages of 25 and 59 and the seventh leading cause of death overall. Viruses, hereditary defects, and reactions to drugs and chemicals are among the known causes of liver breakdown.

Dr. Sandra Cabot, MD, (The Liver Doctor) author of the book *The Liver Cleansing Diet* states, "If you talk to radiologists and gastroenterologists who are looking at people's livers today they will tell you that the condition 'Fatty Liver' affects more than 50% of people over the age of 50."

Dr. Cabot reports that common causes of unexplained idiopathic liver disease is seen in affluent societies related to diets high in saturated fats, refined sugars, excessive alcohol intake, adverse reactions to drugs and toxic environmental chemicals, and viral hepatitis. Dr. Cabot believes that many "mysterious" diseases where the causes cannot be pinpointed are related to reduced liver function. Many would classify IC as a "mysterious" disease.

There are tests to check for liver function. An ultrasound scan or CAT scan can be performed to evaluate the size and shape of the liver. Blood tests can check the level of serum bilirubin and bile acids that might be elevated in certain types of liver and gallbladder disease. Blood tests to measure the levels of liver enzymes may show abnormally high levels if the liver cells are damaged or ruptured, causing them to release their intracellular enzymes into the blood stream. The liver enzymes are called alkaline phosphatase (ALK.PHOS), gamma glutamyl transpeptidase (gamma-GT), glutamic oxaloacetic transaminase (SGOT), and glutamic pyruvic transaminase (SGPT). In the early stages of liver disease where there is only minimal damage to the liver cells there is often only a very slight elevation of the liver enzymes (SGOT and SGPT). In alcohol excess, a common finding is an elevation of the liver enzyme gamma-GT. In persons with chronic liver disease and some gallbladder disease there is a large increase in the levels of blood fats, total cholesterol, and triglycerides. This is to be expected because the liver is the major organ for overall fat balance and metabolism. According to Dr. Cabot, chronic liver disease passes through a long period of minimal vague symptoms.

Dr. Cabot states that conditions of the immune system such as allergies, hay fever, some types of arthritis and autoimmune diseases will dramatically improve by cleansing and healing the liver. Dr. Cabot reports that if the liver is not an effective barrier, toxins, and incompletely digested food find their way into our blood stream and are carried deeper into the body where they must be dealt with by the immune system. These toxins can then damage the cells of other body organs and the immune system and inflammation in its many forms begins.

To summarize, due to the aging process, poor eating habits, toxic exposures and hectic lifestyles the liver function becomes compromised. How does this effect IC? We know that most persons with IC are sensitive to many allergies, foods, chemicals, additives, toxins, drugs, and hormone fluctuations. We learned earlier in the Chapter Defining Interstitial Cystitis that according to Dr. Theoharides, drugs, chemicals, hormones, toxins, free radicals, antigens have the ability to trigger mast cell secretion. Recall that mast cell secretion with the release of histamine is what leads to the pain and inflammation in the bladder.

It follows, if the liver is compromised, it will not be capable of effectively filtering, detoxifying, and neutralizing the triggers of mast cell secretion. We would see a continued presence of IC symptoms when the liver is weak. In addition, the liver is a vital organ that produces our natural antihistamines. If the liver is not functioning at full capacity, this ability to produce natural antihistamines will be diminished. You should see a reduction of IC symptoms once the liver is cleansed, detoxified, and supported nutritionally. A strong and vital liver will completely detoxify mast cell triggers (for example, neutralize drugs, toxins, additives, and break down estrogen) and produce natural antihistamines.

According to the late Dr. Henry G. Bieler, MD, in his book, *Food is Your Best Medicine*, the liver is the *second* line of defense against disease (the *first* line of defense he states is digestion). Dr. Bieler states that as long as the liver function is intact, the blood stream remains pure. When it is impaired, the toxins enter the circulation and cause irritation, destruction and eventually death.

"Of all the alkaline elements of the body, sodium is the most important. It is my belief that the liver is the storehouse of these elements, especially of sodium. It is the element found in the greatest abundance and is the most needed in maintaining the body's acid-base balance. Sodium is found in every cell of the body; also, there are large concentrated sodium-storage centers to be used in case of emergency. These concentrated areas have a great buffer value; in addition, much acid and corrosive poison can be neutralized and stored in them, more or less temporarily. Among the important sodium storage reservoirs are the muscles, brain and nerves, bone marrow, skin, gastric and intestinal mucosa, the kidneys and the liver, which is by far the most important; it is richest of all the organs in sodium, its chief chemical element. Therefore, as the largest storehouse of sodium the liver is clearly the body's second line of defense.

"When the liver is depleted of sodium in order to neutralize acids, its function may be so severely inhibited that illness results. Are you aware that if the liver could keep the blood stream clean by filtering out damaging poisons, man could live indefinitely, barring physical accidents? It is only when the liver's filtration ability is hindered that the poisons get beyond the liver and into the general blood circulation. Only then do the symptoms of disease occur. And that is why you must guard your liver so carefully.

"If, then, sodium is so important to good health, how do we obtain it? How can we observe it? Sodium, the body's vital element is derived from the sodium compounds in the diet. The richest source is in the vegetable kingdom...an individual who eats few vegetables and salads and much over-cooked meat frequently has a sodium-starved liver.

"After digestion of any meal, all of the blood from the intestines circulates through the liver, entering it by way of the large portal vein which flows directly into it. The useful elements from the digested food are taken to the liver which (1) synthesizes new body tissues, (2) prepares fuel for oxidation, and energy, (3) and stores excess nourishment for future use.

"Toxins and other harmful substances are neutralized by the liver and eliminated by the excretory secretion of the liver. This secretion is called bile. Sometimes the power of the liver to neutralize these toxic substances completely is curtailed because of insufficient alkalinity. The bile is then released to the small intestine in a toxic state. During the coursing of this toxic bile through the small intestine, if it has not already caused enough nausea to be eliminated quickly by vomiting, much of the harmful material is reabsorbed. At the same time it may cause various degrees of intestinal inflammation.

"The presence of toxic bile in the intestine can also upset its digestion of useful food, giving rise to toxic indigestion...In some respects bile is comparable to urine. Normally, it is clear bright yellow, alkaline in reaction and non-irritating to the tissues which confine it. When pathological, it changes to darker colors, being most toxic when dark green or black, at which time it has an intense acid and corrosive action on adjacent tissues. This dark green bile can do nothing but harm. Normal alkaline bile is non-corrosive and compatible with almost all food. But as the liver is gradually depleted of its sodium—leached out for the neutralization of toxins—the normal sodium salts of the bile acids are formed with greater difficulty...When there is a too rapid drain of the liver's available sodium, the liver cells die." [1]

The Symptoms of an Unhappy Liver

Symptoms of liver dysfunction may occur even though all blood tests of liver function are "normal." The tests that doctors use routinely to check the liver are not very sensitive—they check for liver *damage* rather than *function*.

Common symptoms due to poor liver function are:

❦ Poor digestion, abdominal bloating, nausea especially after fatty foods, weight gain around the abdomen and diarrhea and/or constipation. Irritable bowel syndrome, associated with abdominal swelling and flatulence, is often due to a sluggish liver. If you wake up in the morning with bad breath and/or a coated tongue, your liver definitely needs help.

❦ Unpleasant mood changes: quick to anger, depression, "foggy brain" and impaired concentration and memory. If the liver is sluggish, excessive amounts of toxic metabolites find their way into the blood stream and can affect the function of the brain.

❦ Allergic conditions such as hay fever, hives, skin rashes and asthma

❦ Headaches. Unfortunately, pain killers can cause further stress on the liver as the liver is the organ that breaks down all drugs.

❦ High blood pressure and/or fluid retention. These may be difficult to control with drug therapy. A liver cleansing diet has been known to bring down high blood pressure to completely normal levels without any drugs being required. *Never stop your medicines without medical supervision.*

❦ Hypoglycemia or unstable blood sugar levels. An unhappy liver can cause fluctuations of blood sugar level with low glucose levels causing fatigue, dizziness, light-headedness, and craving for sugar.

❦ Inability to tolerate fatty foods, gallbladder disease and gallstones. If you feed your liver too much saturated or damaged (rancid) fat, it will try to pump it out of your body through the bile which flows into the gallbladder and then the small intestine. This will raise the cholesterol content of your bile and can result in gallstones (made of hard cholesterol) and gallbladder inflammation. If your liver is not working efficiently, it will not manufacture enough bile salts to keep biliary cholesterol in solution, so gallbladder stones may result.

❦ Fatigue and chronic fatigue syndrome. When tired people cannot find a cause for their ill-health, they are usually eating too much saturated and damaged fats and not enough raw vegetables, fruits, and sprouts.

❦ Excessive body heat, which may be associated with sweating or body odor.

❦ Lowered tolerance to alcohol and various drugs such as antibiotics.

❦ High cholesterol levels, cholesterol can only be removed from the body by the liver in the form of bile and a high fiber diet.

Liver Tonics

Dr. Cabot suggests that liver tonics are helpful for the liver in many ways and can be obtained in powder and capsule form. A good liver tonic needs to contain a synergistic mixture of natural ingredients that work together to support liver function. There are many liver tonics available, from Swedish bitters to tinctures containing various herbs, and these types of tonics have been used for centuries. It is important to use a powerful liver tonic that contains the most essential natural substances for healthy liver function. Such a powerful liver tonic is able to support the detoxification pathways in the liver which breakdown toxins. It is also able to improve the structural and functional integrity of the liver cells and liver filter. Dr. Cabot has designed excellent liver tonics called Livatone and Livatone Plus. Livatone does not contain the B complex vitamins. Livatone Plus does contain B complex vitamins.

I prefer the powder form of Livatone Plus mixed in water. Many persons with IC take plenty of pills already, so the powder form means fewer pills to swallow. It can be added to a vegetable juice instead of water if you wish.

Livatone Plus

Livatone Plus contains the following natural ingredients:

- Glutamine
- Glycine
- Taurine
- Cysteine
- Vitamin C
- Vitamin E
- Natural Carotenoids
- Thiamine (Vitamin B1)
- Riboflavine (Vitamin B2)
- Nicotinamide (Vitamin B3)
- Calcium Pantothenate (Vitamin B5)
- Pyridoxine (Vitamin B6)
- Cyanocobalamin (Vitamin B12)
- Folic Acid
- Biotin
- Inositol
- Lecithin
- Zinc
- St Mary's Thistle (Milk Thistle)
- Cruciferous Vegetables
- Green Tea

The following is a description by Dr. Cabot about the ingredients in Livatone Plus:

Amino Acids

Specific amino acids are essential for the liver to breakdown toxins and drugs and also for the efficient metabolism of nutrients by the liver.

Glutamine

This amino acid is required for phase two detoxification in the liver and is required in increased amounts by those who consume excessive alcohol. It is able to reduce the craving for alcohol. Glutamine supplementation is helpful for intestinal disorders such as peptic ulcers and LGS. *Leaky gut increases the workload of the liver and may cause many health problems.* Glutamine is converted in the body into the powerful liver protector glutathione.

Glutathione is essential for liver phase two conjugation reactions used during detoxification of drugs and toxic chemicals. Glutathione is a potent antioxidant that is produced in the healthy liver where it neutralizes oxygen molecules before they can damage cells. Glutathione levels decline with age, and this may accelerate the aging process. It is not worth taking glutathione supplements, as they are expensive and usually poorly absorbed. It is far more effective to increase glutathione levels by giving the liver, the raw materials it needs to make its own glutathione, namely, the amino acids glycine, glutamine and cysteine.

Glycine

This amino acid performs more biochemical functions than any other amino acids. It is required for the synthesis of bile salts and is used by the liver to detoxify chemicals in the phase-two detoxification pathways.

Taurine

Inadequate levels of taurine are common in persons with chemical sensitivities, allergies, and poor diets. Taurine is the major amino acid required by the liver for the removal of toxic chemicals and metabolites. It is required for the healthy production of bile, and the liver uses it to conjugate toxins and drugs to excrete through the bile. It is found in animal protein such as meat, seafood, eggs, and dairy products but not in vegetable protein. Taurine is often deficient in strict vegans.

Cysteine

Cysteine is an amino acid that contains sulphur and is needed by the phase-two detoxification pathway. It is a precursor of glutathione, which is needed to breakdown pollutants and toxins and has powerful antioxidant effects.

Antioxidants

Antioxidants destroy free radicals and help to detoxify and protect the cells of the body, including the liver cells, from toxins.

Vitamin C

Vitamin C is the most powerful antioxidant vitamin for the liver and reduces toxic damage to the liver cells from chemical overload. It neutralizes free radicals generated during the phase one detoxification pathway in the liver.

Vitamin E

Natural vitamin E is biologically more active than synthetic vitamin E. Vitamin E is a powerful antioxidant that protects fats from damage. Since cell membranes are composed of fats, vitamin E is the best protector of cell membranes. Thus vitamin E can help to protect the membranes surrounding liver cells.

Natural Carotenoids

Carotenoids such as beta-carotene are most commonly found in fruits and vegetables and are most significant for human health. It is important to take only natural sources of beta-carotene and other carotenoids. Beta-carotene is converted in the body to vitamin A and yet has none of the toxic side effects of high doses of vitamin A.

B Vitamins

Thiamine (Vitamin B 1)

This B vitamin has antioxidant properties and is helpful in reducing the toxic effects of alcohol, smoking, and lead. Thiamine protects against many of the metabolic imbalances caused by alcohol. Deficiency of thiamine will often lead to poor mental function.

Riboflavin (Vitamin B 2)

This B vitamin is required during phase one detoxification in the liver and is crucial in the production of body energy.

Nicotinamide (Vitamin B 3)

This is also known as Niacinamide and is required by the liver's phase one detoxification system. It is needed for the metabolism of fats and helps to keep cholesterol levels under control.

Calcium Pantothenate (Vitamin B 5)

Several studies have found that pantothenate can lower cholesterol (by an average of 15%) and triglycerides (by an average of 30%) in those with elevated levels of these blood fats. A study showed that pantothenate speeds up liver detoxification.

Pyridoxine (Vitamin B 6)

Vitamin B 6 is required for effective phase one liver detoxification, and is essential for physical and mental health. Vitamin B 6 inhibits the formation of a toxic chemical called homocysteine, which accelerates cardiovascular disease.

Solving the Interstitial Cystitis Puzzle

Cyanocobalamin (Vitamin B 12)

Supplements of this powerful vitamin are essential for those who are strict vegetarians or those with nervous complaints. It is a great energizer of the nervous system and can reduce depression and fatigue. It is required for phase one detoxification of chemicals in the liver, and can help people who are allergic to sulphites, which are common food and wine additives. A study showed that vitamin B 12 can effectively block most of the adverse reactions to sulphites such as hay fever, sinus, headache, and bronchial spasms. B 12 is required for the liver to perform methylation, which inactivates the hormone estrogen and enhances the flow of bile.

Folic Acid

Folic acid is required for the phase one detoxification pathway in the liver and for cell repair and division. Some studies have shown that folic acid exerts an anti-cancer effect.

Biotin

Biotin is one of the B vitamins and is produced in the intestines by friendly bacteria. It is found in foods such as nuts, whole grain foods, vegetables, brewer's yeast, and in supplement form. Liver cells that lack biotin will be deprived of the energy they need to detoxify chemicals and drugs. Deficiency of this vitamin is not rare and can cause hair loss, dry flaky skin, rashes, and fatigue. Those with a poor diet or long term antibiotic use are at risk of deficiency.

Inositol

Inositol is important in fat metabolism and helps to remove fats from the liver. Deficiency of inositol can increase hardening of the arteries, increase blood cholesterol levels and lead to hair loss, constipation, and mood swings. Excessive consumption of caffeine can reduce the level of inositol in the body.

Lecithin

Lecithin contains healthy fats that are required for the functional and structural integrity of cell membranes. Lecithin is composed of the B vitamin choline, along with linoleic acid and inositol. A choline deficiency promotes liver damage and can be corrected with lecithin supplements.

Zinc

The mineral zinc has antioxidant properties and is part of the powerful antioxidant enzyme called superoxide dismutase (SOD). Zinc is vital for the efficient functioning of the cellular immune system needed to fight infections from viruses, parasites, and fungal microorganisms.

St. Mary's Thistle (Milk Thistle)

Milk thistle, also known as "Silybum Marianum," is an herb with remarkable detoxifying and liver protective effects. It is a very well known liver herb, having been recommended in herbal texts since the late 1600s. Its most active constituent is silymarin, which is a bioflavonoid. Research has shown that milk thistle can protect against some severe liver toxins. Liver disorders in humans have been treated with silymarin with promising results. Most liver toxins produce damage to cell membranes via free radical generation. Silymarin functions as an antioxidant and reduces damage to cell membranes. It prevents the formation of leukotrienes, which are dangerous inflammatory chemicals produced by the immune system. Silymarin can increase the quantity of the powerful liver protector glutathione and improves protein synthesis in the liver.

Cruciferous vegetables

Cruciferous vegetables such as broccoli, cauliflower, cabbage, Brussels sprouts, kale, bok choy, mustard greens, and radish contain important substances such as indoles, thiols, and sulphur compounds, which enhance the liver's phase one and two detoxification pathways. Broccoli has a particularly good effect and enhances glutathione conjugation of toxins. There is evidence that cruciferous vegetables are able to reduce the risk of cancer, and the American Cancer Society has been saying, "A defense against cancer can be cooked up in your kitchen."

Green tea

Green tea exerts strong antioxidant actions and is also able to inhibit cancer cell growth. The Chinese, who are large drinkers of green tea, have a 60% less chance of esophageal cancer. Parts of Japan where people drink a lot of green tea have a lower incidence of many types of cancers, including stomach, esophageal, and liver cancer.

Dr. Cabot suggests the following dosages for Livatone Plus

Livatone Plus contains all of the preceding ingredients finely ground and mixed together in either powder or capsule form.

This is more economical and convenient than having to take them all individually. The tonic can be taken in a dose of one teaspoon mixed in fresh juice just before meals, twice daily, or two capsules just before food, twice daily. Take this dosage for eight to twelve weeks. Then go on to a maintenance dose of one teaspoon daily, or two capsules daily, which can be continued for as long as needed. Some people find that they need to stay on a liver tonic in a maintenance dose permanently because of dysfunctional liver problems. Those who have a very dysfunctional liver, a fatty liver, or problems with excessive weight can continue safely on the higher dose. Children over 3 years of age can take the powder in a reduced dosage of 1/4 to 1/3 of a teaspoon, mixed in fruit juice twice daily, before meals. *When beginning any liver tonic for the first time, always commence with a low dosage, say one quarter of the recommended dosage; ½ a teaspoon of powder daily or 1 capsule daily, and stay on this low dose for the first week. Beginning with the maximum dose of a liver tonic may stimulate the liver's release of toxins too quickly, which could cause nausea, vomiting, or headaches and other symptoms of a healing crisis.*

I prefer to use Livatone Plus in the powder form so the dosage is easier to adjust than taking the capsules. I have observed that taking this liver tonic will definitely improve your liver function, but I can also say that for many of you it might make your bladder uncomfortable initially. This is due to toxins being released from the liver and probably some of the ingredients. You may wish to start by cutting Dr. Cabot's recommended doses in half. For example, instead of starting with ½ teaspoon of the powder in water once a day as she suggests, start with only ¼ teaspoon once a day and work you way up to full the full dose of one teaspoon twice a day for eight to twelve weeks. Then go on a maintenance dose she recommends on the container. If you can tolerate this tonic, take as directed for eight to twelve weeks. If you are too uncomfortable with the liver tonic you may wish to take smaller doses of this tonic for a week or two and then give yourself a rest for a week. Then resume the tonic. Gradually building up the dose and taking periods of rest.

If you find Dr. Cabot's Livatone Plus liver tonic too strong, Dr. Myers suggests the following supplements for liver cleansing and detoxification:

1. Livaplex made by Standard Process. Livaplex contains some animal products. Standard Process products are only dispensed by health care professionals, but can be purchased over the Internet.

2. Livotrit Plus is made by Biotics Research for liver detoxification. Biotics Research suggests taking Livotrit Plus with Beta-TCP. Beta-TCP helps open up the biliary tracts and aids in the flow of bile. Biotics Research products are only dispensed by health care professionals but can be purchased over the Internet.

Since Standard Process and Biotics Research use only natural whole foods in their supplements; they are generally well tolerated with persons with IC. Since these products are made from *whole foods* they are "recognized" and well utilized by the body because they are *not synthetic. If* you are a strict vegetarian go with the Biotics Research liver tonics as these contain no animal products.

Another product I use and recommend is an herbal tea by Crystal Star. It is called Liv-Alive tea. It is usually well tolerated. The nice thing about Liv-Alive tea is you can adjust the potency of the tea my making it weaker or stronger related to your IC reaction. You may want to start making this tea weak and increase the strength with time. It is an excellent remedy for detoxing and strengthening the liver gently. Follow the instructions for brewing on the box.

See Chapter Nourishing Ourselves with Herbs for more information on herbs to heal the liver.

Heal and Soothe the Liver
Massage

Here are some suggestions you can do at home that help heal and soothe the liver and the organs in the abdomen. You can gently massage the liver and abdomen. Let's visualize where the organs are located for this massage. The liver is tucked up under the lower right rib cage and the lower edge of the liver may be felt under the ribs. The stomach and spleen rest on the left side under the left rib cage. The pancreas is located between the stomach and liver in the upper abdomen. The small and large intestines are in the lower abdomen and the bladder behind the pubic bone. The kidney and adrenal glands are located below the rib cage, one on each side of your mid-back.

First lie down on your back and get comfortable. You may do this without clothing and use massage oil if you like. A drop or two of lavender oil mixed in almond oil is relaxing and balancing for this massage or choose an essential oil that makes you feel good and you are not sensitive to. Sandalwood is another good oil for the bladder and kidneys.

You can start by gently pumping up and down over the liver with the palm of your hand. Then with palm of your hand massage with gentle but firm pressure over the liver in a circular clockwise motion. Then reverse directions and massage over the liver counter clockwise. This is very relaxing and soothing. Do this gentle liver massage for a few minutes. Visualize healing energy for the liver and gallbladder.

Try this while lying down and relaxing, too. Again, you may do this abdominal massage without clothing and use massage oil if you prefer. Gently massage your entire abdomen starting about an inch from the navel and gently but firmly with the palm of your hand massage outward in a circular clockwise motion working your way up to the edge of the rib cage and down to the pubic bone. You may wish to place one hand over the other to apply firm but gentle pressure over the organs in the abdomen. Gently massage in this circular motion clockwise for a couple of minutes while you visualize healing energy to all the organs in the abdomen; the liver, gallbladder, pancreas, stomach, spleen, small and large intestines as well as the bladder, kidneys and adrenal glands. After you have massaged the abdomen clockwise then gently repeat this massage going counter-clockwise all the while visualizing healing energy to these organs.

Yoga

Spinal Twist: Always check with your health care provider if you have a history of neck or spinal injuries or weakness before performing this exercise. Here is an easy yoga exercise that is very good for the liver. Wear loose comfortable clothing. Find a quiet place where you won't be disturbed for a few minutes. Sit cross-legged on the floor (sit on a cushion if this position causes a strain to your legs or knees). Keep your spine straight and your chin slightly pulled in so you head is in alignment with the spine. Gently grasp your hands on your shoulders with the fingers in front and the thumbs in the back. Raise your elbows so they are horizontal. Then close your eyes and gently twist left while you inhale through your nose then gently twist to the right and exhale through the nose. Repeat this pattern for a few minutes as tolerated, twisting left and then to the right. All breathing should be done through the nose. Obviously, if you have nasal congestion then you will breathe through your mouth until your congestion improves. Remember, inhaling left and exhaling right as you twist. This will gently massage the liver and internal organs and help with detoxification. Lie down and rest a few minutes after the exercise. Don't over do this exercise or you may start to experience nausea. Drink plenty of water after doing this exercise as tolerated.

Coffee Enemas for Powerful Liver Detoxification

Many persons with IC complain that they cannot drink coffee anymore. Well, there is one way you can have your coffee, but it is from the other end in the form of a coffee enema. Organic coffee taken by enema is a powerful detoxification tool. Coffee enemas have been used for at least 100 years and studies show that a caffeine solution administered by enema stimulates the production of bile and helps to detoxify the liver. A coffee enema floods the lower colon and the caffeine is absorbed through the veins in the lower colon and then into the portal vein and then to the liver. The caffeine that enters the liver through the portal vein causes the blood vessels and bile ducts in the liver to dilate and release bile along with toxins into the bowel. According to Dr. Lark, "a coffee enema that lasts 10 to 12 minutes can facilitate significant purging of toxins from the liver and colon." [2]

When planning to do a coffee enema, give yourself about an hour to prepare the coffee and administer the enema. The caffeine taken by coffee enema is not assimilated the same way coffee taken by mouth is. You do not get a caffeine rush. If I drank coffee made with three tablespoons of coffee, I would definitely be jittery and up all night. However, I have done these enemas many times. Several times I took the coffee enema I did it in the early evening, fell asleep easily, and slept very soundly. After administering the coffee enema, I felt a soft gentle healing flow of energy around the area of the liver and gallbladder. It felt soothing, relaxing, and cleansing. Some people say that after the enemas they feel relaxed and fall asleep easily. Some of the coffee enemas I took however did seem to stimulate me. It was not a wiry jittery nervous feeling; I felt just more energized. For this reason, I recommend doing coffee enemas in the morning or early afternoon so if the procedure does energize you, your sleep will not be disturbed.

What you Need to Do a Coffee Enema:

- Enema bag (never share your enema bag...only one per customer)
- Lubricant such as K-Y® Brand Jelly, Slippery Stuff®, or vegetable oil
- Organic *caffeinated* drip ground coffee
- Spring water free of chemicals
- Old towel to place under you
- Some pillows for comfort under your head
- A timer or clock to mark the time
- Bring reading material, listen to music/meditation tape, or simply relax

How to Make the Coffee

Place three tablespoons of loose organic caffeinated drip ground coffee in one quart of spring water. Use a ceramic or stainless steel pan *not* aluminum. Boil the loose coffee grounds in the water for five minutes then lower the heat and simmer for 15 minutes. Strain the coffee and let it cool to body temperature.

How to Do a Coffee Enema

Put the enema bag and the end of the tubing in the sink in the bathroom and close the clamp. Pour about 4 to 6 ounces of the warm strained coffee into the bag. Open the clamp over the sink and allow the coffee to flow to the tip of the catheter to remove the air from the tubing. Place some lubricant on the tip of the catheter. Hang the enema bag on a towel rack or door handle. Lie down on your towel on your right side in a fetal position with your knees drawn up, and gently insert the lubricated catheter tip into the rectum a few inches. Hold the catheter in place with one hand and release the clamp with your other hand to allow the fluid to flow into the colon. Breathe deeply and try to relax. If you experience discomfort or fullness close the clamp. Retain the fluid for ten minutes to ensure the caffeine reaches the bile ducts in the liver. After ten to twelve minutes, expel the enema in the toilet as a normal bowel movement. If you have an immediate urge to release the enema, do so, and then repeat the procedure until you have used all the coffee fluid.

Helpful Tips

Here are some tips I found useful. It is helpful to take a plain warm water enema to cleanse the colon first of stool. This makes it easier to retain the coffee enemas. In the beginning, take only four to six ounces. With time and practice you will be able to hold more fluid maybe up to eight ounces. If the coffee fluid is warm it is easier to retain then when the coffee has become cold. You may want to reheat the last of the coffee carefully if it feels too cool. It should only be warm to the touch, *never* hot. As with all procedures, supplements, and foods, everyone has different tolerances. You might experience some increase in IC symptoms or you might not. Some report a slight to moderate increase in IC symptoms after the coffee enemas, and drinking more water will diminish these symptoms.

Alternative medical doctors who use coffee enemas with their patients recommend that coffee enemas can safely be taken once a day during a detoxification program. There is no indication that coffee enemas disrupt normal bowel functions. There is little risk of flushing out vitamins or minerals since they are absorbed in the small intestines and this enema is given in the lower bowel.

Some signs of toxicity from releasing toxins too quickly are headaches, fever, nausea, intestinal spasms, and fatigue. I had none of these problems. If you experience these symptoms take the enemas less frequently, or stop and take a break. Persons with inflammatory bowel disease should use coffee enemas cautiously or not at all.

Gallbladder/Liver Flush (see Gallbladder/Liver Flush Chapter on this procedure)

Liver Friendly Foods

Foods on an alkalizing diet are excellent for the liver. An alkalizing diet is a diet rich in vegetables, fruits, and sprouts, and this provides the organic sodium and minerals the liver requires to heal itself and detoxify the body. Here are foods that help support liver health. Remember everyone is different and you must carefully select the foods you are not allergic or sensitive to.

§ Raw vegetables, especially cruciferous vegetables such as broccoli, Brussels sprouts, cabbage, cauliflower, garlic, and onions. Fruits and vegetables with deep bright pigments such as orange, yellow, red, and green are very cleansing: carrots, pumpkin, red cabbage, avocados, olives, and seaweeds. Cooked vegetables should only be lightly steamed. Fresh raw vegetables, fruits, and sprouts are very healing.

§ Legumes which are cooked or sprouted, like beans, lentils, and peas

§ Spices (as tolerated) chili, ginger, coriander, curry, cayenne, turmeric, basil, rosemary, and fennel

§ Sprouts and grasses such as sunflower sprouts, mung bean sprouts, wheat grass, and barley grass are good sources of chlorophyll, which is very liver cleansing. Make sure to eat a variety of sprouts every day.

- No dairy products. They are hard on the liver.

- Whole grains such as amaranth, buckwheat, corn, quinoa, millet, and rice.

- Chicken, preferably free-range, and remove the skin

- Eggs from free-range poultry

- Seafood such as tuna, salmon, sardines, and mackerel

- Avoid eating raw, smoked, or deep fried fish. Note: histamines in foods can pose a problem with IC. You might want to avoid tuna, mackerel, bluefish, mahi mahi, herring, and sardines since these tend to have higher levels of histamines. Shellfish should be avoided since they contain high levels of mercury and toxins. Salmon and trout seem to be well tolerated in persons with IC.

- Spreads such as hummus, tahini, nut butters, honey, natural fruit jams with no added sugar, and fresh avocado

- Cold pressed virgin vegetable and seed oils such as olive, safflower, sunflower, canola, and grapeseed. Buy unrefined oils that are mechanically pressed (genuinely cold-pressed) and kept in dark colored glass bottles to block out the light, since this can reduce rancidity. Keep oils in the refrigerator to decrease rancidity. Use a stir fry "wet method" by adding water or vegetable, chicken, or beef broth to a wok or fry pan, and stir fry for five to ten minutes. Add the oil to the dish after removing from the heat. Avoid foods that are fried since these foods contain harmful trans fatty acids. Avoid foods that have a label that reads, "...may contain partially hydrogenated soybean oil, sunflower oil, safflower oil, or corn oil."

- Salt free or low salt breads from whole grain or multi-grain, especially sprouted grain breads, free of hydrogenated vegetable oils or fats.

- Raw nuts such as almonds, cashews, and walnuts with no added salt

- Raw seeds such as sunflower, sesame, and pumpkin seeds with no added salt

- Beverages such as soy milk, almond milk, rice milk, filtered or purified water, fruit or vegetable juices without added sugar or salt, herb teas, or green tea

Gallbladder / Liver Flush

"For all things produced in a garden, whether of salads or fruits, a poor man will eat better that has one of his own, than a rich man that has none."

— J. C. Loudoun

Your liver keeps your blood clean while your liver and gallbladder secrete bile necessary for digestion. Keeping these organs clean and healthy helps your entire digestive system function better. A gallbladder/liver flush is important to help increase the flow of alkaline bile (pH of 8) into the digestive tract. This flow of alkaline bile helps to neutralize the acid load in the body and rebalance your pH. Bile helps to break down fat in the small intestine and adequate bile helps to neutralize the acidic semi-digested foods that arrive from the stomach into the small intestine. Without adequate flow of healthy alkaline bile food will not digest properly, and this leads to fermentation of food in the digestive tract and increases one's acid load. This leads to irritable bowel problems and exacerbates LGS. The liver flush helps to open the bile ducts by eliminating gallstones. Gallstones can block the flow of bile into the small intestines disrupting the proper digestion of foods. Persons with gallstones and a sluggish liver will probably have headaches, aches, and pains over the liver area and shoulder blades and neck. Every person I have coached so far that has done the gallbladder/liver flush has flushed out gallstones—much to their amazement! When my clients see how many gallstones they pass, they have their significant others do the liver flush.

By doing a liver flush, it should dramatically improve digestion, help your energy level, help balance your pH, and eliminate neck and shoulder aches and pains. You might see many gallstones in the stool the next morning and several days after the flush; they can be green, cream, black, red, or brown colored. Gallstones can be the size of sesame seeds, watermelon seeds, or olive pits.

How to Do the Gallbladder/Liver Flush:

§ Eat a no-fat breakfast and lunch, this allows bile to develop pressure. Higher pressure helps to increase the flow of bile and eliminate gallstones. Examples of low fat meals are vegetable juices, vegetable soups, and cooked alternative whole grain cereals with no fat, and plain rice milk, rice cakes, vegetables, fruits, and sprouts. Apples are fine; low acid Gala or red/yellow Delicious apples are usually well tolerated. You may eat apples: whole, fresh, or cooked or a no sugar applesauce. Baked apples or applesauce make a good natural sweetener and apples and apple juice help to soften gallstones.

- Do not eat after 2 pm. You may drink water or fresh apple juice or no sugar added apple juice diluted with water as tolerated.

- Choose a day like Saturday so you will be able to rest the next day, just in case you do not get a restful sleep.

- One hour before retiring to sleep for the night, drink one bottle of cold magnesium citrate. This is a laxative that can be purchased at a drug store. It comes in flavors such as lemon/lime or cherry. I prefer the cherry flavor. Cool this down in the refrigerator as it will taste a little better cold. Try to drink this whole bottle (10 ounces) in 15 to 30 minutes. While many practitioners suggest Epsom salts (magnesium sulfate) mixed in water, I have found Epsom salts taste horrible. Some IC Puzzle members have used one tablespoon of Epsom salts to 3/4 cup of apple juice to improve the taste instead of the magnesium citrate. Magnesium citrate and magnesium sulfate do the same thing. They help to open the bile ducts so stones may be passed easily, but magnesium citrate is more palatable in my opinion. It is *critical* to take magnesium citrate or magnesium sulfate one hour before drinking the mixture of olive oil and *fresh* grapefruit juice.

- One hour after the magnesium citrate and immediately before laying down to sleep for the night, drink this mix: ½ cup of olive oil (light olive oil tastes better) mixed with ½ cup of *fresh* pink grapefruit juice. Fresh pink grapefruit juice is fairly low acid. It is best to mix the olive oil and juice in a jar with a lid, shake vigorously intermittently, and drink with a straw. Try to drink the oil and juice mixture within 5 minutes. My clients are surprised that this flush does not usually cause an IC flare, and they tolerate the magnesium citrate, and *fresh* grapefruit juice quite well. Low acid orange juice or apple juice will do in a pinch, instead of the fresh pink grapefruit juice.

- After drinking the oil and grapefruit juice mixture, immediately lay down in bed on your back with your head elevated on some pillows. If you do not lay down immediately and stay quiet, you may fail to move the stones out. It is important that you lay quietly for at least twenty to thirty minutes. Some health practitioners recommend laying on your right side with your knees tucked up a bit. Either position is fine. After twenty to thirty minutes, you can change positions, but try to stay in bed as much as possible. You might experience some nausea. Try to relax and get some sleep.

- Expect diarrhea in the morning and to see gallstones in the stool. Some clients place a plastic strainer under the toilet seat to catch the gallstones. Alternatively, you may use a flashlight to observe for gallstones floating in the stool. Look for objects that may look like seeds or round stones. Quite often they are green or tan colored. Gallstones are not hard but soft; if you push on them, they break apart easily.

☙ You should repeat the gallbladder/liver flush once every two to four weeks until all the stones are eliminated. Then do a gallbladder/ liver flush once or twice a year thereafter.

I recommend doing your gallbladder/liver flush a few weeks after starting this program before you work on food list *two*. (See the Getting Started chapter.) Even if your gallbladder has been removed or a gallbladder scan shows *no stones*, it is still important to do the gallbladder/liver flushes. The stones are usually in the bile ducts of the liver and need to be flushed out so alkaline bile is allowed to flow freely.

Before doing this flush you might want to test your body through kinesiology to determine if the body can tolerate a liver flush at this time. As with all remedies, there are always some risk factors involved. The reader should be aware of the possibility of passing a large gallstone, which could lodge in the bile duct and might require medical intervention.

Most of my clients or their significant others have reported no problems with the flushes. Only a few have reported some nausea or do not get the best night's rest. Some IC Puzzle members have used a few doses of Nux vom, a simple and safe homeopathic remedy to relieve nausea if it occured with the liver flush. My husband and I had no problems with the liver flushes. We slept quite well, and felt much relief after passing hundreds of stones.

Solving the Interstitial Cystitis Puzzle

OSTEOPOROSIS

"It is bizarre that the produce manager is more important to my children's health than the pediatrician."

— Meryl Streep

Osteoporosis is most prevalent among postmenopausal women. There are approximately 10 million men and women in the United States who suffer from osteoporosis, a chronic bone-wasting disease. One in two women and one in eight men over age 50 breaks a bone because of osteoporosis.

After a hip fracture, many will never recover their mobility, and one in five dies within a year. The bones contain calcium and magnesium two of the body's major alkaline mineral reserves. When the body becomes overly acidic and the diet does not contain adequate alkalizing minerals, calcium and magnesium are released from bones to keep the pH of the blood stable. Although, in the short run, this meets the blood's requirement to maintain the blood pH, bones become porous and brittle over time and dental disease follows. Bone demineralization to alkalize the blood is one reason persons as they age "shrink" in height. One also sees stooped postures or spinal deformities along with periodontal disease with the aged related to demineralization.

Since the prevalence of osteoporosis is not the same across cultures, researchers are discovering differences in diets that they believe influence the development of osteoporosis. Japanese women consume less calcium than women in the United States and are unlikely to use hormone replacement after menopause but have a lower prevalence of fractures.

It is a known fact that when the amount of protein goes up in the diet, the rate of calcium that is excreted increases. Eating more than *three* ounces of animal protein a day will cause a loss of calcium from the body. Researchers have found that the type of protein matters when it comes to calcium loss. They found that animal sources of protein cause a much greater loss of calcium than vegetable protein.

This has been confirmed in a study of 755 Japanese men and women. The Japanese diet was low in animal protein, high in vegetables, and rich in plant protein such as soy. Researchers found that consuming animal protein was associated with an increase in calcium excretion. The study found no significant relationship between calcium excretion and the consumption of plant protein found in soy and vegetables.

Foods, Elements, and Activities that Interfere with Calcium Absorption and Utilization Contributing to Osteoporosis

1. Eating more than three ounces of animal protein a day will cause a wasting of calcium from the urine.

2. A high salt intake (table salt or sodium chloride) will cause a wasting of calcium.

3. Caffeine, alcohol, and smoking will cause a wasting of calcium.

4. Sugar will cause a wasting of calcium.

5. Foods high in oxalates such as spinach, kale, beets, and rhubarb interfere with the absorption of calcium.

Paleolithic Model

Until man began to cultivate grains and raise livestock 10,000 years ago, people rarely, if ever, ate grains or drank animal milk. According to Eaton and Konner, we simply do not have the genetic make up to tolerate grains and milk products.

1. Whole grains contain phytic acid, which is found in the bran of whole grains (except rice). Phytic acid binds to a variety of minerals including calcium, iron, zinc, and magnesium to form insoluble salts, called phytates, which are then wasted from the body. Probably because grains are a relatively new food, from an evolutionary perspective, it appears that we have not yet developed digestive tracts which can break down phytates.

2. In addition, dairy consumption also has an adverse effect on calcium utilization by affecting the vitamin D receptor sites on cells. Adequate vitamin D is needed to utilize calcium in the body.

3. Lack of adequate sunlight or foods high in vitamin D decrease utilization of calcium.

4. Sedentary lifestyles also interfere with mineralizing our bones. Our ancestors were probably much more active than we are. Impact stress on bone, as in walking and jogging, tends to increase production of calcitonin, which leads to increased deposition of calcium in the bones.

From an alkalizing perspective, having your calcium, iron, zinc, and magnesium bound with phytic acid from whole grains (except rice) and your vitamin D adversely affected by the consumption of dairy products means dairy and grains should be eliminated or used minimally since they interfere with the alkalizing process. Almost everyone I work with can not tolerate grains or dairy, at least not in the beginning of an alkalizing program. In addition, grains and dairy are very common allergens when allergy testing is preformed. (See chapters on Vitamin D and the Paleolithic Model.)

Hormones

"If your thoughts are thoughts that draw low-frequency energy current to you, your physical and emotional attitudes will deteriorate, and emotional or physical disease will follow, whereas thoughts that draw high-frequency energy current to you create physical and emotional health."

—Gary Zukav

Many persons with IC complain that ovulation and/or menstruation, pregnancy, perimenopause, or menopause may exacerbate their IC symptoms. Others report that their cycles do not affect their IC, while some report feeling better or worse after starting or stopping hormonal therapy.

I do not believe that hormone imbalances are the *cause* of IC. I do feel that hormonal imbalances may be another *piece* of the IC puzzle.

Let's review the hormonal cycle of menstruation. The first day of bleeding or menstruation is day one of the cycle. Estrogen* and progesterone are at their lowest levels on day one. Soon estrogen begins to rise. Increasing levels of estrogen thickens the uterus preparing for fertilization. The rise in estrogen also thickens the bladder lining. Estrogen levels reach a peak at ovulation, which is around day 14 of the cycle. There is only a small amount of progesterone present in the first two weeks of the menstrual cycle.

When an egg is released during ovulation, estrogen levels rapidly fall and progesterone levels begin to rise in preparation for pregnancy. Estrogen

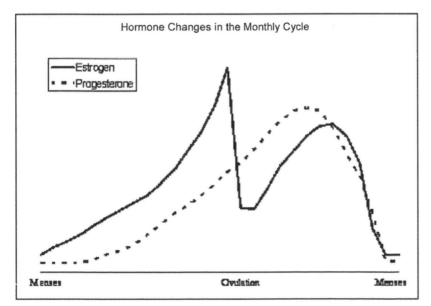

* The term *estrogen* actually refers to a group of hormones, including estrone, estradiol, and estriol.

levels remain at a lower level than that of the first half of the menstrual cycle. During this second half of the menstrual cycle, estrogen and progesterone levels reach a peak around the same time, about the third week of the menstrual cycle. If the egg has been fertilized and implanted, the progesterone levels remain high. If the egg has not been fertilized, estrogen and progesterone decline. The decline of progesterone causes shedding of the uterine lining, and this begins a new menstrual cycle.

Some IC patients say they feel best during their menstrual period when hormone levels of estrogen and progesterone are low. Other patients experience bladder pain during their periods, and many IC patients complain of IC symptoms a few days prior to the onset of bleeding. A number of IC patients also report pain just after a period and/or around ovulation. An explanation for the fluctuation in an individual's IC symptoms could be attributed to differences in hormonal imbalances.

Increased IC Symptoms around Ovulation and Just Before Menstruation

An explanation of increased IC symptoms around ovulation and just before menstruation may be attributed to the spike of estrogen seen just before ovulation. Estrogen falls quickly just after ovulation and then estrogen rises again with a spike just a few days before the period. Estrogen then falls just before the next period. Higher estrogen levels during these spikes provoke mast cell secretion with histamine release contributing to an increase in bladder inflammation.

Increased IC Symptoms During and after Menstruation

Dr. Neal Barnard, MD, author of *Foods That Fight Pain*, discusses menstrual pain related to hormone changes and prostaglandins. I believe this information may shed more light on the relationship of hormone fluctuations, prostaglandins, and interstitial cystitis.

"Chemicals called prostaglandins…these chemicals are made from traces of fat stored in cell membranes and…they promote inflammation. They are also involved in muscle contractions, blood vessel constriction, blood clotting, and pain.

"Shortly before your period begins, the endometrial cells that form the lining of the uterus make large mounts of prostaglandins. When these cells break down during menstruation, prostaglandins are released. They constrict blood vessels in the uterus and make its muscle layer contract, causing painful cramps. Prostaglandins also enter the bloodstream, causing headache, nausea, vomiting, and diarrhea." [1]

"This explains why nonsteroidal anti-inflammatory drugs work for menstrual pain. Ibuprofen (Motrin), naproxen (Anaprox), and other NSAIDs reduce the production of prostaglandins…Rather than focus on the prostaglandins themselves, it may help to focus on the cellular 'factories' that make them. After all, we know that birth control pills reduce menstrual pain, apparently by reducing the growth of the endometrial cell layer. The smaller this layer of cells is, the less tissue there is to make prostaglandins."[2]

If we look at the above explanation by Dr. Neal Barnard, MD, regarding increased pain and menstruation, we can see that an increase in prostaglandins during and just after menstruation may explain why some persons experience more IC symptoms at this time. It is this author's opinion that an increased amount of circulating pain-producing prostaglandins that enter the bloodstream around menstruation can have a negative impact on IC. Higher levels of prostaglandins may contribute to increased muscle cramping of the bladder as well as decreased blood circulation to the bladder related to blood vessel constriction.

Dr. Barnard encourages diet changes in persons with a history of menstrual pain related to elevated estrogen and prostaglandin levels. To reduce estrogen and prostaglandin levels he recommends a total vegetarian diet, which is low in fat since fat drives up estrogen levels. He suggests eating a diet high in fruits and vegetables, whole grains, and legumes, and to avoid completely all animal products. He finds this helps to reduce menstrual pain by decreasing estrogen levels and conversely lowering prostaglandin levels during the menstrual cycle. Incidentally, by eliminating meat and dairy products, you decrease arachidonic acids from animal products as well as reduce your acid load. Arachidonic acids are omega-6 fatty acids found in meat and dairy products that will increase PGE 2, a prostaglandin that increases inflammation in the body. (See chapter on Essential Fatty Acids.)

Progesterone and Estradiol Ratio

Valuable information can be derived by observing the ratio between progesterone to estradiol. If the ratio of progesterone to estradiol is low, there is increased risk of infertility and dysfunctional uterine bleeding.

A decreased ratio of progesterone to estradiol has also been associated with increased kinin release, which results in increased release of the inflammatory prostaglandins and of histamines.

Menopause

Briefly, menopause or "change of life" is the time when a woman stops ovulating or menstruating. When a woman stops ovulating, her ovaries decrease the production of the hormones estrogen and progesterone.

Hormone—or the lack thereof—affects the urinary system as well as the gynecological systems of a woman's body. Estrogen can drop by as much as 75% during menopause.

Estrogen helps stimulate the production of secretions that support the urinary system and the lubrication of the vagina. With the lack of estrogen, one gets drying and thinning of the vagina and decreased secretions that protect the urinary system making the bladder more susceptible to infections.

Talking with an understanding gynecologist about hormone testing and replacement therapy is an option that may increase the protective cellular layer inside the bladder and help with vaginal dryness. There are also different foods that are sources of natural plant estrogens. A good source book for natural supplements during menopause can be found in *Prescription for Nutritional Healing*, by James Balch, MD, and Phyllis Balch, CNC.

My Experience of Hormone Replacement

I can share my own experience of hormone replacement with you. I initially took FemHRT, a synthetic hormone replacement, due to perimenopausal symptoms starting around age 48. I found my hot flashes, irritability, and insomnia disappeared with FemHRT. Hormone replacement did not affect my IC.

I have since switched to a completely natural hormone replacement that my holistic medical doctor suggested. She suggested I try natural sublingual (under the tongue) hormone replacement. These hormones are absorbed directly into the bloodstream and does not require the liver to detoxify them. I was interested in hormone replacement that was "natural" and would not put undue strain on the liver. In addition, after switching from the synthetic hormone replacement FemHRT to natural hormones, I felt more "alive." I realized that the FemHRT took away my perimenopausal symptoms, but it also made me feel "numb." I did not understand this difference until I switched to a natural hormone replacement.

The natural hormone drops consist of estrogen and progesterone replacement taken twice a day under the tongue. You are not supposed to eat or drink for at least 15 to 30 minutes after taking these drops. Biest, stands for two estrogens: Estriol 80% and Estradiol 20%. Some physicians believe that Biest has an even lower incidence of cancer risk because it contains no Estrone. Studies have shown that estrone may accumulate in the reproductive tissues (breast and uterus) with age, and it is thought to be the main cause of breast and uterine cancer. This estrogen is referred to as natural because Biest is chemically *identical* to the estrogens produced by the body. They are made from the fats of wild yams and soy plants. Soy allergic individuals have taken these natural estrogens with no adverse effect. The production of Biest and progesterone process is highly purified to remove the protein portion of the plant, and it is the protein that triggers allergic reactions.

Contrary to popular belief, humans cannot convert wild yam and/or soy to hormones when taken internally or applied topically. Studies have shown that the human body only uses one specific sterol to make these hormones—cholesterol. From cholesterol our body synthesizes hormones such as pregnenolone, cortisol, DHEA, estradiol, progesterone, and testosterone.

The dose of Biest varies between individuals. Some persons may need as little as 0.625mg and others may need as much as 10mg. If the dose is too high (estrogen dominance), PMS symptoms can get worse and symptoms such as headache, water retention, breast tenderness, irritability (mood swings), and spotting will occur. Remember, too, that estrogen dominance will contribute to mast cell breakdown and secretion and increase inflammation, obviously this is something we do not desire. If the dose of Biest is too low then menopausal symptoms can get worse. Contact the pharmacist or your doctor to adjust your dose.

The second sublingual hormone is Natural Micronized Progesterone. Progesterone is needed to help balance and regulate the negative effects of estrogen and premenstrual syndrome. PMS is a symptom of low progesterone, which can be observed in women of any age from puberty to perimenopause. Other symptoms of low progesterone are depression, fatigue, headaches (*especially migraines*) uterine cramping, and fluid retention. Progesterone benefits are as follows: it is a natural anti-depressant, restores libido, decreases PMS, facilitates thyroid hormone action, is a natural diuretic, helps prevent breast and uterine cancer, stimulates osteoblasts or bone building, helps with infertility or embryonic survival. Again, this *natural progesterone* is identical to the progesterone produced by the human body and it is synthesized in the lab from the sterols (fat) of wild yam and soy plants. Some persons may need as little as 5 mg a day or as much as 400mg a day. Most persons take 25 to 100mg twice a day. Too much progesterone and you may see the following symptoms: fatigue, depression, breast tenderness, water retention, or acne. If you have any side effects, contact your physician or pharmacist so they may alter your dosage.

The pharmacy that makes the natural hormone replacement Biest and Natural Micronized Progesterone is Clark's Pharmacy, Inc. Bellevue, Washington. Mark Clark is the pharmacist and he is a fantastic resource. He is well-versed in holistic medicine and is a delight to work with. You do need a physician or a naturopath's prescription to take these natural hormone drops. Another plus with these natural sublingual hormones is that your hormones levels can be tested and the doses can be titrated to help you feel good.

Progesterone and Cortisol

The body can convert some progesterone to cortisol, testosterone, or estrogens when levels of those hormones are low. Progesterone has been described as a "feel-good" hormone, and low levels can cause irritability and anxiety. Cortisol is produced by the adrenal glands. Cortisol will block the histamine response to allergens and help us cope with stress. When our adrenal glands are weak, they are unable to produce enough cortisol to reduce inflammation and deal with stress. What the body will do when the adrenals are unable to meet the demand for cortisol production is use progesterone to make cortisol. When this happens, we do not have adequate progesterone available to balance estrogen. This leads to estrogen dominance which encourages mast cell secretion.

We know that it is the degranulation of the mast cells in the IC bladder and the release of histamines that can cause pain and other symptoms of IC. Since cortisol is a natural antihistamine, natural progesterone supplementation may help to correct hormone imbalances and increase cortisol levels.

The liver functions in balancing hormone levels by breaking down estrogen to a weaker form of estriol. If the liver is weak, as I believe it is with IC, then this will also contribute to hormone imbalances such as estrogen dominance. Estrogen dominance is a trigger for mast cell secretion.

In the Leaky Gut chapter we noted that a proper balance of healthy bacteria in the gastrointestinal tract (probiotics) helps to break down hormones such as estrogen. Recall that dysbiosis and LGS will contribute to hormone imbalances, especially estrogen dominance.

Black Cohosh Herbal Therapy by Shira Lee

Women who have found a correlation between urinary tract symptoms and endocrine imbalance can look to black cohosh for natural healing. Also called *Cimicifuga Racemosa,* the roots and rhizomes of this plant have been used as a medicinal ally to women of all ages since the 1600's throughout North America.

Numerous studies done in Europe as well as in the United States give us promising news for peri-menopausal women who are seeking a gentle natural alternative to synthetic hormone replacement therapy. Scientists, looking for that magical one active ingredient that can justify the hormone balancing results that they are witnessing with this plant, have encountered nature's mysterious and alchemical ways. They can basically say that this herb has "estrogen-like activity."

"Clear attribution of biological activity to a single chemical component remains illusive. It is believed that at least three different chemical fractions soluble in alcoholic extracts may contribute to positive benefits in the treatment of menopausal symptoms." [3]

During menopausal years, regular use of black cohosh over a few months duration can bring balance and ease. Some of these benefits include: a reduction in severity of hot flashes and night sweats, headache relief, decrease in mood swings, and increase of vaginal lubrication. Please note that this herb is not recommended for menopausal women who experience menstrual flooding.

Women who experience hormonal imbalances during other stages of their reproductive years can benefit from use of black cohosh as well. Pre-menstrual tension and menstrual cramps can be eased by use of this herb. It is calming and relaxing to the nervous system and to the reproductive system as a whole. Women who have irregular cycles, painful breasts, or other endocrine-related health challenges might find relief through regular intake of black cohosh root tincture. Midwives and doctors have used *Cimicifuga Racemosa* throughout history to assist just before and during childbirth. *Women in the first trimester of pregnancy should NOT use this herb, as it helps the uterus to contract.*

Many of us with chronic health challenges can celebrate the pain relieving properties of black cohosh. Those who suffer with discomforts from arthritis, fibromyalgia and rheumatic pain can give thanks after a few weeks of taking this plant in tincture form. It's calming and anti-spasmodic qualities benefit us beyond a symptomatic level. This herb restores a core energy which is fundamental to long-term deep healing of the body.

Try adding a few drops of the tincture, made from fresh black cohosh roots to your herbal tea each day, and watch the changes that arise through the nourishment that this herb provides. Perhaps that nagging lack of sleep or the uncomfortable muscle spasm in the back of your neck will gradually fade away. For those with IC, urinary frequency and urgency may well become a memory.

For more information on herbal assistance through menopause, consider Susun S. Weed's, *New Menopausal Years.*

ESSENTIAL FATTY ACIDS[1]

"Margarine is one molecule away from being a plastic."

— Unknown

Fats we consume in our diet have a profound effect on all parts of our bodies since every cell membrane of the body is constructed from fat. The wrong fats and oils can present tremendous problems for the body by increasing pain and inflammation. Conversely, proper essential fatty acids can reduce pain and inflammation. An interesting fact to note is the brain is 60% fat! This information gives a new meaning to the term "fat head." Many persons with IC complain of brain fog and depression. Examining and balancing your essential fatty acid intake will go a long way to reducing pain and inflammation as well as help clear up your thinking and elevate your mood.

"From the retina of your eye to the nerve centers that control the movement of your arms, brain fats are required. The nerves that give you the ability to see, hear, smell, touch and taste require brain fats. The nerves that allow you to run, jump, throw, play the piano, paint a picture, laugh at a joke and fall in love all depend upon *specific* fats."

We need the right balance of "correct" fats to help keep our mind and nervous system functioning as well as decrease inflammation in the body.

"Scientists have studied the brains of persons with multiple sclerosis; they found that the brain tissue was very low in important fatty acids such as DHA. They also found low levels of omega-3 fatty acids in the blood and almost no omega-3 fatty acids stored in fat tissues.

"Doctors in Australia who studied the blood of people with moderate to severe depression found that the balance of essential fatty acids was significantly altered; the level of the omega-3 fatty acids was too low. This adds to the growing body of data suggesting that depression may be closely linked to dietary fat.

"Purdue University researchers found that individuals with symptoms of hyperactivity and attention deficit had lower levels of the omega-3 fatty acid DHA in their blood. Behavior and school performance as well as violence and aggression may also show similar links to dietary fatty acid."

Over the last one hundred years the types of fats we consume has been altered dramatically. This is because we have switched to animal fats, warm weather oils, and processed foods. Our ancestor's ratio of dietary fats of omega-6 fats to omega-3 fats was once 1:1. Today scientists estimate the ratio of omega-6 fats to omega 3 fats to be as high as 30:1. The breast milk of some women contains a ratio as high as 45:1 of omega-6 to omega-3 fats.

"We are beginning to learn that if you want a brain that functions to its full potential and provides a lifetime of vital service, you will pay close attention to dietary fat."

Fat is not all bad. We need fat to make the cell membrane of every cell of our body. This is why strict low fat diets can be detrimental to over all health. What is more important is proper fats in the diet. Even cholesterol is important to make certain hormones without which our body would become diseased. We use fat to combat inflammation, to clot our blood and to contract and relax blood vessels. Women with insufficient fat tissue cannot conceive and bear children.

"Too much fat in whatever form can lead to disease. Too little fat in whatever form can lead to disease. The kind of fat and the balance of various fats are the critical features that determine how fat contributes to disease."

"If you vary the balance of your fats too far one-way or the other the make-up of your cells changes. For most of your cell membranes, the fatty acids must come from the oils in your diet. You cannot make them." Essential fatty acids are needed to make a healthy brain and nervous system and healthy cell membranes throughout the body. In addition, fatty acids are crucial as messengers. "They tell the immune cells to wake up or settle down. They tell the blood vessels whether to narrow or widen. They tell the blood platelets whether to stick together or separate, thus affecting the clotting of the blood. The messengers regulate inflammation."

Some messengers are formed from omega-6 fatty acids while others are formed from omega-3 fatty acids. In many cases the messengers that are formed from omega-6 fats perform the opposite function from the omega-3 fatty acids. The balance of fatty acids within the cell membranes of your body is determined largely by your diet. When your diet is balanced in omega-6 and omega-3 fatty acids then your cell membranes are balanced as well.

"Fatty acids that form the structure of your cell membranes become messengers when a call to action is sent out. This call can be in the form of trauma, a virus, a bacteria, a free radical, a toxic chemical, a heavy metal, or some other trigger. Once the call to action has been sent, your cell's fatty acids are released from the membrane and are chemically transformed into highly active hormonelike substances. Once the hormonelike messengers are released they exert powerful and profound effects on a vast array of functions..."

"These messengers are given the name prostaglandins...we know that prostaglandins are produced throughout the body. Prostaglandins (PG) are formed directly through a series of steps from dietary fatty acids. Those that we are concerned with are called PGE1, PGE2 and PGE3.

"**PGE1** is formed from dietary linoleic acid. This is the fatty acid predominant in corn oil, sunflower oil, sesame oil, and safflower oil. **PGE2** is formed from the fatty acid arachidonic acid. This fatty acid is found only

Solving the Interstitial Cystitis Puzzle

rarely in plants and is most common in animal meat. **PGE3** is formed form the fatty acid EPA (eicosapentaenoic acid), found in salmon, mackerel, herring, sardines, and other fish. Another form of PGE3 is formed from the fatty acid DHA (docosahexaenoic acid)."

PGE1 (linoleic acid) tends to have anti-inflammatory properties and is immune enhancing.

PGE2 (arachidonic acid) is highly inflammatory. It causes swelling, increased pain sensitivity and increased blood viscosity—blood is "thicker." Some of the other compounds associated with PGE2 can cause blood platelet clumping, spasm of blood vessels, and accumulation of inflammatory cells in an area and over the long term can change the way in which nerve cells communicate. PGE2 also will cause an overactive immune system within the nervous system causing the immune cells to attack the host. Leukotrienes are also made from arachidonic acid. Leukotrienes are even more potent inflammatory substances. They are 1,000 to 10,000 times more inflammatory than histamine. Leukotrienes signal white blood cells to travel to an area, which is good when you need them, but if they are in excess they create a lot of damage. PGE2 is important within limits, but when the fatty acids are out of balance by consuming a diet high in animal fats this is when PGE2 can become the "bad guy."

PGE3 (EPA and DHA) tends to have mild anti-inflammatory effect and immune enhancement. It is thought to counter the affects of the powerful inflammatory PGE2 substances.

If the fatty acids get out of balance then one fatty acid tends to dominate. The most common imbalance in the current American diet is high arachidonic acid intake (animal products) and then an increase in PGE2 (inflammation and auto-immune diseases).

"For example, if you consume a diet high in arachidonic acid, this fatty acid becomes predominant in the cell membranes. When an event happens in the body that might trigger inflammation, the inflammatory portion, of which arachidonic acid is a part, works very effectively. However, once its work is done and the process needs to be subdued, there may not be an adequate balance of other fatty acid messengers to do the job. In one sense, the cells are 'primed for inflammation' with inadequate messengers to properly shut off the system."

Dosage of Essential Fatty Acids: A healthy ratio of omega-6 fats to omega-3 fats is 1:1

Here is a following list of food sources for essential fatty acids and their prostaglandin (PG) messengers.

PG Series	Fatty Acid	Fatty Acid Family	FoodSources
1	Linoleic	n - 6	sunflower, safflower, sesame, corn
1	gamma-Linolenic	n - 6	primrose, borage, black current seed oil
2	Arachidonic	n - 6	animal meat, milk, eggs, squid, warm water fish
3	alpha-Linolenic	n - 3	flax, canola, pumpkin, chia, walnut
3	EPA or DHA	n - 3	cold water fish

Dr. Schmidt suggests these five steps to help preserve blood flow:

1. Keep Triglycerides between 40 and 170
2. Keep total cholesterol between 160 and 200
3. Raise HDL cholesterol above 35
4. Keep omega-3 fatty acid intake adequate
5. Consume modest saturated fat and keep total fat between 20 and 30 percent.

Dosage of Daily Essential Fatty Acids

"If we look at the typical American diet, it is rich with animal fat, high omega-6 fatty acids, and low in omega-3 fatty acids. This is precisely the formula one would use if the wish was to promote inflammation and alter brain chemistry in a negative way...Our goal should be to keep the level of arachidonic acid in balance with other fatty acids. This means we should consume foods that are low in arachidonic acid and low in linoleic acid, while balancing our omega-3 fatty acid intake."

Signs of fatty acid imbalance are dry skin and dry hair, dandruff, excessive thirst, **frequent urination**, brittle nails, irritability, hyperactivity, attention deficit, "chicken skin" on the back of the arms, soft nails, dry eyes, alligator skin, learning problems, allergies, poor wound healing, lowered immunity, frequent infections, weakness, patches of pale skin on the cheeks, fatigue, cracked skin on heels or fingertips

One can test for fatty acid imbalance where the red blood cells are analyzed for their fatty acid content. The laboratory reports on the major saturated and unsaturated fatty acids, the ratios between omega-6 and

Solving the Interstitial Cystitis Puzzle

omega-3 fatty acids and relative percentages of each unsaturated fatty acid. I recommend testing for fatty acid imbalances and follow up with a dietician to help you balance *your* fatty acid status. See appendix D for a list of labs.

Fats that contain mostly unsaturated fatty acids are usually liquid at room temperature (flax, sesame, sunflower, walnut, and soybean). Saturated fats are solid at room temperature such as fats of beef, lamb, pork, suet, lard, and some dairy products. According to Dr. Schmidt, it is important that red blood cells be analyzed rather than serum or plasma because red blood cell information gives a better reflection of what is happening in the body. In addition, it is important to consume adequate amounts of co-factors to help in the balance of fatty acids. These co-factors are B vitamins, vitamin C, magnesium and zinc.

The following are food suggestions to help balance essential fatty acids.

Eat fish twice a week: salmon, herring, trout, bluefin, caviar, mackerel, sardines, eel, anchovies, albacore tuna. Salmon and trout are the best tolerated by persons with IC due to the low level of histamines in these fish. Do not eat shellfish as they are high in toxins.

Choose fowl (organic, skinless, free range preferable): turkey breast chicken breast, duck, partridge, pheasant, and other wild game.

Limit beef and pork. Choose very lean, less than 10% fat.

Eggs: Organic eggs from free range chickens raised on DHA Gold feed contains more DHA in the eggs than normal chickens. This should be noted on the label in your health food store.

Dairy products: Choose low fat dairy products if you are not allergic to them. Low fat cheese and low fat yogurt.

You must avoid trans fatty acids or anything with a label that reads fried, hydrogenated or partially hydrogenated. A chemist once stated that margarine is "one molecule away from being a plastic." Avoid the following foods: anything fried in oil or deep fat fried such as French fries, deep fried fish burgers, candy, potato chips, tortilla chips, corn chips, deep fried chicken, cake, doughnuts, mayonnaise (unless it is made from canola oil or a healthy omega-3 oil) margarine, and shortening. If you want to eat chips, look for ones that say baked, they usually are not deep-fried in oil. Olive oil or canola oil make healthy salad dressings and are usually well tolerated by persons with IC.

By decreasing your animal product intake such as beef, pork, poultry, eggs and dairy, you will be decreasing your acid load as well as decreasing the omega-6 fatty acid foods which are high in arachidonic acid and contribute to an inflammatory state. Exchange meat servings for two servings of fish a week. Here are some ideas to obtaining and maintaining quality oils in your diet.

1. Get your oils from *whole foods* where possible, such as from fish, whole flax seeds which you can grind with a coffee grinder in small quantities as needed, seeds and nuts especially, sesame seeds, pumpkin seeds, walnuts, sunflower seeds, soy beans, and green vegetables.

2. Use oils that are certified organic since they will not contain chemicals that are applied in the growing process.

3. Use oils that are stored in dark glass bottles. Essential fatty acids are subject to rancidity when exposed to air, light, and heat.

4. Keep the bottles in the refrigerator and take out a small amount you may need and let it warm to room temperature. Oils that are high in monosaturates such as olive oil do not need to be refrigerated.

5. Use *unrefined* oils. Refined oils are commonly extracted with toxic solvents. Always buy extra virgin organic olive oil to avoid toxic solvents.

6. Oils should be cold-processed and expeller pressed.

7. Avoid oils, seeds, or nuts that taste bitter; they are probably rancid.

8. It is *best* to never heat or cook with oil.

Wet Sauté Cooking Method

Heating oils to a high temperature is how oils become damaged. A method to cook foods without heating oil is to use the "wet sauté" method. Place a small amount of spring water, low salt vegetable, chicken or beef broth in a pan or skillet and heat just below boiling. Add the food you desire to sauté. After the food is cooked, add the oil you desire to the food so the oil is not heated but adds flavor and calories.

Cooking Oils

According to Dr. Schmidt, the oils that one can heat for cooking are peanut oil, pistachio oil, coconut oil, ghee, sesame, butter, and olive oil. For those of you concerned about your saturated fat intake coconut, ghee and butter are considered saturated fats.

Summary

These oils are high in omega-3 fats and ones that we need to concentrate on to turn our inflammatory condition around.

Canola oil derived from a hybrid from the rapeseed plant. It is sometimes called rapeseed oil "…however, canola oil and rapeseed oil are fundamentally different. Rapeseed oil is high in a fatty acid called erucic acid, once believed to be associated with toxicity to heart cells. Modern canola oil contains less than two percent erucic acid, a level not associated with clinical problems." It is best to buy organically produced canola oil since these products are routinely tested to ensure that oil with chemical residue is not used. Canola oil is used in salad dressing, mayonnaise, and vegetable spreads. Do not use it for high temperature cooking. Canola oil and olive oil appear to be the best tolerated oils for persons with IC in the beginning of alkalizing.

Flaxseed oil and flax seed meal. Flaxseed oil can be used daily as a reliable source of omega-3 fatty acids. Flaxseed oil *must* be refrigerated and lasts only two to three months after it is opened. Ground flax seeds is another way to increase omega-3 intake. You can bake with flax seeds. You cannot bake or heat flaxseed oil. Test this oil carefully with IC. *It has been my observation that flaxseed oil and flax seeds can cause increased IC symptoms.* Even so, continue to test this oil every other month or so since with long term alkalizing, food tolerances increase over time.

Fish oils and eating fish high in omega-3 fatty acids decreases inflammation such as salmon, herring, trout, bluefin, caviar, mackerel, sardines, eel, anchovies, and Albacore tuna. Warm water fish such as lake trout, walleye, haddock, and northern pike have smaller quantities of healthy omega-3 fatty acids. Fish oil capsules may be used if one does not prefer to eat fish. Do not use fish oil capsules for infants or young children. Vegetarians can take DHA (healthy Omega-3 fatty acid) in supplements derived from algae. Fish oil and algae capsules should be refrigerated. I recommend a pure fish oil supplement by Pharmax. This oil has absolutely no "fishy" taste. One teaspoon contains DHA 750 mg, EPA 1,050 mg, Total Omega-3 2,250 mg and Natural mixed tocopherols 25mg. You can purchase Pharmax Pure Fish Oil at Clark's Pharmacy. See appendix D for contact information.

Be careful of potentially higher histamine fish such as bluefish, mahi mahi, mackerel, herring, tuna, and sardines. Histamines can be troublesome in the first year of alkalizing with IC. In addition, swordfish and tuna might contain higher levels of mercury. Avoid shellfish completely since they are high in toxins.

You can test any fish you desire, and if it seems troublesome, test again in another few months since alkalizing over time will increase one's food tolerances. For persons with IC, salmon and trout seem to be the best tolerated at least in the first three to six months.

Hemp Seed oil Do not cook with this oil. Refrigerate oil.

Walnut oil Do not cook with this oil. Buy organic. Consume whole fresh unsalted walnuts, if tolerated. Refrigerate oil.

Unsalted pumpkin seeds, soybeans, walnuts, wheat germ, chia, and green leafy vegetables all contain healthy omega-3 fatty acids. I refrigerate the nuts, nut butters, seeds, and oils I use. Buy smaller quantities of oils, nuts, and seeds so they do not go rancid.

Omega-6 fatty acids

The following omega-6 fatty acids need to be balanced in a ratio of 1:1 with omega-3 fatty acids. Most persons with IC will need to focus on decreasing foods and oils high in omega-6 fatty acids and increase their intake of foods and oils high in omega-3 fatty acids.

- Unrefined safflower oil, sesame oil, Evening primrose oil, borage oil, unrefined sunflower oil, rice bran, black currant seed oil
- Very lean meats, poultry
- Free range chicken or poultry raised on high omega-3 fatty acid feed is best
- Chicken eggs from free range chicken fed a high omega-3 fatty acid feed

Most persons with IC will have to concentrate on omega-3 fatty acid oils, nuts, seeds, nut butters, and cold water fish while cutting back on animal meat, dairy, and eggs to help bring back a balance of their essential fatty acids. Oil I use and recommend that is a nice blend of omega-3 and omega-6 fatty acids is Udo's Oil. It is a blend of flax oil, sunflower oil, sesame oil, rice germ, bran oil, evening primrose oil, soy lecithin, and vitamin E. It can be found in the refrigerated section of your health food store.

I use Udo's oil drizzled over vegetables, soups, and salads. In addition, I also incorporate Pharmax pure fish oil, one to two teaspoons a day. Remember, it will take time to eliminate arachidonic acids stores from the cell membranes and rebuild cell membranes with a healthier balance of omega-3 fatty acids. Balancing your essential fatty acids will reduce overall inflammation.

Anti-oxidants

One last critical point I would like to make is to remind the reader that when you increase polyunsaturated essential fatty acids in your diet, it is important that you diet be rich in anti-oxidants especially vitamin E. An alkalizing diet is high in antioxidant foods such as vegetables, fruits, and sprouts, but make sure you have adequate vitamin E (100-800 IU). Anti-oxidants (especially vitamin E) are needed to protect fatty acid molecules and prevent cell damage.

Motherhood and Fatty Acid Status

A balance of the essential fatty acids omega-6 and omega-3 in a ratio of 1:1 is critical in pregnancy and nursing. Remember your child's developing brain and nervous system is built on *your* proper fat intake. Again, the brain is 60% fat. After birth, mother's milk will contain the fats from the her diet. So if you have a child and you are reading this, evaluate not only your essential fatty acid intake but that of your children or grandchildren as well. Consider testing for fatty acid status, and then see a dietician to help you balance the essential fats in your diet.

Solving the Interstitial Cystitis Puzzle

VITAMIN D (CALCIFEROL)

"The sun, with all those planets revolving around it and dependent on it, can still ripen a bunch of grapes as if it had nothing else in the universe to do."

—Galileo

Description

Vitamin D (Calciferol) or "the sunshine vitamin" is not truly a vitamin. In its active form, it is considered a *hormone*. Vitamin D promotes strong bones and a calm nervous system. Vitamin D also affects biological rhythms, behavior, and mood. It is critical to obtain adequate vitamin D. A safe level of vitamin D intake is 400 IU to 800 IU per day. Good sources of vitamin D are food and sunlight. Calcium and magnesium work with vitamin D to enhance each other's absorption and utilization in the body.

Vitamin D is a fat-soluble vitamin and is acquired by exposure to sunlight or food. Good food sources are liver, egg yolks, fish, butter and in small amounts in dark green leafy vegetables. The sun's ultraviolet ray, UV-B, stimulates the body to convert cholesterol found in the skin to vitamin D. The body needs 30 to 60 minutes after sunbathing *(without sunscreen)* to absorb vitamin-D-containing skin oils. It is best to delay showering, bathing, or swimming for one hour after sunbathing. Exposing hands, face, and arms for 10 to 20 minutes, three times a week provides only 200-400 IU of vitamin D each time.

Latitude determines the intensity of UV-B light. Latitudes greater than 30 degrees (both north an south) have insufficient UV-B sunlight two to six months of the year, even at midday. Latitudes greater than 40 degrees have insufficient sunlight to achieve optimum levels of D six to eight months of the year. UV-B is stronger at higher altitudes, such as living in the mountains.

Vitamin D Deficiency

"Lifestyle, skin color, degree of air pollution, and geographical latitude all affect the degree of exposure to the sun, and therefore the amount of vitamin D that can be made by the body. It is also questionable where any vitamin D is synthesized during the winter months and whether the body's stores of this vitamin are able to meet the daily requirements during this period.

"If you rarely spend time in the sun, have dark skin, live in the northern latitudes, avoid fortified dairy products, or have liver or kidney disease, you may be marginally deficient in this vitamin. Recent research indicates that elderly people, also, may be at risk for vitamin D deficiency." [1]

Low vitamin D is associated with several autoimmune diseases including multiple sclerosis, Sjogren's Syndrome, rheumatoid arthritis, thyroiditis, and Crohn's disease. Osteoporosis, fibromyalgia, chronic fatigue, peripheral neuropathy, and Seasonal Affective Disorder (SAD) have also been linked with vitamin D deficiency.

Hypocalcemia (low levels of calcium in the blood), osteomalacia (reduction of the mineral content of the bone), and osteoporosis (reduction in total bone mass) are associated with vitamin D deficiencies as well as mineral deficiencies.

Assimilation and utilization of vitamin D is influenced by certain fats we consume. The fats that help with utilization of vitamin D are saturated fats and the omega-3 fats (flax, canola, pumpkin and walnut oils and cold water fish such as salmon, and trout). Trans fatty acids in fried food and margarine should be avoided. In the Paleolithic model, saturated fats as well as sunshine exposure supplied large amounts of vitamin D. The reduction of both saturated fats and a lack of sun exposure contribute to a current widespread D deficiency.

Dosages

A safe level of vitamin D intake is 400 IU to 800 IU per day. Several studies have indicated that amounts of up to 1,000 IU of vitamin D per day appear to be safe for adults. Symptoms of too much vitamin D are nausea, loss of appetite, headache, diarrhea, fatigue, and restlessness. Higher doses of vitamin D can cause hypercalcemia (high levels of calcium in the blood), which can lead to calcium deposits in soft tissues such as the heart, lungs, kidneys, and the vascular system-deposits that may be *irreversible*.

Without adequate calcium and magnesium, vitamin D supplementation will withdraw calcium from the bone. Do not supplement with vitamin D and do not sunbathe unless you have sufficient calcium and magnesium to meet your daily needs. Adequate calcium is between 1,200mg and 1,500mg, and magnesium intake could be half of that of calcium. Dr. Lark suggests taking calcium and magnesium in a ratio of 1:1 for inflammatory conditions.

If sunbathing is not available due to latitude and seasons, a sunlamp made by Sperti can be used to provide a natural balance of UV-B and UV-A. Used according to instructions, the Sperti sunlamp provides a safe equivalent of sunlight and will not cause burning or heavy tanning. Do not use sun screens, and avoid bathing or swimming for at least one hour after using the sunlamp. Tanning beds are not acceptable.

One additional note will lead us into the Paleolithic model. With the advent of agriculture and animal husbandry about 10,000 years ago there began the cultivation of grains and the raising of animal livestock. It is a fact that whole grains (except rice) contain phytic acid which counters the action of vitamin D (Willis and Fairney, 1972). Phytic acid from whole grains binds with calcium, iron, zinc, and magnesium to make them insoluble salts or phytates, which are then wasted by the body. Recall that calcium and magnesium work with vitamin D to enhance each other's absorption and utilization in the body. *Note that the only common grain with very low phytic acid content is rice.*

In addition, dairy consumption also has an adverse effect on vitamin D by affecting the vitamin D receptor sites on cells. Milk products lower the effectiveness of vitamin D to bind with a variety of cells (including immune cells) and does not allow vitamin D to carry out its important functions. (Perez-Maceda et al. 1991).

Krispin Sullivan, CN, has written a book called *Naked at Noon, Understanding the Importance of Sunlight and Vitamin D.* I strongly encourage the reader to obtain a copy of this book since it contains the most recent research about vitamin D dosages, proper sun exposure, blood testing for vitamin D overdose, or deficiency and chronic diseases related to vitamin D imbalances.

Sunscreen

The following is information from Dr. Susan Lark, MD, on the safety of sunscreens. I suggest applying sunscreen *after* you have sunbathed for the time *you* require for *your* skin type to obtain your adequate vitamin D.

"During a study conducted at the University of Zurich, Switzerland in February 2001, researchers tested six chemicals commonly found in sunscreen. They found that OMC, and four others ingredients commonly found in sunscreen (benzophenone-3, homosalate, 4-methyl-benzylidene camphor, and octyl-dimethyl-PABA) had *estrogenic properties.**

"If you apply substances to your skin that produce estrogen-like effects, it can cause symptoms such as endometriosis, severe PMS, breast cysts, and migraines. In extreme situations, these chemicals can stimulate estrogen receptors, thus possibly increasing your risk of estrogen-dependent cancer. It is even possible for breast-feeding and/or pregnant women to unknowingly pass the hormone to their child. My intent is not to alarm, but rather to inform. If used in small doses, these chemicals may not produce toxic results. But our bodies are exposed to all kinds of toxins, and the cumulative effect can be harmful. If this concerns you, you should avoid substances with estrogenic properties.

"Of the five sunscreen ingredients tested, 4-methyl-benzylidene (4-MBC) was deemed most likely to produce estrogenic effects. For this reason, I would strongly recommend you avoid purchasing products that contain 4-MBC. I would also suggest that children, cancer patients, and anyone with a weakened immune system avoid using products that contain the forbidden five.

"Even sunscreen products with the 'organic' classification can contain estrogenic ingredients, so you really have to read the labels closely. Two safe ingredients that offer UVA and UVB (full-spectrum) protection are

Increasing estrogen levels is a mast cell destabilizer, something we don't want for IC.

zinc oxide and titanium dioxide. Products containing these ingredients (and not the others) are few and far between." [2]

Two sunscreens Dr. Lark recommends are Dr. Hauschka's Sunscreen Lotion and Alba Botanica Sunscreen 18 SPF-For Sensitive Skin.

Solving the Interstitial Cystitis Puzzle

PALEOLITHIC MODEL

"The constitution of man's body has not changed to meet the new conditions of his artificial environment that has replaced his natural one. The result is that of perpetual discord between man and his environment. The effect of this discord is general deterioration of man's body, the symptoms of which are termed disease."

— Dr. Hilton Hotema

Dr. S. Boyd Eaton, MD, and Dr. Melvin Konner, MD, in their revolutionary book *The Paleolithic Prescription* (1988) suggest that much of our chronic disease today is due a deviation in diet and lifestyle that is very different than our Paleolithic ancestors. According to Eaton and Konner, 99% of our genetic heritage dates from before our biologic ancestors evolved into Homo sapiens about 40,000 years ago, and 99.99 percent of our genes were formed before the development of agriculture about 10,000 years ago.

Eaton and Konner state that before the advent of agriculture about 10,000 years ago all people were hunter-gatherers; they gathered various fruits and vegetables, and hunted wild game for their meat. In other words, our genetic makeup has changed by only a fraction, while our diet and lifestyles has changed dramatically!

Until man began to cultivate grains and livestock 10,000 years ago, people rarely, if ever ate grains or drank animal milk. According to Eaton and Konner, we simply do not have the genetic make up to tolerate grains and milk products. Whole grains (except rice) contain phytic acid, which is found in the bran of whole grains. Phytic acid binds to a variety of minerals including calcium, iron, zinc, and magnesium to form insoluble salts, called phytates, which are wasted from the body. Probably because grains are a relatively new food, from an evolutionary perspective, it appears that we have not yet developed digestive tracts which can break down these phytates. In addition, dairy consumption also has an adverse effect on vitamin D by affecting the vitamin D receptor sites on cells.

From an alkalizing perspective, having your calcium, iron, zinc and magnesium bound up with phytic acid from grains (except rice) and your vitamin D adversely affected by the consumption of dairy products means dairy and grains should be eliminated or used minimally. Almost everyone I work with can not tolerate grains or dairy, at least not in the beginning of an alkalizing program. In addition, grains and dairy are very common allergens when allergy testing is preformed.

For our Paleolithic ancestors, the ratio of meat, fruits and vegetables varied with geographic location, climate and season.

Paleolithic Factors that Contributed to Good Health Are the Following:

1. They consumed no refined carbohydrates.
2. They ate half as much fat.
3. They consumed very little sugar and it was from natural sources such as honey and fruit.
4. Their sodium intake was one-fourth of ours.
5. They consumed much more potassium than sodium
6. Their calcium intake was roughly twice ours today.
7. Studies of our ancestors' pre-agricultural diets indicate that magnesium was probably consumed at about a 1:1 ratio with calcium.
8. Their diet contained an abundance of micro-nutrients particularly vitamin C, iron, B vitamins and essential fatty acids.
9. They had five to ten times the fiber mostly from fruits and vegetables not from grains.
10. Their diet was bulky, filling, lower calorie, and nutrient dense.
11. They probably had minimal or no alcohol.
12. Hunters would walk or jog for hours tracking game. Women would walk miles every day carrying children and heavy loads gathering fruits, roots, and vegetables. Paleolithic man's strength and stamina was impressive compared to that of contemporary man.
13. In addition, they spent a good deal of time outdoors not fully dressed and exposed to sunshine thus obtaining large amounts of vitamin D (10,000 IU). If they did not live near the equator, they consumed diets rich in vitamin D such as fatty fish and organ meats.
14. Their air, water, and soil sources were pure. Fruits and vegetables they gathered were grown in mineral-rich soil.
15. Socially and emotionally the hunter gathers were cooperative and close. This decreased stress and contributed to feelings of security and companionship.

It is true that the average life span of our Paleolithic ancestors was forty years, but death was mainly from childbirth, infection or trauma. They did not suffer from chronic long term debilitating disease that now plagues most of us starting around middle age (or earlier) such as arthritis, osteoporosis, atherosclerosis, diabetes, hypertension, obesity, chronic lung disease, cancer, autoimmune diseases, and a multitude of inflammatory conditions, IC being one of many.

According to Eaton and Konner, the impact of change on our health goes beyond diet and lifestyle.

1. Industrial and domestic pollution create additional stress from high levels of noise, water, soil and air pollution.

2. Population pressures put a strain on natural resources.

3. Incandescent lighting has changed the quality and quantity of light. This alters our natural rhythm of night and day and affects our *circadian rhythm* sometimes making our "daylight" as long as 16 hours or more. Sleep cycles are disrupted causing a high degree of insomnia for modern man.

4. Background levels of ionizing radiation are at least 50 times higher in Western countries today than that of our remote ancestors.

Sanitation, vaccination, and certain advances in medical care has produced an increase in life expectancy and infant mortality for modern man. However, according to Dr. Eaton and Dr. Konner, we have exchanged acute medical problems (infection and trauma) for chronic ones by ignoring our heritage. The key is to recognize our ancient genetic heritage and integrate essential elements of the Paleolithic model into our modern existence thereby having the "best of both worlds."

ALKALINE WATER

"We only know the worth of water when the well is dry."

— Benjamin Franklin

What Is Pure Water?

We know that all life is dependent on water and that water exists in nature in many forms: clouds, rain, snow, ice, and fog; however, strictly speaking, chemically pure water does not exist for any appreciable length of time in nature. While falling as rain, water picks up small amounts of gases, ions, dust, and particulate matter from the atmosphere. Then, as it flows over or through the surface layers of the earth, it dissolves and carries with it some of almost everything it touches, including that which is dumped into it by man.

These substances include industrial and commercial solvents, pesticides, herbicides, radioactive materials, road salts, decaying animal and vegetable matter, and living microorganisms, such as algae, bacteria, and virus. These impurities may damage growing plants and transmit disease. Many of these impurities are removed or rendered harmless, however, in municipal drinking water treatment plants. Chlorine is the most widely used disinfectant for treating the water supply in the nation, with over half a million tons used annually by the water treatment industry. However, chlorine is an acid-forming element that has long-term negative health risks. It makes sense to filter tap water eliminating this acid-forming element and convert it to health-enhancing pure alkaline water with a pH as high as 9 to 11.

Water is one of the most important elements in the body, which is comprised of approximately seventy percent water. One of the contributing factors of chronic disease is not providing the body with sufficient water. To estimate adequate fluid intake, take your weight, in pounds, divide it by two, and you will have approximately the number of fluid ounces you require daily.

Daily Intake of Water: 140lb ÷ 2 = 70 fl. oz.

Alkaline Water Ionizer

Alkaline water will have a pH above 7. Ionized water is different from the water we drink. It is called "living water" and contains negative ions. It has a different boiling point, freezing point, viscosity, and surface tension. The objective of alkaline water ionizers is simple. The concept is to convert ordinary tap water into alkaline water similar to the natural waters of mountain streams and waterfalls. This water has a negative charge, which increases alkalinity.

Percentage of Total Global Reserve		
	Percentage of All Water	Percentage of Fresh Water
World Oceans	96.5%	0.0%
Glaciers and Permanent	1.7%	68.7%
Ground Water	1.7%	30.1%
Ground Ice and	0.02%	0.9%
Lakes	0.01%	0.3%
Soil Moisture	0.001%	0.1%
Atmosphere	0.001%	0.04%
Swamps	0.001%	0.03%
Rivers	0.0002%	0.01%
Plants	0.0001%	0.003%
Total	100%	100%

In household water ionizers, the water is first filtered through an activated carbon filter that removes chlorine, bacteria, and other pollutants but retaining the dissolved minerals. The water is then subjected to an electrical charge using electrolysis, which charges the water with positive and negative ions. The positive ions are the acidic minerals, which are bled off to one side leaving the beneficial alkaline minerals. The alkaline minerals are the negative ion minerals such as calcium, magnesium, and potassium. These negative ions are extremely beneficial in neutralizing free radicals. Increased alkalinity is beneficial in neutralizing acidity in the body and transporting calcium to the bones. The ionizer does not add any chemicals or minerals to the water. It only splits the minerals already in the water to the alkaline side and the acidic side.

In Asia, they have been using water ionizers for more than thirty years. Ionizers have been tested and approved by independent laboratories to meet FDA standards.

The makers of the water unit state the cost of a water ionizing system is between $500 and $800 to purchase and should last approximately 10 years. The maker's claim no plumber is required, it is simple to install, and the approximate cost of making pure, filtered, ionized water is about 2 cents per gallon. There are companies that produce units that treat the entire home water supply.

Oxygen

According to *Alternative Medicine Digest, Issue #9*, Dr. Hidemistu Hayashi, MD, is one of Japan's foremost microwater (alkaline water) researchers. Dr. Hayashi says that alkaline microwater acts as a powerful antioxidant in the body destroying harmful free radicals. Once the body's cells absorb alkaline microwater it helps dissolve acidic wastes that have accumulated.

An antioxidant quality of ionized alkaline water is hydroxyl ions (OH-). These are oxygen molecules with an extra electron attached to them as are all antioxidants such as vitamins A, C, and E. Hydroxyl ions scavenge for free radicals, which are unstable oxygen molecules that cause damage. Once the hydroxyl antioxidant and free radical have canceled each other, the result is that the body is provided with additional oxygen and therefore more energy.

Oxygen is the most abundant element on earth. Oxygen constitutes about two thirds of the human body and nine tenths (by weight) of the water in rivers, lakes, and oceans. Oxygen destroys cancer cells as well as bacteria and virus invading the body. Oxygen is one of the most exhausted nutrients in our body because of our diet and the earth's oxygen-depleted environment today. Since oxygen is an alkaline element, it helps to neutralize our body's acids. It is vital to human health, perhaps one of our most important nutrients. Alkaline water has excess oxygen, more than the two to one ratio of ordinary water.

Potential Benefits of the Alkaline Water Component of Ionization

- Increases energy level
- Washes acidic waste from the body
- Food cooked with ionized water tastes better
- Ionized water boils faster and cools down faster
- Drinking alkaline water promotes healthier skin and complexion
- Good for animals as well as humans
- Healthy cells live in an alkalized environment
- Promotes overall health and healing by bringing the body into balance

Potential Benefits of Acid Water Component of Ionization—*Do Not Drink*

- Washing with acid water is good for complexion
- Wash food with it to help remove bacteria
- Beneficial as a vaginal douche for Candida
- Makes a good hair rinse
- Extends the life of cut flowers

Testing Water pH and Creating Alkaline Water

To properly test the pH of water it is best to purchase a Hydrion Lo-Ion test kit. This kit is more accurate to test unbuffered solutions such as water.

If the cost of a water ionizer is prohibitive, one can purchase a patented alkaline concentrate—a healthy ratio of potassium and sodium—to provide alkalinity. One alkaline concentrate to consider is Alkalife® a water additive developed by scientist, engineer, and inventor Sang Whang, author *Reverse Aging*. He claims by adding two drops to an 8 to 10 oz glass of drinking water it will change drinking water into alkaline water. You might need to add more than two drops of Alkalife depending on your original water pH. Some persons with IC complain that Alkalife does not agree with their bladders. Like supplements and food, you need to test your tolerance for Alkalife. Some Puzzle members have reported positive results by adding Coral Calcium sachets to water to increase mineral content and raise the water pH. A few persons on a very limited budget have used a dash of sodium bicarbonate (baking soda) or potassium bicarbonate to their drinking water to raise the pH. Again, you need to test water with a Hydrion Lo-Ion test kit.

Mineral Spring Water

When getting started, I recommend drinking a mineral spring water if a water ionizer is too costly. I found the pH of Evian and Arrowhead spring waters test around 7.2 to 7.4. I drink Evian and Arrowhead spring waters and cook with ionized water from my kitchen water ionizer. Some IC Puzzle members have reported they did not tolerate certain mineral waters, so again, test carefully until you find one that is alkaline and agrees with you. *Never* drink carbonated drinks as they usually cause IC to flare. *Never drink plain distilled water because it draws the minerals from your body. It can be used under the supervision of a health care provider to help in a detox program.*

pH of Mineral Waters of the World

Brand	pH
Trinity Springs (USA)	9.6
Noah's California Spring Water (USA)	8.7
Adobe Springs (USA)	8.4
Famous Natural Deep Well Mineral Water (USA)	8.2
Cedar Springs (Canada)	8.1
Famous Crazy Natural Mineral Water (USA)	8.1
Mountain Lite (Canada)	8.1
Naturalle Mountain Spring Water (USA)	8.1
Deer Park (Maryland) (USA)	8.0
Loon County (USA)	8.0
Alaska Chill (USA)	8.0
Crystal Geyser Natural Spring Water (USA)	7.9

Solving the Interstitial Cystitis Puzzle

EartH2O (USA)	7.9
Pennine (United Kingdom)	7.9
Arrowhead (USA)	7.8
Brecon Carreg (United Kingdom)	7.8
Cotswold Spring (United Kingdom)	7.8
Highland Spring (United Kingdom)	7.8
Shepley Spring (United Kingdom)	7.8
Springhill (United Kingdom)	7.8
Sugarloaf Spring Rain (Canada)	7.8
Taiga World (Canada)	7.7
Calistoga Mineral Water (USA)	7.7
Celtic Spring (United Kingdom)	7.7
English Mountain (USA)	7.7
Hawaiian Springs Natural Water (USA)	7.7
Naya (St.André Est) (Canada)	7.7
Stretton Hills (United Kingdom)	7.7
Tipperary (Ireland)	7.7
Zephyrhills (USA)	7.7
Calistoga Mountain Spring Water (USA)	7.6
Blue Keld Spring Water (United Kingdom)	7.6
Carolina Mountain Spring Water (USA)	7.6
Galloway (United Kingdom)	7.6
Giant Springs (USA)	7.6
Hinkley & Schmidt (USA)	7.6
Lauré Pristine Spring Water (USA)	7.6
Mace Sparkling Irish Spring Water (Ireland)	7.6
Mountain Forest Spring Water (USA)	7.6
Pure Montana (USA)	7.6
Diamond Natural Spring Water (USA)	7.6
Monashee (Canada)	7.6
Agua Purificada Aquasystem (Mexico)	7.5
Aveta Celtic Goddess of Healing Waters (Ireland)	7.5
Fiji (Fiji)	7.5
Fountainhead (USA)	7.5
Kootenay Springs (Canada)	7.5
Naya (Mirabel) (Canada)	7.5
North Downs Sprint Water (United Kingdom)	7.5
Vittel (France)	7.5
Ashridge (United Kingdom)	7.4
Buxton (United Kingdom)	7.4
Colfax (USA)	7.4
Glendale Spring (UK) (United Kingdom)	7.4
Palomar Mountain Spring Water (USA)	7.4
Rocky Mountain Spring (Canada)	7.4
Keeper Springs (USA)	7.4
Calistoga Spring Water (USA)	7.3
Cobb Mountain Natural Spring Water (USA)	7.3
Northern Crystal (Canada)	7.3
Sparkletts (USA)	7.3

Strathglen Spring (United Kingdom)	7.3
Wildboarcloagh (United Kingdom)	7.3
Yukon Spring (Canada)	7.3
Mount Olympus (USA)	7.2
Alhambra (USA)	7.2
Ballygowan (Ireland)	7.2
Black Mountain Spring Water (USA)	7.2
Evian (France)	7.2
Findlays (United Kingdom)	7.2
Galway (Ireland)	7.2
Gibraltar Springs (Canada)	7.2
Nash's (Ireland)	7.2
Silver Stone (Ireland)	7.2
Sta. Maria (Mexico)	7.2
Vermont Pure (USA)	7.2
Aston Manor Malvern Springs (United Kingdom)	7.1
Spar Family Value Still Spring Water (Ireland)	7.1
St. George's Well (United Kingdom)	7.1
Aquafina (Canada)	7.0
Colorado Crystal (USA)	7.0
Cristal Springs (Canada)	7.0
Glen Orrin (United Kingdom)	7.0
Mountain Valley Spring (USA)	7.0
Volvic (France)	7.0

Solving the Interstitial Cystitis Puzzle

Solving the Interstitial Cystitis Puzzle

SEX

"The art of medicine consists in amusing the patient while nature cures the disease."

— Voltaire, French Philosopher (1694-1778)

Persons with interstitial cystitis report an increase in pain, urgency, and frequency with sexual intercourse and lasting for several days after intercourse. When starting this alkalizing approach consider choosing alternative sexual outlets other than sexual intercourse. This makes it easier to evaluate the diet and supplements. Once you are stable on the hypoallergenic alkalizing diet, explore different positions, and avoid the most uncomfortable ones at first. As your confidence builds with the diet, you can reincorporate the positions that had caused greater discomfort.

Before starting my alkalizing program, I avoided the male-dominant missionary position because it caused more discomfort. I found these positions to be preferable: woman on top, penetration from behind, or side-lying. This is an individual preference and something you and your partner need to explore together. However, since I have changed to a hypoallergenic alkalizing program, my IC symptoms after sex have disappeared.

At various times in the beginning of my alkalizing program, I used Heel allergy and Heel inflammation homeopathics along with warm baking soda baths if I had discomfort after sex. I used several Heel tablets until I felt more comfortable. Taking a dose or two of sodium bicarbonate/potassium bicarbonate in a 4:1 mixture ¼ to ½ teaspoon helps decrease inflammation. See appendix E for supplements. For others, prescription Pyridium, Pyridium-Plus, or Urised, although not "natural remedies," may provide some analgesic relief. Pyridium should not be taken long term. It may cause hemolytic anemia which means the destruction of red blood cells. More serious effects, if used long-term, include liver and kidney toxicity. Pyridium will turn your urine orange and stains clothing. Pyridium should not be used by people with kidney or liver disease. Uristat is a weaker formulation of Pyridium and can be purchased over the counter however let your doctor know if you use Uristat. Urised is a prescription drug and may help calm hyperactive bladders. This medication may cause urine retention, dry mouth, and turns the color of your urine blue.

I have started an IC Puzzle support group at Yahoo on the Internet since the first edition, and some members suggest using a heating pad for relief; others feel a cold pack is useful. Taking over-the-counter Tylenol occasionally may help. Be careful with Ibuprofen (Advil or Motrin) or aspirin as these can add to your acid load and increase leaky gut problems. Aspirin and Ibuprofen should always be taken with food, but may help decrease pain and inflammation by decreasing prostaglandins. In the beginning of this program, if you participate in sexual intercourse, taking an over the counter antihistamine or a prescription antihistamine might decrease an IC flare after sex. It is best to take the antihistamine 20 or 30 minutes before sex. Some over the counter antihistamines are Benadryl and Claritin. (Do not take Claritin D. The D stands for decongestant and the decongestant may cause a flare.) Zyrtec, Allegra, Vistaril, and Atarax are prescription antihistamines. Antihistamines may cause drowsiness, mucous membrane dryness, and *urinary retention*. Drink adequate fluids and use sexual lubricant to help with dryness. Some persons may not tolerate any of the medications mentioned and find they react to them with more bladder symptoms. Always ask your health care provider if antihistamines are safe for *you*. However, have hope; I cannot emphasize enough that maintaining a hypoallergenic alkalizing diet is what enabled me to resume normal sexual relations. The supplements, medications, and pain relievers are temporary measures.

You might enjoy quiet intimate hand holding walks and mutual massage. Consider creating intimate moments in the bath and shower. A gentle and sensuous approach to intercourse might be more satisfying. Intimacy does not always have to mean sexual intercourse. Cunnilingus and fellatio are not traumatic to the urinary tract, are pleasurable, and add diversity for those who are comfortable with these. Find time for intimate conversations. While healing, communicate openly with each other before you get to the bedroom. This is important for greater intimacy and a healthier sex life.

Adequate lubrication is important to decrease irritation to the urogenital tract especially with vulvodynia and for peri- and post-menopausal women. A lubricant I strongly recommend is Slippery Stuff® gel distributed by Wallace-O'Farrell. It contains no sugar. Many sexual lubricants contain glycerin; glycerin is sugar. Read your labels. Glycerin is defined as follows: glycerol, a sweet syrupy hygroscopic trihydroxy alcohol $C_3H_8O_3$. Glycerin is "food" for yeast.

Slippery Stuff® gel looks and feels like one's natural lubrication and is designed to provide vaginal moisture yet not remain on the vaginal walls to trap harmful bacteria. It is very much like the body's own natural lubrication. It is odorless, tasteless, and since it is naturally water-based and contains no sugar, it prevents bacterial or Candida growth. I reuse a clean plastic vaginal applicator that comes with vaginal anti-yeast cream medication and insert Slippery Stuff gel into the vagina before intercourse. Remember to wash the applicator with anti-microbial soap and warm water between applications, and air dry.

Discover ways that help you both feel loving and intimate while the bladder heals. A book you might find useful is *1,001 Ways to Be Romantic* by Gregory Godek.

Anal Intercourse

The topic of anal intercourse was discussed in the IC Puzzle group this year. I sincerely apologize to any reader who may be offended by this subject matter, however, I feel it is important to have as many options for enjoying intimacy with our partners as we can while we heal IC. For those of you who are suffering and worried about trying another way to have intercourse without bladder repercussions, this is a viable option. And if done carefully, it will not cause bladder or rectum discomfort. And you might even find it pleasurable! Understand, I am not saying this is how you will have to have sex for the rest of your life, but as you are healing IC and want to consider a nice alternative to vaginal intercourse, this is an option. The muscles of the rectum are very strong and snug, so this type of intercourse can be quite pleasurable for the man and the woman. The mouth, vagina, and rectum are made of mucous membranes and are comparable tissues, so the sensation for the man and woman are similar. I want to share some comments made by persons with IC regarding anal intercourse.

    ❖ "I used a tap water enema to clean out my rectum. I did have a little wine that night and he massaged my body gently and I was very relaxed. We went very slowly, we used lots of Slippery Stuff lubricant. I was very relaxed; he used one, then two, then three fingers gently inserted into the anus initially in order to help me not feel too tense or guarded. He was very gentle (and excited so intercourse did not last too long). I used a vibrator to stimulate myself while we had anal intercourse and this may have been a bit of a distraction as well. I must say my orgasm was the most intense I have ever experienced."

    ❖ "I've tried it before...it was a might painful at first...after a while it was a lot less painful and a lot more of a turn on, and I actually had quite an orgasm!!! Wooo Hooo!"

    ❖ "I did find some slippery stuff at a local sex shop, and we also bought my first vibrator. We really took our time, and I was truely amazed with the results. It didn't hurt when we had anal intercourse, and I am fine so far afterwards. If all goes well we will finally have an alternative to oral sex. I don't mind giving that but I have had enough. I think [my partner] will be ok with a change, and he won't be complaining about his lack of sex. I really hope you have included this in your sex chapter as it has proven VERY helpful for us."

First I am going to assume you practice *safe* sex because you are married and know your partner's history. Safe sex whether vaginal or anal includes using a latex or vinyl condom. The following are some tips if you consider anal intercourse: your partner could wear a condom. Mostly to keep him from getting E. Coli in his bladder from anal intercourse. However, a condom does dull the man's feelings making intercourse take longer. Condoms also are more drying to the anal (or vaginal) membranes, so use plenty of lubricant. DO NOT USE VASELINE this creates too much friction. Whether you choose to use a condom or not, here are several things I suggest:

1. The woman should use a plain warm tap water enema to gently clear the rectum of feces, and this makes it cleaner. Also the clearing of the rectum decreases the urge to feel like you need to move your bowels with anal intercourse.

2. The man should drink a glass of cranberry juice before he has anal intercourse, and be sure to urinate soon after intercourse. This helps eliminate any possible lingering E. Coli that might be in his urethra.

3. Both partners could take a shower or bath before anal intercourse, but certainly after intercourse.

4. After anal intercourse, the man should use an antimicrobial scrub such as Phisohex, Hibiclens, or Betadine (found in drug stores) on the shaft of his penis and around the head of the penis to prevent bacterial infection. Be careful not to get the soap into the urethra while scubbing. The man should also use this scrub on his hands and fingers he many have used to help relax the woman's rectum. The man should *gently* scrub for several minutes with these anti-bacterial agents to eliminate microbes from his hands and penis. Test any antibacterial scrub on the man's forearm to test for allergies *before* using on the genitals. Read labels carefully on these antimicrobial scrubs before using.

5. *Never* put the man's penis in the rectum and then into the vagina. You risk getting a vaginal and/or urinary tract infection this way. You could have gentle vaginal intercourse first, then proceed to anal intercourse, this would be safe.

6. Use adequate sexual lubricant. I find Slippery Stuff is very comfortable when I have anal sex.

Note: Contraindications of anal sex are if the woman has irritable bowel syndrome, anal fissures, hemorrhoids, or other colorectal conditions. These conditions should be healed before considering anal sex.

Well, that is what I have to say on this subject. I do hope I have not turned anyone off by this topic but wanted to be helpful and hopeful for those who are worried about their relationships and are afraid. My apologies again to anyone who found this topic offensive. I know I cannot please all of the people all of the time, but my goal for this book, my website, and the IC Puzzle group is to help persons with IC in any way I can.

STRESS

by Wm. Zeckhausen, D. Min.
Pastoral Psychotherapist, Laconia, NH

"Who taught you all this, Doctor?" The reply came promptly: "Suffering."

— Albert Camus, *The Plague*

I have worked 25 plus years as a pastoral psychotherapist. I was diagnosed with IC 3 years ago. For two years, Amrit Willis has helped me, through practical information on diet, and life style, and equally important emotional and spiritual support. She has invited me to contribute some suggestions for addressing the psychological response to living with IC.

The physical symptoms of pain, frequency, urgency, and spasms are too well known by most of us. They, along with the disruption and limitations of normal life before IC, all produce stress. Shame, embarrassment, guilt, anger, fear, panic attacks, and depression may be experienced by many of us, consciously or unconsciously, during the course of the illness, all contributing to stress. As if that weren't enough, unresolved psychological issues from our past might be intensified due to our IC experience.

For those of us who have gone through this torturous journey, it may be very difficult to look objectively at our emotional responses. However, for some of us, to take responsibility for receiving help with our emotional responses to IC might be at least as important as to address the physical problems themselves.

Addressing the various forms of stress that enter our life, besides trying to figure out how to deal with the physical symptoms, might seem too overwhelming a task. In fact, not to do so could turn out to be more overwhelming, as our emotional responses begin to take on a life of their own. All of us have known the experience of feeling overwhelmed before we heard of IC, and eventually have overcome those feelings. Facing our psychological/spiritual response to IC increases the likelihood that we will achieve greater maturity and depth as persons than we had before our IC experience.

The Chinese symbol for crisis consists of two symbols, one meaning danger and the other opportunity. We certainly initially experience IC as a crisis. IC's uninvited and unwelcome symptoms create stress. At some point, sooner, or maybe much later, we are told we have IC. To have a diagnosis may be a relief. Or it may increase our stress. The odds are most of us find that our stress increases and intensifies physical symptoms. And the stress certainly upsets our sense of emotional well being. Researchers speak of challenge, commitment, and control as three characteristics of the stress-hardy personality. To work at seeing IC's intrusion into our life as a challenge rather than a disaster, can help us overcome our fear of IC and its symptoms. Each of us would fill in the details of the challenge for ourself, in some ways similar, in some ways different, from others. But guaranteed is that to whatever degree we shift from perceiving IC in a way that results in our feeling helpless and hopeless, to the perception of IC as challenge, we will enjoy a welcome change in the quality of our life experience, as we are becoming more stress hardy.

I recall every now and then the casual comment by an Old Testament professor 40 years ago, who said, "I don't worry about somebody who falls down. I worry about the person who falls down, and doesn't get up." How many times are we going to fall down? Only as many times as we have the ability to also get up. When captured by despair, fear, or doubt, we might make our mantra the affirmation "I have the staying power, to see this through successfully."

It can be near impossible, when captured by pain, fear, or despair, to think that this isn't only about us. But it isn't. Realize that the grace by which we learn to contain our suffering can provide a powerful model for coping with inevitable crises that enter every life for those people for whom we are important, whether it be a spouse, parents, children, clients, or friends. It is essential in coming to terms with our dis-ease, that we see what we are addressing in such a way that transcends our individual journey.

Psychotherapeutic support with a competent and caring therapist should be very helpful in relieving our psychological/spiritual suffering from this disease. If you are uncomfortable seeking such help, it might be useful to consider it not as confirmation that something is wrong with you, but rather that you are committed to your own growth as a person—a sign that something is very right with you! A therapist can be very helpful in enabling us to find and strengthen inner resources we might not have known we have, in coping with IC. I feel it would be useful to suggest some books to read.

An outstanding book for understanding the effects of stress, as well as how to relieve it, is *Why Zebras Don't Get Ulcers* by Robert Sapolsky. It is regularly highly recommended at therapists' conferences, and it is reader friendly, as its title hints at the humor and imagination that is a delightful part of its style.

Martin Seligman, Ph.D., noted researcher in "learned helplessness" authored the book *Learned Optimism*. In it, he describes cognitive tools to understand an unconscious style of thinking that is pessimistic and likely to lead to depression and effective guidance on how to change. His concepts have been tested by teaching them to group participants who were depressed, while a control group of similarly depressed persons utilized anti-depressant medication.

Solving the Interstitial Cystitis Puzzle

Both groups found relief from depression in a few months. The group on anti-depressants then stopped taking the meds. Their confidence was in the meds. Some of them became depressed again in a few months, and returned to their meds. The group using the concepts to become conscious of pessimistic thinking and how to change to optimistic thinking were relieved of their depression also. The important difference was that their confidence was in conceptual tools they had learned, i.e., their confidence was in themselves, and they did not become depressed again in a few months. Seligman's latest book is titled: *Authentic Happiness*. It integrates what he said in *Learned Optimism* and goes beyond that.

The author of *Kitchen Table Wisdom: Stories That Heal*, Rachel Remen, MD, has Crohn's disease, a chronic condition, and has had numerous surgeries for it beginning in her teens. The book is popular with physicians, and she regularly receives a standing ovation after her keynote presentations at physician's wellness conferences. The book is helpful in discovering the need and means to find positive meaning in our circumstances, rather than succumbing to being a victim.

Although understandable that we should initially experience ourselves as "victims" of IC, it's not healthy to hold onto that perspective. Victor Frankyl, Jewish psychiatrist who lost family members in the holocaust and was himself in a "camp," observed that those prisoners who could create meaning in that horrible and terrifying context had a chance of survival, whereas those who couldn't find meaning in it, inevitably died in the camps. When he was rescued from his camp, he subsequently developed a form of therapy, with adherents around the world, titled *logotherapy*, which means "meaning therapy". When we suffer, discovering or creating a positive meaning in relation to the suffering makes it tolerable, and is likely to reduce stress.

One need not be a "believing" Christian to appreciate words in a letter Paul wrote to a church, found in the New Testament. Paul tells of having prayed that the "thorn in his flesh" might be removed. Scholars to this day can only speculate on what that "thorn" referred to, but IC patients will have no difficulty identifying with the experience of a thorn in the flesh! Paul wrote that the answer he received said in effect that he had to live with it, that God's strength would come through his weakness. Fortunately we have or should have hope and the belief that our symptoms sooner or later can be considerably or entirely removed. But that doesn't happen over night. Part of our learning while coping with our symptoms, may be discovering the numerous ways that out of our "weakness" empathy has been developed for others, as well as discovering and taking in the kindness of others in reaching out to us.

It was helpful for me to shift from feeling like a leper cut off from the rest of humanity and its seeming normalcy to the realization that I had gained an understanding and sensitivity to people with chronic medical conditions and pain that I didn't previously have. The shift from being an outsider to an insider can make a world of difference in the quality of ones life.

A fundamental reliever of stress is to have at least one person and preferably more with whom one has a close and positive relationship. In Dr. Dean Ornish's book, *Love and Survival: The Scientific Basis for the Healing Power of Intimacy,* he is quoted as saying, "I am not aware of any other factor in medicine—not diet, not smoking, not exercise, not stress...that has a greater impact on our quality of life, incidence of illness, and premature death from all causes."

One of the most disempowering and painful experiences is a panic attack subsequently followed by fear of more panic attacks. Our first panic attack may happen as a result of feeling overwhelmed by the problems of IC. We might have had such attacks previously that began to return when we were diagnosed with IC. The miserable inhibiting condition of living in fear of additional panic attacks is completely curable.

A brilliant, clear, and effective book in providing tools for overcoming panic attacks is *Don't Panic: Taking Control of Anxiety Attacks* by Reid Wilson, Ph.D. His information on what creates a panic attack and how to become free of panic attacks includes some of the most practical and understandable material on meditation and diaphragmatic breathing.

His guidance on the patterns of self-talk we engage in, i.e., worried, self critical or hopeless, enabling us to become conscious of each pattern, seeing how any one let alone all three may trigger high anxiety, and modeling a supportive form of self talk that replaces the negative patterns, has been proven with his panic prone patients over the years to be most effective. The section on self-talk, besides pulling the rug on panic attacks, would lead to more effective functioning and deeper confidence for anyone, whether they ever had panic attacks or not.

In the book, *Self Hypnosis: The Complete Manual For Health And Self-Change*, authors Brian Alman and Peter Lambrou, Ericksonian hypnotherapists, have a chapter titled "Pain Control Strategies." It taught me some psychological techniques to diminish my experience of pain that I haven't come across elsewhere and would not have occurred to me. Also helpful are the chapters titled: "Stress Management" and "Freedom from Fears, Phobias and Anxieties."

An insightful book on breathing and utilizing breathing to relieve and resolve negative feelings is *Conscious Breathing: Breathwork for Health, Stress Release, and Personal Mastery* by psychotherapist Gay Hendricks, Ph.D. A complementary book on breathing is *The Art of Breathing* by Nancy Zi.

To repeat, what it takes to be stress hardy: May we encourage each other to regard IC as a challenge, commit ourselves to seeing it through, and learn what we need to about our bodies, our minds, and our spirits in order to gain greater control over our lives.

Solving the Interstitial Cystitis Puzzle

Nourishing Ourselves with Herbs

Written by Shira Lee, M.A.

"Everything on the earth has a purpose, every disease an herb to cure it, and every person a mission."

—Mourning Dove Salish

As we learn to relate to the food we take in as nourishing medicine for our bodies, we can broaden our diet to include healing plants. Healing plants are called herbs, and have been a primary source of medicine for people throughout the world. Almost every culture, for thousands of years, has benefited from the curative properties of plants.

Most herbs are alkalizing, but not all are appropriate for a urinary tract that is sore and inflamed. How can we know which herbs to experiment with? I find it helpful to reach for those which are soothing, mild, and calming. It also helps to see our body as a whole, and consider using herbs that balance our entire system.

Information about herbs and healing can be ambiguous. Some people swear that tinctures are by far the best and only way to take herbs, while others encourage preparing only the dried or fresh herbs in teas. Some "experts" say that comfrey leaf is healing for the bladder, while others tell us not to ingest it. Given this reality, I've decided to write only about herbs that I have personal experience with, and which do not flare my sensitive bladder. The herbs mentioned here are merely a few of the wonderful plants available to us. These assist in soothing, strengthening and balancing our bodies.

I encourage you to cautiously experiment, and whenever possible, to experience plants growing in their natural habitat. Some of the herbs I prepare grow wild near my home. Even if I am not able to wildcraft those herbs, it is a delight to develop a relationship with the plants that are my medicine. I raise some of my own herbs in my small organic garden, and some I purchase as dried herbs, tinctures or capsules. A list of resources for studying, purchasing, and learning to know and love plants is at the end of this chapter and in appendix D. Perhaps some of my favorite herbalist authors will become yours as well.

We can use herbs to assist in cleansing the liver, strengthening the digestive system, and cooling the heat of living an over-stressed life. Herbs also relax spasmodic muscles, calm the nervous system, and soothe the mucous membranes of our organs of elimination. Many herbs help with microbial infections, while others tonify, providing nourishment and extra "oomph" when we are exhausted. Healing plants can be used to balance hormones and moderate histamine reactions. Plant medicines that are helpful for some people are not helpful for others.

When using herbs, it is best to start out with only one or two at a time. Each herb has its own qualities, and affinity with particular body systems. As you take your first sip of nettle tea, for example, close your eyes, and experience the green, mineral-rich brew enriching every cell of your body. With each new plant you include in your diet become aware over time of the subtle shifts and responses in your body.

Some medicinal herbs are most effective when extracted in alcohol. Herbs that are prepared in alcohol are called tinctures. Other herbs are best used from the dried leaves, flowers, or roots. These can be grown or bought in stores that specialize in natural foods. If you live in an area where there is no access to natural food stores, check the resources in appendix D for ways to purchase herbs through the mail or through the internet. Reputable sources of herbs are important. There are certain companies that are particularly conscious about how they wildcraft or grow herbs. Some retail stores will make a special order of herbs for a customer. All one need do is ask.

Healing herbs are often effective when made into a tea from the loose, dried, or fresh plant. Taking time to see, feel, and smell herbs gives us a way to relate to this form of "food" our body is ingesting. We can also control the strength of tea we make. We begin by steeping the herb for only a short while. As long as the dried loose herbs are stored properly in a sealed glass container, they can be stored for one to two years.

Tinctures are practical in that they last for years in amber jars, shielded from light and can be added to hot water or tea. Those with IC need to avoid alcohol, which is the base of most tinctures, so these should only be used consciously and carefully. This means adding the concentrated tincture to very hot tea and allowing the alcohol from the drops to evaporate. Some tinctures use vegetable glycerin as their base, which is very sweet and can be tolerated only by some. According to Herbal Ed of Herb Pharm, vegetable glycerin is not the ideal solvent for some herbs, meaning that the medicinal quality of the herb is lost somewhat in using glycerin as a tincture base. [1]

Dried herbs in capsules should generally be the last choice when taking in herbs. When buying herbs in capsules, the customer can pay up to eighty dollars a pound for an herb, which might otherwise cost from three to twenty-five dollars a pound in bulk. Some herbs need the process of heat to be more effective. In addition, capsules are made from powders that have been sitting around an unknown amount of time and are notorious for being made from lesser quality herbs. The convenience of capsules, however, can be an advantage, and I find myself taking a few healing plants in this form, such as barberry, olive leaf extract, aloe vera, and kava ("Pharma Kava" from Herb Pharm).

When making tea with loose dried herbs, we learn that each part of a plant is prepared differently. The roots and barks of plants, for example, are simmered over time (a decoction). Leaves are never boiled; only steeped in water that has been boiled (infusion). Developing a relationship with the plant we are preparing is a wonderful way to slow down and relate to the natural world. The process of making our own herb tea is a process of self-nurture and care, which in itself cultivates awareness and healing.

Some Herbal Suggestions

Let's start with a plant that almost everyone can recognize at least by its sun yellow flowers or, if in a later stage of its cycle, by its delicate yet strong round seed pods.

Dandelion (*Taraxacum officinalis*): If you aren't on government property, and you aren't breaking the law, go ahead, pick that seedpod. Close your eyes, and as you make a wish, feel the root of this plant reaching deep into the earth, providing nourishment and strength to the soil. As you blow out your wishes and intentions to the universe, and the tiny seeds float around you, celebrate your communion with this plant, which may soon become a good friend.

In this brief discussion, we will focus specifically on the therapeutic qualities of dandelion root. This gentle and cooling root has been used in cultures throughout the world for centuries, especially to heal the liver, digestive system and gall bladder. As an overall body tonic, dandelion root can gently cleanse and strengthen the liver and digestive system. Though dandelion is a strong diuretic, this property is balanced by its high potassium content. Several herbalists write that it is one of the best natural sources of potassium available to us.

As we learn from Amrit, cleansing the liver and balancing the digestive organs is a necessary part of a long term bladder healing program. Dandelion's bitter taste stimulates digestive secretions such as bile, gastric and pancreatic enzymes. In the Western Herbal tradition, dandelion root is prized for its high mineral content, which also gives it a salty taste. Peter Holmes, with his outstanding ability to bridge Eastern and Western Herbal traditions explains:

This quality (high mineral content/salty taste) provides the root with its "detoxicant and regulating effects on the whole body. Chronic and degenerative toxicosis conditions involving the connective tissue and interstitial fluids are addressed...Dandelion works undramatically yet, given time and consistency, deeply in altering mode. The root's resolvent action is tailor-made for those with systemic metabolic and microbial toxicoses presenting damp heat or damp with hyperuricemia [excess uric acid in the blood], depositions (such as stones) or eczema...Chinese Herbalism...values the anti-inflammatory action of this heat and toxins-clearing remedy, and applies them to heat toxin symptoms such as boils, internal abscesses, and throat inflammations. The cooling and detoxicant effects of the root's bitter taste are here put into effect. Modern research supports these uses for dandelion root and, moreover, has demonstrated the immunostimulant and antiviral activity..." [2]

We find dandelion root alive and well in the Ayurvedic tradition as well, where it continues to be used to stimulate the digestive functions and help with detoxifying the liver. [3]

Herbalist Susun Weed gives dandelion root a French accent, and lets the plant speak for herself. "My tonic effect is not just for maintaining your health, eh? I can help you wiz some troubles. Oui. I help you wiz troubles like cancer, heart and lung problems, digestive woes, and painful joints. I tell you, I am ze hot stuff, doctor dandelion, the family doctor supreme…try me as a wise woman's ally when helping yourself or others heal kidney and urinary problems, including all kidney and bladder diseases (oui, even cancer), kidney stones, diabetic kidney problems, gout, dropsy, edema. Renosis, urinary stones and gravel, and ulcers in the ureters, urethra or bladder…I tell you before, I play gentle, eh?" [4]

Dandelion root can be used for treating infections of many kinds. In vitro, the aqueous extract inhibits staphylococcus, streptococcus, Diplococcus pneumoniae, Bacillus diphtheriae, Pseudomonas aeroginosa and Bacillus typhi. It has anti-fungal properties as well. [5]

A tincture made from the fresh roots can be a convenient way to take this herb. Begin with a few drops a day in some mild hot tea or hot water.

The dried roots can also be made into a decoction by simmering a small amount in water for fifteen minutes or so. You can add this dark brew to your favorite tea. I suggest keeping the dosage low and steady. If you ingest large amounts over time, heartburn, nausea or loose stools may result. [6]

Give "doctor dandelion" some time to work gently and deeply. Allow your creative self the enjoyment of combining this nourishing root with other herbs you find soothing and balancing.

Nettle Leaf (*Urtica dioica*): Ahhh, here in the plant universe, we find a friend that can nourish us in more ways than one can count. We can drink nettle leaf tea as much as we like, and have no worries about over-consuming. People all over the world use nettles as medicine as it is truly a gift for the human body. Here is a wonderful example of a food and medicine, as nettle leaves can be picked (carefully, with gloves!) and cooked as a delicious addition to our diet of greens.

For those who worry about the fact that this plant is also called, "stinging nettles", please note, that as soon as the plant is properly dried or cooked, it no longer stings. This plant has become a dear friend, as she grows abundantly along the flowing river where I walk daily, and I delight in seeing her change from a young, vital plant to a towering tree-imitation. She seems to love the wet places that I frequent. Of course I've had my moments of eagerly picking a summer-ripe thimbleberry or reaching to look at a hidden spring wildflower and being stung to my senses by this wild deep-green plant. Nature provides generously, though, as there is almost always a Yellow Dock plant growing within inches or feet; its young leaves are a perfect antidote to the smart of nettle-sting on one's skin.

Nettle leaf is rich in countless easily absorbable nutrients. Some of these include chlorophyll, vitamins A, D and K, calcium, iron, potassium, phosphorus, silica, zinc, and trace minerals. This plant is rich in protein (10.2%), manganese, selenium, and niacin. [7]

Susun Weed, in her book, *Healing Wise*, gives us ample information and inspiration to incorporate nettles into our daily diets. Here are some examples:

"...I have found nettle a powerful ally in restoring and maintaining the vibrancy of my adrenals, my hormonal and circulatory systems, my energetic, bio-chemical, and magnetic fields, and my emotional, sexual sensitivity...

"Ask nettle to be your ally in healing those with gravel or stones in the kidneys or bladder, bloody urine, kidney pains, chronic urinary tract infections, diabetic water retention and kidney stress from insulin, chronic cystitis, dialysis and kidney surgery, stress, allergies, childbirth trauma...

"Nettle...can help the gradual healing of a person with a chronic condition such as Epstein-Barr virus, hay fever, allergies, lymphatic swellings, ARC/AIDS, nerve inflammations (including lumbago and sciatica), persistent headaches, high blood pressure, inexplicable lethargy and exhaustion, repeated bouts of flu and colds, hardened arteries, weakened veins, infertility, rheumatism, joint aches, continuous skin eruptions, and loss of nerve sensitivity...

"Nettle infusions heal kidney cells like nothing else I've ever seen. The usual curative dose is one or two cups of infusion daily for ten to twelve weeks or longer...

"As a tonic for adrenals and kidneys, try a cup daily for six weeks and then three or four cups a week for as long as you like..." [8]

When first introduced to nettles, I learned that it is a wonderful plant for nourishing the blood and helping to grow healthy and glossy hair. It has been known for centuries as an herb to stop bleeding.

Michael Moore gives us an understanding of nettle's alkalizing properties. "Nettle as juice or tea is an especially useful diuretic for those in a relatively 'acid' state, with an increase in nitrogen metabolism, increased hydrogen ion excretion in the urine, and a lower, more acidic pH. This occurs together with an increased stress on the blood-buffering system. Since the blood must maintain its slightly alkaline pH, and since nearly all the waste products the body produces are acid, nettle tea...helps to add electrolytes and alkali to assist the buffering system when under stress, and Nettle specifically helps increase the transport and excretion of blood nitrogen waste products. This makes it very useful in arthritis, eczema, and psoriasis—particularly when the problem is aggravated by anxieties, freak outs or really bad food (and combinations thereof)." [9]

Nettle tea can be used as a douche, eyewash, a gargle or as an enema. This green plant..."will shrink, tighten, and generally act as an anti-inflammatory astringent for simple redness and irritation of the mucosa." [10]

Most herbalists suggest that the best way to consume nettles is by infusing the herb in either hot or cold water. Some experts say to steep the herb for only a few minutes, while others suggest leaving the herb in the water overnight. For a sensitive bladder, I suggest beginning with a hot infusion, steeped for only a short while. This is "playing it safe." As you feel more comfortable with nettles as one of your favorite alkalizing friends, you can experiment with adding more dried herb to your infusions and steeping the herb for longer periods of time. Listen to your body as you enjoy this mineral-rich green drink.

Michael Moore suggests using nettles as a food supplement: "Powder the dried leaves and store them in a closed container in the refrigerator..." [11]

Here's my favorite herbal quote about Nettles: "All over the country people are taking arcane, obscure food supplements, often with little information to go on, and with the side effects and other problems seldom mentioned; and they cost a lot of money. Spirulina and chlorella are algae—dried pond scum that is excellent food for pollywogs, but so high in nucleoproteins (DNA, RNA) that it can cause nitrogen overload, purine buildup, and uric acid excess. Bee pollen is high in sugar and protein, well digested, and gives one a nice lift; but it is also expensive, especially considering what it is: the genetic information of plants mixed with worker-bee spit and enzymes—high in uric acid potential, with the possibility of giving one an allergic reaction to the bee source and whatever pollen they collected. Every year we see some new harebrained food supplement derived from weird sources, containing new stuff that we didn't know we needed (or even existed), and which we can now obtain...usually at great expense. Most of these hustles are elaborations of valid concepts or discoveries that, with flights of marketing fancy, packaging, and product development, are presented as stuff you need (but didn't know until now). This is simply the health food industry's version of the corruption of much of American retailing: marketing and image strategies to create the impression that there is a necessary product inside. It is seldom done with such cynicism; I am sure most folks believe most or all of what they try to sell.

"Nettle powder is something that you can gather yourself in places that you trust, and you can add it to smoothies and salad dressings; put it in bread; add it to your tea, home beer, and so forth. It is green food your body recognizes and can help build blood, tissue, and self-empowerment." [12] *For IC patients, I'd skip the home beer suggestion.*

Licorice Root (*Glycyrrhiza glabra, G. uralensis*): Here we have a sweet friend that has been used throughout the world for thousands of years. Fifty times sweeter than sugar, licorice is one of the most commonly

Solving the Interstitial Cystitis Puzzle

used herbs in China, the United States and in Western Europe. Known as "the great harmonizer," this famous friend helps with many systems of the body.

This herb holds an honorary place in the *Pen Tsao Ching*, the classic book of Chinese herbs written over five thousand years ago! Greek, Roman, German and English herbalists have all used licorice for countless centuries.[13]

Chinese medicine utilizes licorice in many formulas, because of the root's ability to balance disparate qualities of herbs, i.e., bitter and sour, hot and cold, tonifying, and dispersing.

In Western herbology, we can look to this plant for soothing any and all mucous membranes. Sore throats, sore labia, irritated lungs, stomach ulcers, urinary irritation, and inflamed intestines, all respond to the gentle healing qualities of this herb.

Look to licorice root as "An herb primarily for kidney deficiency, with frequent urination, particularly in the evenings before bed, especially for those with constipation and allergies. It will also help lessen chronic urinary tract inflammation."[14]

In 1611, Johann Schroeder "devotes quite some space to explaining how and why licorice 'linders the sharpness of urine' (referring to excess uric acid in the urine), 'tempers the sharpness of the fluids causing urinary stones' and 'heals bladder ulcers.'"[15] Modern herbalists as well, cite the healing effects of licorice on urinary irritation and pain.

Licorice root has become well known for its ability to repair damaged adrenal glands, which can restore overall health in an individual.

"Liquorice is one of a group of plants that have a marked effect upon the endocrine system. The glycosides present have a structure that is similar to the natural steroids of the body...this explains the beneficial action that liquorice has in the treatment of Addison's disease."[16]

Most recently, this popular herb has been found to be highly effective against stomach and duodenal ulcers. This is confirmed in several studies. Clinical reports indicate that a 90 percent success rate can be achieved using licorice preparations for the treatment of stomach and duodenal ulcers.[17] Licorice has a marked antacid effect, and is an excellent antispasmodic for the smooth muscles of the stomach and the intestines.

Some of the many microbial infections that this root can treat are malaria, tuberculosis, Staphylococcus aureus, Escherichia coli, Candida albicans, Streptococcus sobrinus, S. mutans, Salmonella typhimurium, Trichophyton mentagrophytes, T. rubrum, and Toxacara canis.[18]

People with immune disorders have found help from the consistent use of this herb. Licorice root is an immune system regulator. It increases the generation and activity of white blood cells, stimulates interferon production in the body, and enhances antibody formation. "Several trials have shown that it also possesses a distinct immunomodulator activity. That is, if the immune system is overactive, licorice calms it down; if under active, it pumps it up." [19]

Look to licorice root for its anti-infective, anti-inflammatory, and antiseptic effects, which have been known in several cultures for centuries. Presently we also know of its protecting and detoxifying action on liver cells, which highlight its use for infectious hepatitis and other liver disorders.

I suggest caution in using this herb if you have high blood pressure or have a tendency to swell. Do not use during pregnancy.

This is an herb to combine with others. Try a small amount of the cut dried root, simmered in water for ten or fifteen minutes before adding to an infusion. A little will go a long way. Enjoy its sweet taste and its harmonizing effect while you allow licorice root to sing its song slowly and gradually throughout your body cells.

Marshmallow Root (*Althaea officinalis*): Many people healing themselves of interstitial cystitis have already discovered the relief that can be found from regular use of marshmallow root. This is a demulcent herb, which means that the plant is rich in mucilage and can soothe and protect irritated or inflamed tissue.

Michael Moore writes that marshmallow root is probably the single most useful herb he knows for soothing the bladder, ureters, and urethra membranes after recuperating from an infection, stone episode or a bout of interstitial cystitis.

The healing tradition of this herb can be traced back to twenty-five hundred years ago. Throughout time and cultures, people have been using marshmallow root as a nutritional food. The Roman naturalist, Pliny, in the year 77 wrote, "Whosoever shall take a spoonful of the mallows shall that day be free from all diseases."

It is no wonder that the name of this herb "althaea" comes from a Greek word "altho" which means, "to heal". For the past several hundred years, healers have prescribed this herb internally for inflammation of mucous membranes, colds, sore throat, diarrhea, gonorrhea, gastritis, esophagitis, enteritis, and peptic ulceration. Additionally, kidney and bladder disorders of all kinds respond positively to marshmallow root.

The anti-inflammatory properties of marshmallow root combine well with its anti-microbial properties to fight respiratory infections, including bronchitis. This would be a good choice of an herb in treating Crohn's disease and irritable bowel syndrome as well as urinary tract infections. When dealing with difficult infections, it would be wise to include stronger anti-microbial herbs as well, such as echinacea (tincture), goldenseal, oil of oregano, or olive leaf extract.

This plant can also be used externally as a wash or poultice for conditions that include pain, irritation, and bruising. One can use marshmallow for relief of the discomfort of vulvodynia by putting the tea on a cloth for the external genitalia or by inserting the cool tea internally as a douche.

For internal use, one may prepare the tea with either hot or cold water. Add four teaspoons of the dry cut herb to a quart of water. Simmer slowly for ten to twenty minutes, then strain. You can drink this herb throughout the day. Cold water infusions are made by soaking the same amount of herb in a quart of water overnight. Strain in the morning and enjoy this cooling, nutritious brew throughout the day. Tincture of marshmallow can be added to hot water or tea as well. I suggest using a teaspoon of tincture per cup of tea.

For those who prefer capsules, you can experiment. Some people do not benefit as well from this form of marshmallow, but it doesn't hurt to experiment. This is a mild, harmless food, which children and the very ill can consume safely.

In the twenty-five hundred years that this herb has been used, no harmful effects have been reported.

Slippery Elm Bark (*Ulmus fulva*): Nature generously offers us another demulcent, which is very similar in properties to marshmallow root. This is a soothing, nutritious food that can be used for all ages and is easily assimilated. People from an array of cultures have been using this herb for at least fifteen hundred years.

Suck on slippery elm lozenges for sore, inflamed throats, and drink the tea or take capsules of this herb for every inch of your alimentary canal all the way down to your bottom where slippery elm can relieve the pain of hemorrhoids. People who suffer from problems of the stomach and intestines, including ulcers, gastritis, and Crohn's disease can give thanks for the cooling, soothing properties of this long-used herbal ally.

Bladder pain and irritation can be soothed with this herb as well. Slippery elm is alkalizing to the whole body. If you've had too much coffee to drink, relieve the burning in the stomach, intestines, or bladder with slippery elm tea.

Slippery Elm is helpful for people who live with chronic diseases of all kinds. Because of its ability to provide nourishment, it helps with debility and fatigue. For external use, make a tea, and after it has cooled, apply to swollen, irritated mucous membranes. I add it to a mouth rinse I make for sore and inflamed gums. For burning bladder pain, think of using anti-inflammatory slippery elm in combination with marshmallow and other herbs. Make a tea with the cut dried herb, or take slippery elm in capsules, several each day.

Alfalfa leaf (*Medicago sativa*): Alkalize, you say? Well, get out some alfalfa tea, and start drinking! Or, if you prefer, find some good quality alfalfa tabs. For a low price and not much effort, you'll have a new food to help you get that pH paper reading up in the dark greens and blues.

I was inspired to take alfalfa by my chiropractor whose fibromyalgia symptoms disappear when he takes his alfalfa tabs. Another friend's chronic knee pain goes away when she remembers to drink her alfalfa tea regularly. Alfalfa helps heal interstitial cystitis and other related health challenges through its nourishing and restoring qualities.

"By causing systemic altering and regulating changes, Alfalfa herb is also recognized today as a remedy for chronic and degenerative disorders. Alfalfa's wide gamut of components ensures a resolvent, detoxicant and dissolvent action that goes hand in hand with its primary nutritive function...The saponins and phytoestrogens lower blood lipid levels (an antilipemic action) and one of its proteins is considered antitumoral. The remedy has also shown liver and small intestine-protective activities, especially when caused by chemical damage...These are just some examples of the mechanisms of its systemic detoxicant effect."[20]

This well known herb is abundantly rich in chlorophyll and eight essential digestive enzymes. Its high mineral and vitamin content allow this plant to be helpful for anyone needing a boost with digestion and nutrition. According to Thomas Bartram, a well known British herbalist, alfalfa leaf stimulates growth of supportive connective tissue and is useful for collagen diseases including arthritis. This plant is also helpful with rheumatism, dyspepsia, backache, chronic ulcers, and infections of sinus, ear, nose, and throat. [21]

Alfalfa is a wonderful cleanser as well as an herb to help with depression and pain. For those who have trouble with regular elimination, I suggest a steady intake of alfalfa in tea or tablet form as an alternative to the harshness of purgative and strongly laxative herbs.

This is an herb that is safe to use during pregnancy. Some women may find alfalfa helpful in regulating the endocrine system. Generally, use of the leaf has no precautions. In the mountain of herb books in my library, I have found only one caution mentioned for the leaf of this plant and that is in Susun Weed's revised *New Menopausal Years*. She mentions that menopausal women who have trouble with profuse bleeding should avoid the use of this herb as it may be thinning to the blood. [22]

The only other caution in using alfalfa is in regard to the seeds and sprouts. Alfalfa seeds contain a toxic amino acid called canavanine, which has been associated with an activation of systemic lupus erythematosus. Eating a few alfalfa sprouts should be fairly safe; moderation in this case is suggested.

Welcome alfalfa leaf as a nutritious part of your growing herbal pantry, and watch the gentle shifts that this healing plant can bring to you and to your loved ones.

Chamomile (*Matricaria recutita, M. chamomilla, Chamomilla recutita*):
Let's peek around in an herb garden, recognizing the gentle soothers our
bodies long for. Look here, we come upon some delicate daisy-like flowers
waiting to be picked and made into a healing relaxing brew.

"Slow down," says my friend, with the golden-ochre centers and tiny,
delicate white petals. This plant almost took over my entire garden one
year when I lived in the hot foothills of the Sierra Nevadas and had decided
to add chamomile to my herbal family. Since moving to a cool coastal climate
where I prefer to grow edible greens and a variety of botanicals, I've learned
to purchase chamomile dry by the pound and enjoy simply remembering
what it was like to pluck each individual chamomile flower for my daily
teas.

Chamomile has been the friend who takes my hand when the mind is
going far faster than the body can go. You know who I mean; the one who
whispers gently and softly into our ear, "take a break," or "remember to
breathe deeply into this moment." Chamomile blossoms beckon me into the
softer quieter me who knows without a doubt that going too fast is only
going to sabotage the greater healing I long for.

I learned to like the taste of chamomile only after some time, and even
still, I prefer that she shares the pot with other botanical medicines.
Peppermint or spearmint, nettles, and licorice are often some of my choices.
Some people enjoy the nutty, sweet, unique taste of this flower on its own.

Cystitis sufferers benefit from chamomile's ability to relax spasmodic
muscles. Chamomile is a remedy that helps those who feel tense,
oversensitive, weak, and in pain. This plant is analgesic, anti-inflammatory,
and a mild sedative. If you've had too many trips to the bathroom all night
and your nerves feel like sandpaper the next day because of lack of sleep
and pain, choose chamomile.

For those who suffer from irritable bowel conditions, gastritis, ulcers, or
simply a nervous tummy, pour some chamomile tea to harmonize, heal, and
stop the pain. Many people suffer from acid reflux, and chamomile might
be just the tea to keep the digestive energies moving down in the direction
they should go.

Think of chamomile when you suffer from menstrual cramps or when
you need some help in relieving your body of a Candida overgrowth. Most
premenstrual and menopausal symptoms such as headache, irritability,
insomnia, moodiness, and depression can be relieved with chamomile
infusion

This gentle plant can help with acute health challenges, such as fevers,
flu, enteritis, throat inflammations, and infections of the eye, mouth, and
gums. Calm the spasms of a persistent cough with quieting, relaxing
chamomile blossoms.

Chronic muscle aches and spasms that accompany fibromyalgia and chronic fatigue immune dysfunction syndrome (known as myalgic encephalomyelitis in Europe and Canada) can respond well to regular daily infusions that include chamomile blossoms. For a real treat, add chamomile tea to your bathwater before you get in for a soak.

In several other Western countries, this herb is given far more respect as a phytomedicine (herbal medicine) than it is in the U.S. "According to a recent article by Ivan Salamon (1992) M.recutita [chamomile] is included in the pharmacopaeias of twenty-six countries. Writing on the plant in the June-August 1992 issue of the Australian journal *Focus on Herbs*, Salamon also noted that in Czecho-Slovakia, a common folk saying has it that 'an individual should always bow before the curative powers of the chamomile plant.'" [23]

Generally, this herb is quite safe for the most sensitive among us. Unless you have a serious allergy to members of the aster family (which is quite rare) allow yourself to discover the lovely ritual of slowing down with chamomile tea. Put one to two teaspoons of dried blossoms in your teapot for each mug of tea and add almost boiling water. Allow to steep about five to ten minutes and enjoy. Watch the stress find its way out of your mind and body, and feel that easy smile come across your face.

Cornsilk (*Zea mays*): Those silky threads from garden corn may be the medicine you've been looking for. Many people with cystitis have already discovered the relief that this herb can bring to a burning, sore urinary tract.

Cornsilk was used among the early pioneers in the United States for acute urinary tract infections. It is also used in Chinese medicine and has maintained its reputation among doctors of Oriental medicine.

Urinary and kidney complaints of many kinds can be eased by cornsilk tea. It is a soothing urinary demulcent, a diuretic and an analgesic to inflamed or injured urinary tract mucosa. Consider using this herb for any type of cystitis, urinary retention, pus in the urine, or incontinence. Other conditions that are relieved by cornsilk are prostate gland enlargement, irritation of the urinary tract by phosphatic and uric acids, urethritis, and expulsion of gravel or stones.

Peter Holmes writes of the usefulness of this herb in treating what Oriental medicine calls, "gallbladder damp heat" and "gallbladder fire." This can include acute or sub-acute gallstone attacks. Chinese medicine also uses this herb for jaundice. [24]

Cornsilk is most helpful when used fresh. The best tinctures of cornsilk are made from the fresh plant. Dried cornsilk tea can also be used. No need to measure...this is a mild remedy that can be used freely, as it brings soothing relief. If you have an allergy to corn, you might want to use marshmallow root instead of cornsilk. These herbs have similar soothing properties for short term pain relief and long term healing of interstitial cystitis.

Aloe Vera (*Aloe barbadensis*): Aloe vera is probably the most well-known plant in the interstitial cystitis healing community. This plant has been known to assist in relieving more maladies than one could list in a brief summary. Please be aware that the part of the plant that we are discussing here is from the tubular inner cells found in the central pulp of the aloe leaf. Medicines made from the outer leaf (Aloe latex, A. ferox) are a very strong laxative herb.

Aloe gel is used externally for burns and tissue trauma. It is cooling, protecting, soothing, and disinfecting. This is a wonderful plant to have growing in your kitchen for first aid. Aloe gel is antiseptic and antifungal as well, so it can be used on painful or itching rashes and fungal infections including Candida albicans. Irritations in the delicate genital and rectal areas of the body can be soothed by this curative plant. Aloe is anti-inflammatory and moisturizing. Aloe juice is known to help with inflamed gums and other discomforts in the mouth.

Internally, many people with interstitial cystitis are experiencing relief from taking aloe vera capsules. There have been some small studies done with freeze dried aloe vera that show positive results in healing the symptoms of interstitial cystitis.[25] Because this disease is multi-causal and each person's biochemistry is unique, there is no one plant that has proven a cure-all for IC. When we look, however, at all the healing qualities that this famous plant embodies, it is no wonder that relief can often be found through continual long-term use of this herb.

The freeze-dried aloe is often preferred amongst people who live with IC because in this form there is no added citric acid, a necessary preservative found in the fresh juices and gels. Citric acid is one of the ingredients that most people with IC need to avoid. For those who are not bothered by citric acid, several brands of the fresh, organic juice can be purchased in natural food stores or through the internet.

For women with IC and vulvodynia who are able to be sexually active, I suggest integrating the cool aloe gel as part of sexual play and penetration to help soothe and cool any inflammation in the pelvic area. Applying the juice or gel after sexual activity as a compress to the vulva or as a douche intravaginally can prevent post coital pain in some situations.

Aloe vera is a bactericidal against *staphylococcus aureus, streptococcus viridans,* and five strains of *streptococcus mutans*, which is the cause of dental plaque.[26] We can welcome its demulcent, analgesic, antiviral, and antibiotic properties for a variety of discomforts and ills. Aloe contains eighteen amino acids and vitamins and is a wonderful detoxifier.

People with digestive disorders including gastritis, peptic and duodenal ulcers, irritable bowel syndrome, and chronic candidiasis have found benefit from drinking the fresh aloe vera juice or taking the freeze dried capsules. I have spoken to people who have had relief from fibromyalgia and arthritis-related discomfort with the regular ingestion of this herb.

There are several companies that sell whole freeze dried aloe vera in capsule form. Some of these companies grow their aloe vera organically. I suggest doing a price and quality comparison before purchasing these capsules, paying attention to any additives that might cause irritation or allergy.

Meadowsweet (*Filipendula ulmaria,* also known as *Spiraea ulmaria*): For those of us who have difficulty taking aspirin and non-steroid anti-inflammatory drugs, we have some good news in the form of meadowsweet. The aerial parts of this plant have been used since the middle ages, predominantly in Europe.

Aspirin actually derives its name from the older botanical name of this herb: *Spiraea ulmaria.* In 1839, a German chemist discovered that meadowsweet's flower buds contain salicin, the same chemical that had been isolated from white willow bark eleven years earlier. Experimentation was done, and aspirin is the result; the drug is made from a combination of synthesized ingredients, including acetylsalicylic acid. Long term use of aspirin can lead to gastric ulceration and bleeding, but meadowsweet does not produce these side effects. This beautiful, aromatic plant actually works as a gentle digestive remedy for acidity and stomach pain. A few experts refer to this plant as "the herbalist's bicarbonate of soda."

Meadowsweet is a urinary tract analgesic and antiseptic. It dries what Oriental medicine calls "dampness," a condition common to almost everyone with pelvic disorders. This herb stops discharge, bleeding, and promotes tissue repair.

I like the gentleness of meadowsweet. Very sensitive individuals, children, and the elderly can generally benefit from this herb. It is not going to be a replacement for codeine or heavy narcotic-based pain relievers. Meadowsweet is a deep-acting remedy when used continuously.

The pain relieving properties of this herb are not limited to the urinary tract. It is well known, especially in Europe, as an herb to relieve rheumatism of the joints and muscles and for gout. It is listed as an antiphlogistic (an agent that prevents or counteracts inflammation and fever) in the conservative *PDR for Herbal Medicines*, a publication that is based on scientific research of herbs in Europe. Commission E, the expert panel that evaluates herbal medicines for the German counterpart of the FDA approves this herb as a treatment for the common cold. [27]

Meadowsweet is helpful in relieving diarrhea; it is effective against *Shigella dysenteriae.* For those who suffer from urinary tract infections, it has been shown to be active against *Escherischia coli.* For any of these conditions, I'd suggest adding this herb as a tincture or tea in combination with other effective herbs.

182   *Solving the Interstitial Cystitis Puzzle*

Generally, this herb is used as a tincture, so be sure your tea or water is very hot when you add several drops of meadowsweet tincture. Allow the alcohol to evaporate before drinking.

If you have a true serious aspirin allergy—not just a queasy tummy from taking aspirin—, I would suggest not taking this herb. If you are in a lot of pain, it is fine to take this herb in addition to a stronger over the counter or prescription pain medication. If you have asthma, this plant is contraindicated.

Skullcap (*Scutellaria lateriflora, S. galericulata*): I'll confess, I've hardly spoken to anyone over the past few years who hasn't exhibited at least some signs of nervous exhaustion. It seems to come with the territory of living in the twenty-first century. If your phone machine is blinking, your e-mail box has over fourteen unread messages, your car ignition has a glitch sometimes, and you haven't found time to call your dentist to make the appointment for that achy back molar, not to mention the bladder spasms that came on last night that just don't go away, I think it's time to introduce you to another dear friend. Please, meet nerve restorative extraordinaire; skullcap. Here is a plant that will, over time, offer you freedom from spasmodic pain, nerve exhaustion, and sleepless nights.

Okay friends, let's put some water up to boil, and while the heat's on, we can explore some of the gifts this member of the mint family has to share. You say you haven't time, Johnny has to get to baseball practice and it's your turn to drive? You can't stop now, the deadline's due on your present project at work? That's the time to stop, breathe deeply and softly into your belly, and make some skullcap tea. Okay, you're really in a jam? Put some tincture in the hot water, but do yourself a favor, take it!

Medicinally, we use the aerial parts of this plant, which were also used by the nineteenth century Eclectic physicians, forerunners of our present-day naturopathic doctors. These healers prescribed scullcap for insomnia, nervousness, intermittent fevers (malaria), convulsions and the delirium tremens of advanced alcoholism. Until 1947, this plant was listed as a standard drug in the *National Formulary*, the pharmacist's reference. [28]

Today we use this herb in many of the same ways. We can use skullcap along with other relaxing herbs, such as hops, valerian, passionflower, or chamomile. Skullcap doesn't just relax the nervous system; it also nourishes and strengthens the nerves. It can be a botanical to turn to, not only with interstitial cystitis pain, but also with chronic headaches, muscle spasms and exhaustion. People who live with M.E. (myalgic encephalomyelitis, also called chronic fatigue immune dysfunction syndrome) can benefit greatly from the consistent use of this herb.

Skullcap is a good friend in the case of premenstrual tension, depression, insomnia, and nervous stress following bereavement or shock. It has been used for seizures, including epilepsy, as well as hysteria.

This is a gentle herb. One can find countless tincture and tea preparations containing skullcap. One of my favorite combinations is "Avena-Skullcap Compound", made by Herb Pharm in Southern Oregon. Avena (oats) works quite well with skullcap, nourishing and building the nervous system. I suggest a compound such as this for those discontinuing use of alcohol, cigarettes, or any kind of drug withdrawal. Think long, slow, and steady when using scullcap in these ways.

In purchasing this herb, it is especially important to be aware of the quality of one's herbal source. This herb has often been cut with inferior products. Additionally, skullcap herb, once dried, does not maintain its medicinal potency for more than about six months. I suggest a tincture made from fresh skullcap, used either alone or in a combination as mentioned above, added to your hot tea of choice.

If using the dried herb in tea, enjoy combining skullcap with other nourishing plants, such as peppermint, chamomile, licorice, and nettles. Put half a teaspoon of dried skullcap in your teapot for each cup of tea and steep about ten minutes. As we pour our cup of skullcap tea, let's watch the steam dance gracefully up into the air, disappearing with our unnecessary tensions. Relax and enjoy.

Kava (*Piper methysticum*): So, you've made a gentle brew, containing some of the above-mentioned teas, including chamomile and skullcap, but you say your nerves are still a bit on edge? It is one a.m. and you can't fall asleep, your bladder is still burning? I suggest you try kava. People have been doing so for three thousand years, with a very positive response. Please note that this herb has nothing to do with coffee...kava is an herb that lives somewhat on the opposite end of the spectrum from coffee. In fact, one of its many benefits is its ability to relax those edgy nerves that a person can get from having one too many lattés.

I know I am not the only person who has difficulty with the side effects of prescription and over the counter pain relievers and muscle relaxants. Here is an herb that I have had no trouble taking, and which helps relieve muscle spasms, insomnia, and general up-tightness. In Europe, this medicinal botanical is an approved phytomedicine prescribed for anxiety and depression.

This herb originates from the South Pacific, where it has been used as part of a ceremony, usually involving a circle of people drinking a brew of kava from a coconut shell. Ceremonial use of kava has helped to enhance sociability and group harmony, and has served the purpose of settling disputes and facilitating reconciliation. Aside from its use as a ceremonial beverage, kava has also been used medicinally in South Pacific cultures.

People with chronic urinary disorders can benefit greatly from kava's antispasmodic, antimicrobial, and antifungal properties. This herb specifically helps with pain and spasms of the urethra and bladder. People who live with interstitial cystitis often suffer from difficulty falling asleep because of pain and stress, layered with the anxiety, muscle tension, depression and exhaustion that accompany these challenges. Kava, also called, "kava kava", can help with all of these related health issues. For people with problems involving urinary incontinence, kava is a perfect remedy.

"As a soothing relaxant to urinary functions, kava root will also reduce urinary irritation and pain, whatever the cause, including prostate congestion, cystitis, uricosuria, or just plain stress. Severe vaginal and anal itching are also included in its action…Its urinary restorative effect includes an excellent astringent mucostatic (or mucus decongestant) action. For those with simple, chronic urinary incontinence with dribbling, irritated urination arising from an underlying bladder Qi deficiency, Kava is absolutely pertinent. Anti-incontinent, analgesic and anti-inflammatory actions here successfully operate in concert…"[29]

Recent clinical studies have shown kava to be a safe, non-addictive, anti-anxiety medicine, as effective as prescription anxiety agents containing benzodiazepines such as Xanax and Valium. While benzodiazepines tend to promote lethargy and mental impairment, kava has been shown to improve concentration, memory, and reaction time for people suffering from anxiety. Benzodiazepines are infamous for being addictive with complications in withdrawal. Kava has been clinically demonstrated as a means of achieving a state of relaxation without adverse side effects.

Kava can be helpful with digestive stress, including indigestion, distended painful abdomen, and stomach ulcers. Allow yourself some kava in cases of headache as well as neck and back pain. There have been problems with inferior kava products being marketed. Be sure your kava is of high quality. The medicinal kava being described here is made from the extract of dried four to eight year-old rhizome and roots of the *Piper methysticum* plant. Usually this plant is harvested from the South Pacific or from Hawaii.

The tincture of kava has a very numbing, strong taste, so if you choose to take it in this form, I'd suggest NOT adding your tincture drops to a whole cup of tea…try adding them to a tablespoon or two of hot tea or water. I have had very positive results with Herb Pharm brand "Pharma Kava" capsules. Take two at bedtime for a restful night's sleep. The tincture is a great dental numbing agent as a hold-me-over if you have a toothache while you wait for your dentist appointment.

If you take more than just a little bit of kava, I suggest you do not operate a motor vehicle. I'd also suggest you not take this herb if you are taking psychiatric drugs or consuming more than a small amount of alcohol. Huge doses over a long period of time can create strange skin reactions, which disappear as soon as you stop taking the herb. With moderation and gentleness, this herb can be of great assistance for many of the ailments that come with living in this century.

Editor's Note: According to Ray Sahelian, MD, in the last few years there have been several reports of individuals in Europe with liver damage while consuming kava on a regular basis. Recently a few reports of liver damage occurring in kava users in the US have also been mentioned in the media. As of now, there have not been any scientific published studies that have proven liver damage occurs in subjects consuming kava. Those who have been taking kava regularly (daily) for many months or years should seek advice from their doctor who will most likely ask that the kava be stopped and liver enzymes tested. This is a blood test that is done routinely. Until we know the full details about the safety of kava, it is best to consult with an herbal expert about using kava on a regular basis.

Milk Thistle (*Silybum marianum*): Two thousand years ago, people didn't have to worry about dealing with the fumes of a diesel truck idling in front of them on a highway. Neither did their livers have to process one of the forty chemicals present in indoor carpeting, including styrene, formaldehyde, vinyl acetate and propylene glycol. [30] Yet, the seed from *Silybum marianum* was used even then as a treatment for liver conditions.

We do not need to be a scientist to realize the dangers of being exposed to countless toxic chemicals. Those of us who are part of the IC Puzzle group online have begun to compare notes and have realized that bladder flares are often associated with common chemical exposures. This can include well meaning friends and family members wearing fragrances in our homes, the simple painting of a bathroom, or use of a laundry detergent with hidden toxins.

Everyone's liver needs help these days. Milk thistle is specifically an herb that can decongest, restore, detoxify, and protect the liver. Milk thistle's softening and dissolving actions can be helpful in the hardening-type of hepatic disorders, such as sclerosis and stone-formation.

It is the silymarin in milk thistle that is so effective in guarding the organ from damage by pollutants, viral invaders, and other toxins. This is a medicinal botanical that has passed the scrutiny of scientists with good grades: milk thistle deters toxins from penetrating liver cells, guards against free radical oxidation, and lowers fat buildup in the organ. Studies in Europe have demonstrated milk thistle's ability to relieve symptoms associated with cirrhosis, viral hepatitis, jaundice, and poisoning.

What a gift we have in milk thistle! It offers us assistance in digesting fats, synthesizing proteins, and protecting the gall bladder. For those with allergies of all kinds, milk thistle will help reduce reactions. Milk thistle has anti-inflammatory properties and is a good friend in those pre-menstrual moments (and days).

Some authors suggest that this herb is best taken in capsule form or as a tincture. Apparently the plant is not very soluble in water. Milk thistle is somewhat warming in its thermal nature, which means that it should be taken carefully at first by those with sensitive bladders. Begin slowly by taking only a few drops of the tincture or one capsule a day. Allow your body's response to determine your daily dose if you find that this is your medicine.

Other herbs and healing suggestions

Additional herbs that may be helpful for those living with interstitial cystitis and related health challenges are those that are specifically for fighting infections. These are stronger herbs and not generally medicines that people consume without a break. Not all antimicrobial botanicals are listed here, and not all of these will be appropriate for everyone. I will mention some of them briefly and hope that you will seek further support regarding use of these herbs from your naturopathic doctor, acupuncturist, or other health professional.

Interstitial cystitis has been associated with a variety of microbial imbalances, including bacterial, viral, and fungal infections. These are botanical medicines that are helpful for some people.

Pau D'Arco (*Tabebuia spp.*): This is an antifungal which has been used as a tea for chronic Candida albicans infections. Simmer the bark in water for about twenty minutes and strain. Drink a few cups of this tea a day. Pau d'arco can be used as a douche or as a rinse on male and female genitalia. A salve of this herb can be applied to fungal infections anywhere on the body. This tea is relatively high in tannins, so go cautiously at first.

Oil of Oregano (*Origanum vulgare*): Oil of oregano is not exactly the herb you sprinkled in your spaghetti sauce in the days when you could eat such things. What is labeled as "oregano" in the supermarket culinary herb section is usually a variation of marjoram or thyme. The oil of oregano mentioned here for internal use is also not the "essential oil," which should only be used topically.

Oil of oregano is a completely natural substance derived from wild oregano species, and sold in a concentrated form. There are many studies described in recent literature which support the potency of this oil as a germ killer, anti-inflammatory, and as a pain killer.

This medicinal plant oil is antiviral, antibacterial, antifungal, and antiparasitic. I've had good results using oil of oregano capsules to treat urinary tract infections. Positive results have been reported by people who live with fibromyalgia, chronic fatigue immune dysfunction syndrome, and other related health challenges.

"A recent study compared the anticandida effect of oregano oil to that of caprylic acid. The results indicated that oregano oil is over 100 times more potent than caprylic acid against candida." [31]

Entire books have been published describing the potency of oregano oil in relieving the pain and cause of countless health disorders. One of these is *The Cure is in the Cupboard*, by Cass Ingram. All of the recently published materials describing the benefits of oil of oregano emphasize the importance of the quality and source of this curative plant. I found that taking the potent oil alone caused burning on my tongue and mouth. Since taking the oil in soft gel capsules, I have had no problem, as long as it is taken with food.

Olive Leaf (*Olea europea*): Perhaps a dove has arrived into our lives, bringing a healing message through the olive branch it offers. This plant is famous throughout time and over continents. The olive leaf has been used as medicine throughout the Middle East, the Mediterranean region, as well as in Peru, Chile, and elsewhere in South America.

It was at the end of the nineteenth century that scientists discovered a phytochemical in the leaves called oleuropein, which helps to explain the effectiveness of this plant in treating a broad number of disorders.

Olive leaf extracts are being used to treat bacterial, viral, and fungal infections with impressive results. For people who have stubborn cases of candidiasis, the use of this plant has been found helpful, especially when rotated with other natural anti-fungal botanicals, such as grapefruit seed extract, oil of oregano, and berberine-containing herbs, such as barberry or goldenseal.

Many other infections can be treated with olive leaf extract. Because it is eliminating viruses, bacteria, and fungi, it can create a "die-off" reaction, which can include headaches, and general malaise. I suggest beginning with just one capsule a day of this herb and gradually increasing the dose. Some people can take two capsules a few times a day. For others, this would be too potent. Taking this herb in tea or tincture form is also effective.

Barberry (*Berberis vulgaris*): Here is an herb that is considered one of the best remedies for correcting liver function and promoting the flow of bile. What I love about barberry is that it is gentle, and easy on digestive systems that don't handle stronger liver-cleansing protocols. For people who feel weak or debilitated, and know they need to work on cleansing the liver, I suggest making acquaintance with barberry. It is the root bark of this plant that is used medicinally.

For those with interstitial cystitis, barberry can clear toxins gently, as well as treat infections, either acute or occult, that may be contributing to discomfort. Like other herbs that contain berberine, barberry has been found to be effective against viruses, candidiasis, amoebas, bacterial infections and parasites. Barberry is similar to goldenseal in many ways, yet it is easier on the stomach, and can be taken for longer periods of time, without destroying the fragile balance of the intestinal tract. Other similar berberine-containing herbs are oregon grape, phellodendron huang bai, and coptis huang lian (the latter two are used in Chinese medicine).

Solving the Interstitial Cystitis Puzzle

Barberry is a good choice of plant remedies for inflammation of the gallbladder or for gallstones. Any congested state of the liver, including jaundice, can respond favorably to barberry. Additionally, barberry acts against malaria, diarrhea, constipation, acute gastroenteritis, and salmonella and can help to reduce an enlarged spleen.

Amrit's emphasis on liver congestion as the culprit in many health challenges can allow us to understand why barberry is helpful with a variety of disorders. I suggest considering the use of barberry for arthritic conditions, cysts, headaches, and fatigue.

I've had good results using capsules of barberry powder, yet this plant can also be prepared as a decoction. A teaspoon of the root bark for each cup of tea can be simmered for fifteen minutes or so. It can also be taken in tincture form, adding the drops to very hot water.

For chronic conditions, I suggest taking this herb for a few weeks at a time at most, and then take a break before continuing again. This botanical can be alternated with other antimicrobial herbs for stubborn conditions, such as systemic yeast infections.

* * *

By now your pantry is probably getting a bit full. As you enjoy the process of integrating healing teas into your daily rhythm, I encourage you to continue drinking plenty of clear alkaline water. Most teas have some diuretic properties. Their cleansing and nourishing qualities can be wonderfully helpful for chronic health challenges, yet they are not a replacement for water. Even if urinary frequency is a problem, drinking these alkalizing mineral-rich fluids will help you in the long term to heal the causes of interstitial cystitis.

When the weather is cold in the coastal area where I live, drinking plain cool- temperature water doesn't always sound so appealing. I make a very light broth with vegetables that work for my body, such as celery, carrots, maybe some potato peels for potassium, and a leaf from a bok choy plant. I simmer the veggies in water for fifteen or twenty minutes and drink this broth after it's cooled down to just slightly warm. This is a replacement for water, as it contains no diuretic herbs. Usually I make enough broth for one or two days at a time.

Herb teas can be refrigerated for about two days. Be sure not to overcook the tea when you are warming up your brew. After some time of experimentation, try creating a combination of herbs that will be your own personal blend. I have my own "Good Morning Blend" and some other healing combinations, which sit out on the counter for me to see. These teas help me to slow down and take in some of the lovely nutrients that nature provides. Pour a cup for a loved one as well, and enjoy a few precious moments of shared comfort and healing.

References and Suggested Reading:

Bartram, Thomas,

> *Bartram's Encyclopedia of Herbal Medicine*. New York: Marlowe and Co., 1998

Buhner, Stephen Harrod,

> *Herbal Antibiotics*. Pownal, Vermont: Storey Books, 1999

Castleman, Michael,

> *The New Healing Herbs*. New York: Bantam Books, 2002

Duke, James A.,

> *The Green Pharmacy Herbal Handbook*. U.S.A.: Rodale/Reach, 2000

Foster, Steven, and Chongxi, Yue,

> *Herbal Emissaries; Bringing Chinese Herbs to the West*. Vermont: Healing Arts Press, 1992

Foster, Steven,

> *Herbal Renaissance*. Salt Lake City: Peregrine Smith Books, 1993

Gladstar, Rosemary,

> *Herbal Healing for Women*. New York: Fireside/Simon and Schuster, 1993

Hoffman, David,

> *The Holistic Herbal*. Dorset, England: Element Books, 1988

Holmes, Peter,

> *The Energetics of Western Herbs*, vol. 1 and 2, Revised Third Edition, Boulder: Snow Lotus Press, 1998

Hsu, Hong-Yen,

> *Oriental Materia Medica; A Concise Guide*. Long Beach, California: Oriental Healing Arts Institute, 1986

Lawson, Lynn,

> *Staying Well in a Toxic World; Understanding Environmental Illness, Multiple Chemical Sensitivities, Chemical Injuries and Sick Building Syndrome*. Chicago: Noble Press, 1993

Moore, Michael,

> *Herbs for the Urinary Tract*. New Canaan, Connecticut: Keats Publishing, Inc. 1998

Medicinal Plants of the Pacific West. Santa Fe, New Mexico: Red
   Crane Books, 1995

Murray, Michael, and Pizzorno, Joseph,

Encylopedia of Natural Medicine. Revised second edition, Rocklin,
   California: Prima Communications, Inc., 1998

PDR for Herbal Medicines. First Edition, Montvale, New Jersey:
   Medical Economics Company, 1998

Tierra, Michael,

Planetary Herbology. Santa Fe, New Mexico: Lotus Press, 1988

Weed, Susun,

Healing Wise. Woodstock, New York: Ash Tree Publishing, 1989

New Menopausal Years; The Wise Woman Way. Woodstock New York:
   Ash Tree Publishing, 2002

See appendix D for Herbal Resources

* * *

Shira Lee, MA, offers intuitive counseling, flower essence therapy and self-
healing support. She is available for e mail and telephone consultations.
She can be reached at gentlybe00@yahoo.com

Shira Lee
PO Box 1036
Mendocino, CA 95460

Solving the Interstitial Cystitis Puzzle

An Alkalizing Program

"Let thy medicine be thy food...and thy food thy medicine."

— Hippocrates

Although doctors are generally trained to use drugs, surgery, and the latest laboratory technologies, nutrition therapy is a real orphan in the medical community. In other words, to quote Abraham Maslow, "It is tempting, if the only tool you have is a hammer, to treat everything as if it were a nail." Nutraceuticals or the use of foods to heal has been overlooked in the treatment of IC. Diet changes and allergy elimination diets in the treatment of IC have been explored and with good results, but they have not gone far enough.

It is interesting to note, thus far, that doctors have reported an improvement of symptoms in IC patients who observe certain food restrictions. The reported restrictions are many including acid-forming foods, acidic foods, allergens, and foods containing acids, such as chocolate and coffee. In addition, we know very well in the IC community that alkalizing substances such as Tummy Tamer or Coffee Tamer (calcium carbonate, potassium hydroxide, magnesium hydroxide) and simple baking soda (sodium bicarbonate) will diminish some symptoms of IC. The healthiest route to take is to decrease acids by decreasing acid-forming foods and making lifestyle changes. We need to increase foods, supplements, and activities that promote alkalizing. This of course requires work on the part of the patient, and there are no "quick fixes" or "magic bullets."

One could say with IC, and likely other conditions, we have borrowed on our bodies' alkaline mineral reserves that we are essentially "bankrupt." With an alkalizing diet and lifestyle, we can restore, replenish, and eventually start a "savings account" of alkalizing minerals.

Alkalizing is 80:20

Essentially, in my researching an alkalizing program for healing, studies recommend to consume 80% alkalizing foods and 20% acid-forming foods. Foods that are alkalizing and should make up 80% of your diet are fruits, vegetables, and sprouts, which contain calcium, potassium, magnesium, iron, and organic sodium plus other trace minerals and vitamins.

Foods that are acid-forming and will make up the other 20% of your alkalizing diet are meats and animal products, grains, legumes and most seed and nuts. Animal products contain high levels of sulfur and phosphorus that when metabolized are converted to strong sulfuric acid and phosphoric acids. Grains, legumes, nuts, seeds, carbonated drinks and dairy contain high levels of phosphorus and are converted after metabolism to strong phosphoric acids.

Understand that eating a high acid diet is not the same thing as eating an acid-forming diet. Although they are high in citric acids, citrus fruits when they are metabolized create an alkali ash in the body. In other words, fruits help to neutralize body acids. The potassium and organic sodium they contain is especially useful in neutralizing acids. However, the acid in foods troubles persons with IC, so there is a dilemma here. We need the alkaline elements found in fruits to help neutralize the body's acids, but we cannot tolerate the citric acid, at least not initially. It has been my observation for me and others that after three to six months on an alkalizing diet, the diet becomes much broader with more fruits, vegetables, and sprouts tolerated.

Note:

Many of the toxic chemicals that enter the body are fat-soluble hence they tend to be stored in fat tissue where they may stay for years. Toxins will be released during times of exercise, stress, fasting, or detoxification. This is something to remember when starting any kind of detox program. An alkalizing program is a detoxification program. For some of you it is best not to go too fast.

I discovered certain fruits less troublesome in the beginning of my alkalizing program; however, *my* list of fruit that I tolerated may not be *your* list of fruits that you will tolerate. If yeast is not a problem for you, *small* amounts of dried fruits are usually well tolerated and can help add calories. Once I was on my hypoallergenic alkalizing program for a few months and my urine pH indicated my body trend was more alkaline with a pH between 7.0 and 7.4, I was able to consume citrus fruits and spicy foods with no "flare-ups." I was not taking any alkalizing supplements to tolerate these foods. We will review certain foods that may cause less discomfort for you in the Getting Started chapter.

When making food choices, eat a variety of the freshest, organic seasonal vegetables and fruits as possible, preferably raw or lightly steamed, from the neutral to highly alkalizing categories listed in the appendix A. Farmer's markets are good places to shop as well as your local health food store. Home gardens are wonderful if you have time and space. Choose unprocessed organic foods without additives, hormones, and chemicals whenever possible and affordable since these substances are toxins and acid-forming. I wash and slice vegetables for a relish tray with dressing or hummus that I serve with evening meals along with a cooked vegetable or two and an entrée. Consider experimenting and adding new vegetables, fruits, and sprouts to your diet. Avoid or use minimal natural sugar (honey or organic maple syrup) and salt (sea salt) since they are acidifying as well. Cooking fruits and vegetables decreases their alkalinity and destroys helpful anti-inflammatory enzymes, and over-cooking causes them to be acidifying.

Briefly, I will present five essential alkalizing elements and the benefits they provide in the body, remembering there are other vitamins, minerals,

Solving the Interstitial Cystitis Puzzle

essential fatty acids, and trace elements required, too. This is why it is so critical to eat a well-balanced hypoallergenic alkalizing diet. Please see chapters on Vitamin D and Essential Fatty Acids.

"Every human being or animal that dies of 'natural causes' dies of a mineral deficiency."

— Nobel Prize nominee, Dr. Joel Wallach

Autonomic Nervous System

The sympathetic nervous system (SNS) in the body controls our fight or flight response mechanism. The parasympathetic system (PSNS) in the body controls our rest and digestive response mechanism. It works like this:

- Calcium: Stimulatory mineral for the Sympathetic Nervous System
- Magnesium: Inhibitory mineral for the Sympathetic Nervous System
- Potassium: Stimulatory mineral for the Parasympathetic Nervous System
- Sodium: Inhibitory mineral for the Parasympathetic Nervous System

Note:

Too much calcium and sodium are stimulating. Note that magnesium and potassium are relaxing to the body. Most Americans do not get sufficient calcium and consume too much inorganic sodium, and we are especially deficient in magnesium, potassium and *organic* sodium.

"Eight out of the top ten causes of death in the United States are the result of diet related degenerative diseases."

— Former US Surgeon General, Dr. C. Everett Koop, MD

Calcium
Stimulatory Mineral for the Sympathetic Nervous System

Calcium has a *stimulatory* effect on the sympathetic nervous system, responsible for fight or flight. Calcium is one of the alkaline elements needed to help neutralize and buffer our body's acids. It is called the "king" of the alkalizing elements since it is found in the highest proportion in the body. In a 154 pound person there is approximately 1160 grams of calcium. Calcium is necessary with phosphorus* to help build and maintain strong bones and teeth. About 99% of the body's calcium is found in the bones and teeth. Adequate calcium is needed also for proper muscle contraction, nerve conduction, and blood clotting.

Proper absorption of calcium also depends on adequate amounts of vitamin D. Adequate amounts of the fat-soluble vitamin D can be ingested (400-800 IU) or acquired by adequate exposure to sunlight. Without adequate vitamin D, the body is unable to utilize calcium. It is critical that vitamin D is consumed from foods or obtained from sun exposure. (Please see chapter on Vitamin D.)

Note:

Our bodies' utilization of the calcium in food can be adversely affected by the presence of two chemicals called phytic acid and oxalic acid. Phytic acid is found in the bran portion of grains. Rice has only a small amount of phytic acid in it. Oxalic acid is present in significant quantities in spinach, rhubarb, and dark green leafy vegetables. The magnitude of the effect depends on the amount of these acids we consume, and a higher intake of calcium may be necessary if large quantities of foods containing oxalic and/ or phytic acids are eaten. Diets high in protein, salt, sugar, caffeine, and alcohol will also increase the requirement for calcium.

Paleolithic Model Note:

Until man began to cultivate grains and livestock 10,000 years ago, people rarely, if ever ate grains or drank animal milk! According to Eaton and Konner, we simply do not have the genetic make up to tolerate grains and milk products. Whole grains contain phytic acid, which is found in the bran of whole grains. Phytic acid binds to a variety of minerals including calcium, iron, zinc, and magnesium to form insoluble salts, called phytates, which are wasted from the body. Probably because grains are a relatively new food, from an evolutionary perspective, it appears that we have not yet developed digestive tracts which can break down these phytates. In addition, dairy consumption also has an adverse effect on vitamin D by affecting the vitamin D receptor sites on cells.

From an alkalizing perspective, having your alkaline minerals such as calcium, iron, zinc, and magnesium bound up with phytic acid from grains and your vitamin D adversely affected by the consumption of dairy products means dairy and grains should be eliminated or used minimally since they interfere with the alkalizing process. Individuals I work with can rarely tolerate grains or dairy, at least not in the beginning of an alkalizing program. In addition, grains and dairy are very common allergens when allergy testing is performed.

Too much phosphorus—found especially in carbonated beverages, meats, dairy, grains, and nuts —interferes with calcium absorption. It is recommended that phosphorus not exceed the amount of calcium taken. In order to utilize calcium well, in addition to vitamin D, we need 1 gram of phosphorus and 0.5 grams magnesium for each 1 gram of calcium. We normally get plenty of phosphorus—usually too much. Although we need phosphorous, it is very abundant in our diets through a high intake of grains, carbonated drinks, dairy, and meats, which then drives up our requirements for calcium and magnesium. Too much phosphorus in the diet will increase the excretion of calcium.

Solving the Interstitial Cystitis Puzzle

Calcium, Magnesium, and Mast Cells

Calcium and magnesium compete for the same absorption sites. "Magnesium helps to relax muscles and to stabilize mast cells, preventing them from bursting and releasing a flood of histamine, thereby triggering an allergic reaction. In contrast, calcium stimulates mast cells to release histamines. In individuals with inflammatory conditions (like IC), the normal calcium to magnesium ratio of 2:1 can be modified to 1:1 or even 1:2." [1]

Calcium and magnesium are important to properly maintain the heart and blood vessels. A low level of calcium intake and calcium depletion is associated with increased risk of high blood pressure, fragile porous bones, osteoporosis, abnormal heartbeat, dementia, convulsions, nervous conditions, muscle cramps, and numbness of the arms and legs.

When you have an inadequate intake of calcium, the body will take the calcium from the bones usually starting with the spine and pelvis first; this is what thins the bones and contributes to osteoporosis and causes us to "shrink" as we age. Dental problems and loss of teeth can be traced to inadequate calcium intake and /or calcium depletion.

Foods High in Calcium

Dairy foods are highest in calcium with the exception of cottage cheese. However, there is much controversy in using dairy as a good source of calcium. Besides the fact that dairy is a common allergen and interferes with vitamin D activity, *pasteurized* milk products have such a high level of phosphorus and animal protein that they actually end up being slightly acid-forming and not a good source of calcium. "Calcium is necessary for the maintenance of optimal bone health. However, calcium intake accounts for only about 11% of calcium balance. The most important factor in calcium balance is calcium excretion which is most adversely affected by protein and sodium. The more protein and sodium you consume, the more calcium you need. Thus people living in countries consuming a high protein, processed food diet (i.e. typical North American diet) require more calcium ... Great plant sources of calcium include fortified soy milk, dark greens*, raw almonds, sesame seed paste, legumes, figs, and blackstrap molasses...50-70% of the calcium from most low oxalate vegetables is absorbable as compared to 32% in cow's milk." [2]

Raw milk products or those that are not pasteurized are considered neutral. Generally avoid dairy products for your calcium intake. You will actually lose more calcium from your body when using pasteurized dairy products. There are two reasons for this: (1) More sodium, potassium, and calcium are required to buffer the acids from dairy products than we obtain from drinking or eating dairy products. This is because dairy products are

...low-oxalate greens are best—oxalates found in spinach, Swiss chard, rhubarb and beet greens bind with the calcium in these foods making it unavailable for absorption.

high in phosphorus and protein. (2) In order to assimilate anything with phosphorus, we need twice the amount of calcium; eating dairy forces the body to find calcium wherever it can such as bones and teeth. There is one exception to this: whey. Whey is the by-product of making cheese. The phosphorus and acids remain in the cheese, making whey a valuable food especially high in organic sodium.

Better alternatives for calcium are low acid calcium fortified orange juice or calcium fortified alternative milk products such as rice, soy, and almond. You can also use calcium fortified alternative milk products (soy, rice, and almond) as cheese and yogurt. I use organic vanilla rice milk, plain rice milk and almond milk. The company Soyco makes good soy, rice and almond cheeses such as Swiss, mozzarella, and American. Silk makes a nice tasting vanilla soymilk. Plain rice, soy, and almond milk are surprising sweet. If you are really limiting your sugar intake, read the labels on alternative milk products. Many alternative milk products do not add sugar, but some do. The company Westsoy has even come out with Tropical Whip Soy milk blended with fruit juice and fruit puree (a good idea for a fruit smoothie in the morning if you tolerate this brand). The alternative suggestion of Tropical Whip Soy is only for those who have alkalized for at least six months or longer. You will not tolerate these in the beginning. I just want the reader to understand that your diet can be tasty and enjoyable in time with variety. A good alternative milk and cheese product to test when you are getting started should be made from rice provided you do not test allergic or sensitive to rice.

It is a good idea to test and explore different brands of alternative milks and cheeses that agree with you and that you find enjoyable. Not all alternative milks and cheeses taste the same. I tested a few brands before I found the ones I enjoyed. The exception I make with dairy is I will use one cup of organic vanilla or fruit yogurt or kefir for a protein source and an additional way to increase healthy bacteria (probiotics) in the gastrointestinal tract.

To review: foods, elements, and activities that interfere with calcium absorption and utilization.

1. Whole grains contain phytic acid, which is found in the bran of whole grains. Phytic acid binds to a variety of minerals including calcium, iron, zinc, magnesium to form insoluble salts, called phytates, which are then wasted from the body. Probably because grains are a relatively new food, from an evolutionary perspective, it appears that we have not yet developed digestive tracts which can break down these phytates. Rice is low in phytic acid.

2. Lack of adequate sunlight or lack of foods high in vitamin D will decrease utilization of calcium.

3. In addition, dairy consumption also has an adverse effect on calcium

utilization by affecting the vitamin D receptor sites on cells. Adequate vitamin D is essential to utilize calcium in the body. Pasteurized dairy products are acid-forming.

4. Eating more than three ounces of animal protein a day will cause a wasting of calcium from the urine.

5. A high salt intake (table salt/ sodium chloride or natural sea salt) will cause a wasting of calcium.

6. Caffeine, alcohol, and smoking will cause a wasting of calcium.

7. Sugar will cause a wasting of calcium.

8. Foods high in oxalates such as spinach, beets, kale, and rhubarb bind with calcium and interfere with the absorption of calcium. (See oxalate food list in the Getting Started Chapter.)

9. Sedentary lifestyles also interfere with mineralizing our bones. Our ancestors were probably much more active than we are. Impact stress on bone, as in walking and jogging, tends to increase production of calcitonin, which leads to increased deposition of calcium in the bones.

10. Mental and physical stress and diuretics cause a loss of calcium.

11. Proper magnesium intake to utilize calcium is necessary.

Mineral Supplements

Calcium absorption is reported to be inefficient with only 20 to 30% absorbed. Your body can only absorb approximately 500mg of calcium at a time therefore, it is recommended to take calcium in divided doses with meals and at bedtime. If you take buffered vitamin C, count the milligrams of calcium and/or magnesium in the buffered supplement so your calcium and magnesium intake are roughly 1:1.

The use of mineral supplements is recommended, since the average daily intake of calcium for most Americans is only about 400mg to 500mg per day. Most Americans have a negative balance of calcium. If the average intake of calcium is 500mg and one consumes meat, coffee, sodas, alcohol, and leads a stressful life, this will create the excretion of calcium in the urine.

Note: *Too much calcium without an adequate balance of magnesium causes constipation, so you need to balance your calcium and magnesium.*

The calcium supplement I recommend for IC is by Healthy Life Harvest called Aloe Vera with Coral Calcium. Each capsule contains high grade whole leaf aloe vera powder, and bio-available, ionic coral calcium as well as 72 trace minerals. Dr. Halstead believes that the micronutrient trace mineral components of coral calcium exert important biological effects. The aloe plant is a natural anti-inflammatory, antibiotic, and antifungal agent but only when used in its whole-leaf form. Aloe Vera is high in muccopolysaccarides and has been shown to have healing properties for the gastrointestinal (GI) tract and benefits the immune system. This special IC formula is prepared to maximize absorbability. Suggested dosage is four capsules one to two times a day thirty minutes before meals. Take with 6 to 8 ounces of water. Four capsules contain 616 mg of coral calcium, vitamin D3 (cholecalciferol) 120 iu, magnesium (from coral, citrate, oxide) 172 mg, plus whole leaf aloe vera powder. These coral mineral supplements have been tested and are reported to *not* be a source of toxic heavy metals or other organic pollutions.

Some individuals with interstitial cystitis I have worked with have had dramatic symptom relief just from adding Healthy Life Harvest Aloe Vera with Coral Calcium, which is encouraging, and which adds to other anecdotal evidence of the effectiveness of aloe vera and coral calcium. A fact: many people claim a benefit from taking coral calcium. More research is required to assess these reports of benefit. We look forward to clinical testing with coral calcium to assess its long-term effectiveness. As an aside, clinical studies have indicated a risk for men prone to prostate cancer who take high doses of calcium supplements.

Note: If you are truly allergic to fish and shellfish discuss taking marine coral minerals with your healthcare provider first, as you may be allergic to coral mineral supplements.

Healthy Life Harvest Aloe Vera with Coral Calcium is not *critical* for recovery, but it is an excellent *natural* source of calcium, magnesium, and trace minerals if you tolerate this. The key to recovery from IC is a hypoallergenic alkalizing diet with adequate vitamins, essential fatty acids, and mineral intake, especially alkalizing minerals.

If for some reason, you do not tolerate Healthy Life Harvest Aloe Vera with Coral Calcium, then test good calcium, magnesium, and vitamin D supplements that *you* tolerate and provide the dosages of calcium, magnesium, and vitamin D discussed in this book. Calcium sources from bone meal contain too much phosphorus, an acid-forming element. Do not take these. Dolomite is a calcium supplement that is the least absorbable form of calcium. Antacids are not recommended since most contain high levels of the toxic element aluminum. The best forms of calcium supplements to take (other than natural coral calcium) are calcium carbonate, calcium lactate, and calcium citrate. I have noticed that some persons with IC do not always tolerate calcium citrate, so test carefully. Twin Labs, Allergy Research Group, Solaray, and Thorne are reliable companies that make excellent supplements quite often tolerated by persons with IC. You may have to go through a few brands before you find the ones that agree with *your* body. Obtain your trace minerals from plenty of sea vegetables, sea vegetable salt such as nori, kelp, dulse, and seaweed.

The best and safest way to get adequate calcium is from *food*. High calcium foods are sea vegetables such as dulse, kelp, Irish moss, seeds, and most greens. Other good food sources for calcium are beans, tofu, figs, and hazelnuts. 1/2 cup of cooked broccoli, 1 oz. of almonds (about 30 almonds), or 1 tablespoon of molasses provides about 100mg. of calcium.

Calcium has no known toxic effects. *Mental and physical stress and diuretics cause a loss of calcium from the body.* Supplementation of up to 2,500mg of calcium a day is considered safe. Suggested calcium doses for the following conditions: [3]

Broken bones and fractures	1,000mg-2,000mg
High Blood Pressure	1,000mg-1,500mg
Osteoporosis	1,200mg-2,000mg

The development of kidney stones in connection with high calcium intake is rare. [4]

Daily Recommended Intake (DRI) of Calcium [5]

๑ Age 51 and over: 1,200mg because of reduced rate of absorption

๑ Adults ages 19 to 50: 1,000mg

๑ During pregnancy and lactation: 1,000mg for women 19 and older; 1,300mg for women 18 and younger

๑ Preteens and teens ages 9 to 18: 1,300mg

๑ Children ages 4 to 8: 800mg

๑ Children ages 1 year to 3: 500mg

๑ Infants ages 6 months to 1 year: 270mg

๑ Newborn to age 6 months: 210mg

"You can trace every sickness, every disease, and every ailment to a mineral deficiency."

— Two-time Nobel Prize winner, Dr. Linus Pauling

Magnesium
Inhibitory Mineral for the Sympathetic Nervous System

Magnesium *inhibits* the sympathetic nervous system, responsible for fight or flight. In other words, magnesium has a calming effect on the body.

Nearly 70% of the body's supply of magnesium is located in the bones while 30% is found in the cellular fluids and some soft tissue. A 154-pound person would be comprised of about 21 grams of magnesium.

Magnesium is involved in the electrical stability of the cells, neurotransmission, and helps regulate the acid-alkali balance in the body. *Magnesium stabilizes mast cells and decreases the release of histamines, making this an important mineral when healing IC.* Evidence suggests that if calcium intake is high, magnesium intake needs to be high or there will be a deficiency of magnesium. Magnesium helps to promote absorption and metabolism of other minerals such as calcium, phosphorus, sodium, and potassium.

It is estimated that the typical American diet barely meets the recommended daily amount of magnesium. Magnesium deficiency can easily occur because magnesium is refined out of many foods during processing. Cooking foods removes the minerals. A deficiency can occur in people with diabetes, persons on diuretics and digitalis medications, the elderly, those with pancreatitis, alcoholism, pregnancy, and those on low calorie diets and high carbohydrate diets.

Magnesium deficiency is thought to be closely related to coronary (heart) disease and strokes. Symptoms of a deficiency include gastrointestinal disorders, irregular heart rhythm, lack of coordination, muscle twitch, tremors, weakness, apprehension, personality changes, confusion, depression, and irritability.

Potassium and magnesium (along with organic sodium) are some of the most important minerals for rebalancing the electrical properties of the cell and eliminating excess acidity and help to balance calcium.

Green Drinks

Magnesium is found chiefly in fresh green vegetables and is an essential element in chlorophyll. I like to add *Veggie Magma*™ (a green powdered vegetable juice supplement) to low sodium V-8 juice for a great energy boost. There are many powered green supplements and tablets on the market. Another good natural alkalizer high in magnesium is *fresh* wheat or barley grass. It is best to start with only one ounce of *fresh* wheatgrass or barley grass a day and gradually increase to a couple of ounces a day. If you take more than one ounce to start, you may feel nauseated since these grasses will detoxify you. Initially, I suggest you try only a small amount of the wheat or barley grass—maybe just a few sips. Some people do not mind the taste. Wheatgrass has a very sweet saccharine-type taste that some like and others dislike. I, myself, do not prefer the taste of fresh wheatgrass but take an ounce or two a day since it is very healing, energizing, and alkalizing. Intermittently, I take a break from fresh wheatgrass for a few weeks and then resume using it.

Many health food stores carry fresh or frozen wheatgrass and barley grass and the green powder/tablet supplements. Robeks and Jamba Juice stores will usually sell you fresh wheatgrass by the ounce, and you can order a flat of the fresh wheatgrass to take home and juice. A flat of wheatgrass will give you about 10 to 12 ounces of fresh wheatgrass and lasts about a week. You must water the flat gently everyday, and keep in a cool place. Once the grass in the flat grows too tall and starts to droop and the bottom of the grass turns yellow, the grass is getting too old. If you cannot juice and drink the entire flat and you find it is growing too fast, cut down the remaining grass, juice it, and freeze it in ice cube trays. I just use a large pair of scissors to cut the fresh wheatgrass. Freeze the wheatgrass juice and pop out one cube at a time and you have about one ounce of wheatgrass. Let the frozen cube of wheatgrass gradually thaw at room temperature; do *not* microwave the wheatgrass cube or the juice. *You must have a juicer that will specifically juice wheat grass. I do not recommend the hand-crank grass juicers. You will probably get tired and not efficiently extract all the juice from the grasses with a hand-crank juicer.* I recommend and use the Omega 8001 juicer. It juices hard and soft fruits and vegetables and juices wheatgrass or barley grass. In addition, you can make fresh nut butters and (vegetable) pastas! The Omega 8001 costs around $200.

You can also grow your own flats of fresh wheatgrass or barley grass at home by purchasing a wheatgrass kit and growing the grass from seeds. I ordered a kit over the Internet and did grow a few flats, but due to time constraints, I prefer to run over to Robeks or Jamba Juice for a quick ounce or two of wheatgrass with an orange juice chaser. Fresh is the most potent and the best for healing. Green wheatgrass or barley grass drinks and green supplements might be tolerated in the beginning of the hypoallergenic alkalizing program, but some have a reaction to these supplements. There are a few reasons for these reactions. Rarely, one may be allergic to the "grasses." Wheatgrass and barley grass because they are still a grass do not contain gluten. Technically, they are not a grain so it is not an allergic reaction to a grain. In addition, green supplements will increase the rate of detoxification and may cause more bladder discomfort. You may need to test several different green supplements until you find one that agrees with you. Hold on to the supplements and test them every month or two since tolerance will increase with time. It could take you three to twelve months before you can tolerate the green supplements just discussed. Do not give up testing and trying to add these drinks and supplements! They will hasten your recovery.

Supplements

Of magnesium supplements, the magnesium found naturally in coral calcium is well absorbed. Magnesium oxide supplement contains the greatest percentage of magnesium and is usually well tolerated by most persons with IC; however, we are all different so you must test carefully. Magnesium carbonate contains about 40% magnesium. Other forms of magnesium which have lower amounts of magnesium are magnesium citrate, magnesium malate and magnesium aspartate. I personally supplement with Healthy Life Harvest Aloe Vera with Coral Calcium and Twin Labs magnesium oxide. I keep my calcium and magnesium ratio 1:1 as suggested by Dr. Lark. Again, too much calcium and not enough magnesium will cause constipation.

The best and safest way to obtain adequate magnesium is from *food*.

Besides the green drinks and supplements listed earlier, other excellent sources of magnesium are soybeans, spinach, pumpkin seeds, squash and sunflower seeds, egg yolks, figs, apples, and nuts, especially cashews and almonds.

Suggested magnesium dosages that appear valuable for the following conditions: [6]

Angina	500mg-1,000mg
Fibromyalgia, chronic fatigue	6-12 tablets of magnesium malate (6 tablets supply 300 mg of magnesium, 1,200mg malic acid)
High blood pressure	500mg-750mg
Osteoporosis	500mg-1,000mg

Large amounts of magnesium (3,000-5,000mg) have a laxative effect and cathartic effect. *Mental and physical stress and diuretics cause a loss of magnesium from the body.*

Toxicity symptoms have been noted in subjects treated with 9,000 mg of magnesium or in persons with kidney failure. [7]

Daily Recommended Intake (DRI) of Magnesium [8]

჻ Adult males ages 31 to 70: 420mg

჻ Adult females ages 31 to 70: 320mg

჻ Adult males ages 19 to 30: 400mg

჻ Adult females ages 19 to 30: 310mg

჻ Pregnancy: add 40mg to comparable age

჻ Lactation: same as comparable age

჻ Males ages 14 to 18: 410mg

჻ Females ages 14 to 18: 360mg

჻ Children ages 9 to 13: 240mg

჻ Children ages 4 to 8: 130mg

჻ Toddlers ages 1 year to 3: 80mg

჻ Infants ages 6 months to 1 year: 75mg

჻ Newborn to 6 months: 30mg

"I give you all the seed-bearing plants that are upon the earth, and all the trees with seed-bearing fruit; this shall be your food."

— Genesis 1:29

Potassium
Stimulatory Mineral for the Parasympathetic Nervous System

Potassium has a *stimulatory* effect on the calming parasympathetic nervous system. In other words, potassium has a relaxing effect on the body.

Potassium is an essential alkaline ion that is found mostly *inside* the cells (98%). A person weighing 154 pounds would be comprised of approximately 150 grams of potassium. Potassium and sodium together help regulate the distribution of body fluids. It unites with phosphorus to send oxygen to the brain, keeps skin healthy, stabilizes blood pressure, and works with sodium to keep the heartbeat regular. Potassium has been used to prevent and treat high blood pressure and has proved effective in treating allergies. In metabolic acidosis, H+ (hydrogen ions or acids) enter the inside of the cells while K+ (potassium ions) are "kicked" out of the cell and excreted in the urine. This is how the cells become acidic over time, and we deplete our alkaline buffer system, especially potassium. Bicarbonate raises the pH and reverses this H+ and K+ exchange process.

Potassium and magnesium (along with organic sodium) are some of the most important minerals for rebalancing the electrical properties of the cell and eliminating excess acidity and help to balance calcium.

Hypokalemia or low potassium can be caused by acute dehydration, adrenal insufficiency, and chronic renal failure. A low intake of potassium and a high intake of sodium can lead to hypertension. The excessive use of table salt depletes the often-scarce potassium supplies. Diarrhea can deplete potassium levels and potassium stores decline with age. A potassium deficiency can result from an inadequate intake of fruits and vegetables. *Mental and physical stress, diuretics, and diabetic acidosis can cause a large loss of potassium.*

Some signs of potassium deficiencies are nervous disorders, insomnia, constipation, slow, irregular heartbeat, and impaired glucose metabolism.

Kidney failure or an inability to urinate causes toxicity. Do not take supplemental potassium without checking with your physician if you are taking any kind of prescription drug. Do not take any potassium supplement if you have kidney disease, heart disease, or Addison's disease. Do not use potassium supplements if you have a stomach or intestinal ulcer or chronic diarrhea.

The best and safest source of potassium is *food* which includes all vegetables, especially green leafy ones, orange juice (low acid orange juice for persons with IC), bananas, avocados, potatoes (especially the skin), garlic, dried fruit especially dates, figs, and apricots.

Potassium toxicity is seen when daily intakes exceed 18 grams or 18,000mg of potassium or with kidney failure. [9]

Dietary Goals of the United States for Potassium

- Adults and children ages 10 to 18: 2,000mg
- Children ages 6 to 9: 1,600mg
- Children ages 2 to 5: 1,400mg
- Toddlers ages 1 year to 2: 1,000mg
- Infants 6 months to 1 year: 700mg
- Newborn to 6 months: 500mg

"Sowe Carrets in you Gardens, and humbly praise God for them, as for a singular and great blessing."

—Richard Gardiner, 1599

Sodium
Inhibitory Mineral for the Parasympathetic Nervous System

Sodium *inhibits* the calming parasympathetic nervous system. In other words, sodium has a stimulating effect on the body.

Sodium is an essential mineral and is found in every cell in the body, but is predominately found in the extracellular fluids (fluids *outside* the cells). In a 154 pound person the approximate amount of sodium found in the body is about 63 grams.

Sodium functions with potassium to maintain the body's acid-alkali balance. The usual intake of *inorganic* sodium in America far exceeds the need. Sodium chloride (usually in the form of table salt) is an *inorganic* salt and it is very difficult to break these *inorganic* bonds. Sodium chloride has the opposite effect of *organic* sodium. An excess of *inorganic* sodium leads to the loss of potassium and calcium in the body and contributes to mineral loss and imbalances. Diets that have an excess amount of *inorganic* sodium chloride contribute to the rising incidences of liver, heart, and kidney disease.

The simplest way to reduce *inorganic* sodium intake is to eliminate the use of table salt. Processed foods are often very high in *inorganic* sodium chloride. Table salt (including natural sea salt) actually takes *organic* sodium out of the body, and causes more damage than any other substance. Stay away from table salt and use minimal amount of natural sea salt.

Food Is Your Best Medicine—Dr. Henry Beiler, MD

"Of all the *alkaline* elements of the body, sodium is the most important. It is my belief that the liver is the storehouse of these elements, especially of sodium. It is the element found in the greatest abundance and is the most needed in maintaining the body's acid-base balance. Sodium is found in every cell of the body; also, there are large concentrated sodium-storage centers to be used in case of emergency. These concentrated areas have a great buffer value; in addition, much acid and corrosive poison can be neutralized and stored in them, more or less temporarily. Among the important sodium storage reservoirs are the muscles, brain and nerves, bone marrow, skin, gastric and intestinal mucosa, the kidneys, and the liver, which is by far the most important; it is richest of all the organs in sodium, its chief chemical element. Therefore, as the largest storehouse of sodium the liver is clearly the body's second line of defense."

"When the liver is depleted of sodium in order to neutralize acids, its function may be so severely inhibited that illness results. Are you aware that if the liver could keep the blood stream clean by filtering out damaging poisons, man could live indefinitely, barring physical accidents? It is only when the liver's filtration ability is hindered that the poisons get beyond the liver and into the general blood circulation. Only then do the symptoms of disease occur. And that is why you must guard your liver so carefully."

"If, then, sodium is so important to good health, how do we obtain it? How can we observe it? Sodium, the body's vital element is derived from the sodium compounds in the diet. The richest source is in the vegetable kingdom…an individual who eats few vegetables and salads and much over-cooked meat frequently has a sodium-starved liver…"

"But as the liver is gradually depleted of its sodium-leached out for the neutralization of toxins- the normal sodium salts of the bile acids are formed with greater difficult…When there is a too rapid drain of the liver's available sodium, the liver cells die." [10]

Dr. Regan Golob states, "The more meat you eat, the more sodium you lose from the body's alkaline reserve. If all the sodium is used up, the body goes to the bones for calcium as the next best mineral with which to neutralize acid, until you have osteoporosis and/or arthritis."

"When all the alkaline reserve (sodium, calcium, magnesium) is used up, the body goes into survival mode and gets rid of excess protein (acid) by eliminating it directly as ammonia and protein in the urine. So, when you smell ammonia in the urine, at any age, stop all flesh protein, eat only fruits and vegetables, and drink lots of filtered water."

Organic sodium is needed for utilization of oxygen. Lack of *organic* sodium can cause the following problems: a weak liver condition, indigestion, weak muscles and tissues, cracking joints, arthritis, osteoporosis, difficult breathing, catarrh or mucous, lack of saliva, lack of hydrochloric acid, sleepy during the day and awake at night, patient feels good one day and bad the next, slow digestion, constipation, gas in stomach and bowels, palpitation, weak eyesight, nerves on fire, judgment unreliable, stiff joints, bloating, gas, dry skin, confusion, frontal headache, offensive breath, poor concentration, weak heart, emotional up's and down's, poor complexion. Lack of *organic* sodium is the forerunner of most chronic and degenerative diseases because it is one of the most important, if not the most important buffer of acids for the body. 99 people out of 100 are lacking *organic* sodium.

Organic sodium is found in sea vegetables such as, raw kelp, raw wakame, and vegetables such as celery, carrots, boiled beet greens, Swiss chard, spinach, dandelion greens, white cooked corn, raw Chinese cabbage, jalapeno peppers, chili powder, dried apple rings, goat's milk, sheep milk, organic goat milk whey, sea vegetable seasoning.

National Research Council Recommended Daily Sodium Intake

๖ Healthy adults: 1,100mg to 3,300mg

๖ Children ages 10 to 18: 500 mg

๖ Children ages 6 to 9: 400mg

๖ Children ages 2 to 5: 300mg

๖ Children ages 1 year to 2: 225mg

๖ Infants 6 months to 1 year: 200mg

๖ Newborn to 6 months: 120mg

"The whole is greater than the sum of its parts. Unlike supplements, fruits and vegetables contain a variety of nutrients, which cannot be extracted."

— Dr. T. Colin Campbell, PhD

Iron

Iron is a mineral concentrate that is found in the largest amount in the blood. In a 154 pound person there is approximately 3 grams of iron in the body. Iron is the main carrier vehicle for getting oxygen to all the cells of the body and helps in buffering acids in the body. Iron is needed to make hemoglobin, which carries oxygen from the lungs to all the tissues of the body. Oxygen is an alkalizing element.

Symptoms of deficiency as well as anemia may include constipation, lusterless or brittle nails, spoon-shaped nails, nail ridges that run lengthwise, difficulty breathing, tiredness, apathy, reduced brain function, pale pallor and heart enlargement.

Vitamin C increases the absorption of iron. Persons with IC need to take buffered vitamin C or a non-acidic vitamin C. Allergy Research Group makes a good, buffered vitamin C and Solaray makes a non-acidic vitamin C. You can find these brands at your health food store or on the Internet. You will need to test carefully when you incorporate vitamin C into your regimen.

Foods rich in iron are very lean meats, leafy green vegetables (especially spinach), wax beans, yellow beans, French green beans, sprouts, raw coconut milk, avocado, dried raw kelp, raw wakame, succotash, whole grains, dried fruits especially dried peach, legumes, and molasses.

Recommended Daily Allowance (RDA) of Iron:

- Males ages 19 to 70: 10mg
- Females ages 51 to 70: 10mg
- Males ages 9 to 18: 12mg
- Females ages 9 to 50: 15mg
- Pregnancy: 30mg
- Lactation: 15mg
- Children ages 6 months to 8 years: 10mg
- Newborn to 6 months: 6 mg

"The best interest of the patient is the only interest to be considered."

—Dr. William J. Mayo

Daily Values for Everyone

The 1990 Nutrition Labeling and Education Act brought us Daily Values on food labels beginning in 1994. Before this time, our food labels listed percentages of the US RDA. Actually, the Daily Values combine the old US RDA, renamed Reference Daily Intake, and a set of standards called Daily Reference Value (DRV) for other nutrients. The only term that appears on the label, however, is Daily Value. This information is presented below.

Daily Values = Daily Reference Values + Reference Daily Intakes

Dietary Guidelines

"On February 23, 1999 a coalition of more than 20 groups, including the American Heart Association, The American Cancer Society, The Produce for Better Health Foundation (PBH), the American Institute for Cancer Research, the Boys & Girls Clubs of America, the American Diabetes Association, and the American Association of Retired Persons urged the government to make fruits and vegetables the center of the American diet. This message was primarily directed to the members of the Dietary Guidelines Committee, who are making up the nutritional guidelines to be revised for the year 2000.

"The groups say there is strong evidence that if people eat more fruits and vegetables, lives and a considerable amount of health care dollars will be saved. According to this group, five of the top ten causes of death in the United States are diet related—heart disease, cancer, strokes, diabetes, and other forms of atherosclerosis, and diet plays a preventive role in birth defects, cataract formation, hypertension, asthma, diverticulosis, obesity, and diabetes.

A Guide to Natural Healing

"Talking about Americans... 'Dinnertime is vegetable time; over 75% of all vegetables they eat are consumed at this time. But, even though dinnertime is the most popular time for eating fruits and vegetables, only 28% of the foods they eat at dinner are fruits, vegetable, or 100% juices. The average American's annual fruit and vegetable deficit is serious,' ... 'Most of us have an annual fruit and vegetable deficit ranging from 219 to 1,629 servings—that's per person. It really adds up." [11]

Attack on the Food Pyramid

"With obesity reaching epidemic proportions in the U.S., some critics say it's the government's food pyramid that should go on a diet. The pyramid, dating back from 1991, pictorially reflects the U.S. Department of Agriculture's guidelines on what Americans should eat every day to maintain a healthy weight. From a broad base of six to eleven servings of food in the grains and carbohydrates group, the pyramid narrows upward to fewer servings of vegetables and fruits to fewer still of such foods as milk and meat. Finally, at the pyramid's pointed top are fats, oils and sweets, which consumers are advised to "eat sparingly." While the government has stood by this regimen for eleven years, some critics say it's no coincidence that the number of overweight Americans has risen 61% since the pyramid was introduced-and almost instantaneously appeared on the sides of pasta boxes, bread wrappers, and packages of other food products in the pyramid's six to eleven servings category. David S. Ludwig, an obesity researcher at Children's Hospital in Boston, says the pyramid and guidelines focus too much on reducing fat. He says people are getting fat because they are eating too many refined carbohydrates, such as white bread, that make them even hungrier later so they overeat. The habitual consumption of foods with refined carbohydrates "may increase risk for obesity, type 2 diabetes and heart disease," he wrote in a May (2002) article in the Journal of the American Medical Association...Beyond the debate over fats and carbohydrates, many nutrition experts say the pyramid needs to better define serving size to be effective. Most people don't realize that a one USDA-size serving is about the size of a minibagel, says Marion Nestle, chairman of the Department of Nutrition and Food Studies at New York University. She also says the pyramid "emphases grain products too heavily without specifying whole grains...They're not talking about white bread." [12]

The position of the American Dietetic Association (ADA) is that appropriately planned vegetarian diets are healthful, are nutritionally adequate, and provide health benefits in the prevention and treatment of certain diseases. According to the ADA, mortality rates are lower in vegetarians for the following diseases: coronary artery disease, hypertension, lung and colorectal cancer, and cross-cultural data indicate lower breast cancer rates. The Vegetarian Diet Pyramid is provided for the reader to review as it relates to chronic disease and nutrition.

I am not suggesting the reader needs to become a vegetarian; I am

Solving the Interstitial Cystitis Puzzle

merely presenting the information available on known diets as they relate to disease prevention.

Researchers from Harvard, Oldways, and the World Health Organization have developed the Traditional Healthy Mediterranean Diet Pyramid. This pyramid reflects the current state of worldwide clinical and epidemiological research on healthy eating and low rates of diet-linked chronic diseases and high life expectancy typical of the Mediterranean region in 1960. The Mediterranean diet pyramid is presented to the reader for review as it relates to lower levels of chronic disease.

The Mediterranean diet breaks down to these basics:

 Low to moderate amounts of cheese and yogurt.

 Minimally processed, seasonally fresh, and locally grown foods.

 An abundance of foods from plant sources including fruits and vegetables, potatoes, beans, nuts and seeds, grains.

 Low to moderate amounts of fish and poultry weekly; limited eggs to zero to four servings per week.

 Fruit as a typical daily dessert.

 Red meat is eaten only a few times per month.

 Olive oil is the principal fat replacing other fats and oils.

 Total dietary fat ranges from 25% to 35% of energy, with saturated fat no more than 7 to 8 percent of total calories.

 Regular physical activity at a level that promotes healthy weight, fitness, and well-being.

When making food selections try to choose a variety of fresh seasonal fruits, vegetables, sprouts, organic animal products, legumes, nuts, seeds, and grains. Learn to incorporate sea vegetables as a condiment and in meals since they are high in organic sodium and potassium and trace minerals. This will increase your intake of essential trace elements. Select as close to eighty percent of your food from the alkalizing categories listed in appendix A of this book, with emphasis at every meal on fruits and vegetables. When choosing fish, consider the high omega-3 sources such as salmon, tuna, mackerel, trout, halibut, whitefish, sardines, anchovy, orange roughie, or bluefish. Eat shellfish rarely since they live in the most polluted waters close to shore and are high in toxins. (Tuna, bluefish, mackerel and sardines may be higher in histamines and should be consumed cautiously for persons with IC.)

If you enjoy eating meat, choose free-ranging organic poultry or meat that has not been subjected to hormones or antibiotics. However, studies show that the amount of animal protein eaten can lower your calcium levels. Animal protein intake over three ounces a day causes a loss of calcium from the urinary tract.

I have designed an Alkalizing Food Pyramid for the reader to explore, which has as its alkalizing base fruits and vegetables as well as sprouted legumes, sprouted grains, sprouted seeds, and sprouted nuts. The remainder of the pyramid is comprised from the food categories that are acid-forming which includes meat, fish, poultry, dairy, grains, legumes, most nuts and seeds, and natural sugars. Fats and oils are considered neutral.

Alkalizing Food Pyramid

It is important to eat a well-balanced diet in order to consume adequate daily trace elements, vitamins, minerals, fiber, and essential fatty acids. One goal of a hypoallergenic alkalizing diet plan is to replace our lost minerals. Youths are naturally quite alkaline, which is why one sees so much exuberance and energy. Theoretically, I suppose, one could regain the vitality of youth by following an alkalizing program. It is important with children to maintain their alkaline stores by encouraging plenty of fresh fruits and vegetables. To alkalize, it is essential to avoid caffeine and sodas and to limit sugary or salty snacks. Refer to the table on page 218 for food substitutions for children and adults to help make a more comfortable transition to a hypoallergenic alkalizing diet.

Foods to Avoid or Limit

The following acid-forming items are consumed in substantial quantities in the typical American diet. These items are troublesome to persons with IC and increase "flare-ups."

Cola drinks (pH 2.5) (addictive, mood and energy altering)

§ Caffeine (50mg per serving) creates a diuretic effect causing the kidneys to excrete the alkalizing elements calcium, magnesium, sodium, and potassium.

§ The diuretic effect of caffeine increases urination and the drying of the mucosa in the vagina, urethra, and bladder.

§ Sugar with caffeine doubles the amount of calcium excreted by the kidneys.

§ Carbonation in soda is formed by adding carbon dioxide and phosphorus. These substances add to the body's acid load.

§ The kola nut of the cola acuminata has a stimulatory effect that intensifies physiological responses to stress.

Coffee (pH 5) (addictive, mood and energy altering)

§ Coffee contains over 208 kinds of acids.

§ Caffeine (100mg per cup) causes a diuretic effect that causes the kidneys to excrete the alkalizing elements calcium, magnesium, sodium, and potassium.

§ The diuretic effect of caffeine increases urination and the drying of mucosa in the vagina, urethra, and bladder.

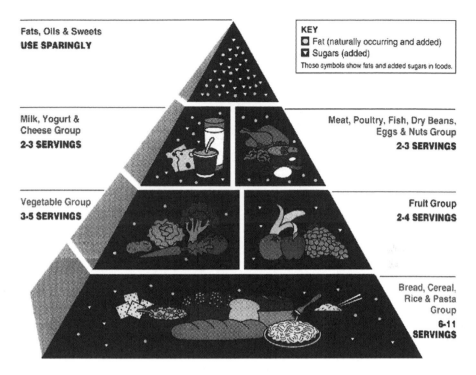

Fats, Oils & Sweets
USE SPARINGLY

Milk, Yogurt & Cheese Group
2-3 SERVINGS

Meat, Poultry, Fish, Dry Beans, Eggs & Nuts Group
2-3 SERVINGS

Vegetable Group
3-5 SERVINGS

Fruit Group
2-4 SERVINGS

Bread, Cereal, Rice & Pasta Group
6-11 SERVINGS

Source: U.S. Department of Agriculture and the U.S. Department of Health and Human Services or USDA and DHHS.

§ Sugar in a cup of coffee doubles the amount of calcium excreted by the kidneys.

§ Caffeine intensifies physiological responses to stress.

Tea pH (pH 6.5) (addictive, mood and energy altering)

§ Caffeine (60 mg per cup) causes a diuretic effect that causes the kidneys to excrete the alkalizing elements, including calcium, magnesium, sodium, and potassium.

§ The diuretic effect of caffeine increases urination and the drying of mucosa in the vagina, urethra, and bladder.

§ Caffeine intensifies physiological responses to stress.

Alcohol (addictive, mood and energy altering)

§ Alcohol has poor nutritive value except calories.

§ The diuretic effect causes the kidneys to excrete the alkalizing elements, including calcium and magnesium.

A Guide to Natural Healing   213

🍸 The diuretic effect also causes drying of the mucosa of the vagina, urethra, and bladder.

Sugar (addictive, mood and energy altering)
🍸 Sugar depletes the body of B-complex vitamins and alkaline minerals increasing acid load, anxiety, and irritability.

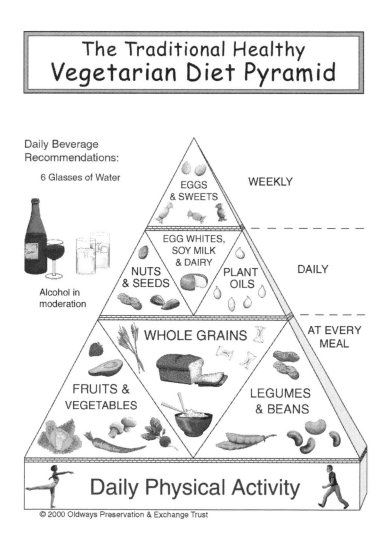

The Traditional Healthy
Vegetarian Diet Pyramid

Daily Beverage Recommendations:

6 Glasses of Water

EGGS & SWEETS — WEEKLY

Alcohol in moderation

EGG WHITES, SOY MILK & DAIRY

NUTS & SEEDS — PLANT OILS — DAILY

WHOLE GRAINS — AT EVERY MEAL

FRUITS & VEGETABLES

LEGUMES & BEANS

Daily Physical Activity

Solving the Interstitial Cystitis Puzzle

Carbonated Beverages

♦ All carbonated or sparkling drinks contain carbon dioxide and phosphorus, which are acid-forming.

Salt

♦ Excess salt (inorganic sodium chloride especially table salt) causes the excretion of potassium.

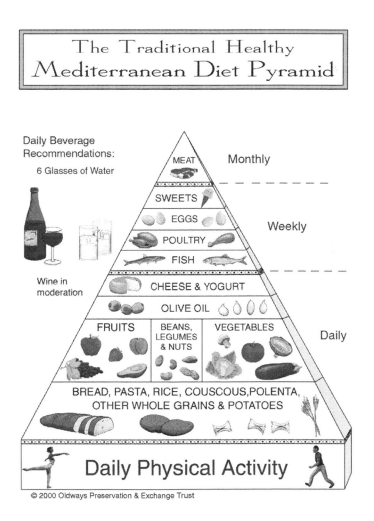

The Traditional Healthy Mediterranean Diet Pyramid

Daily Beverage Recommendations:

6 Glasses of Water

Wine in moderation

MEAT — Monthly

SWEETS
EGGS
POULTRY — Weekly
FISH

CHEESE & YOGURT

OLIVE OIL

FRUITS | BEANS, LEGUMES & NUTS | VEGETABLES — Daily

BREAD, PASTA, RICE, COUSCOUS, POLENTA, OTHER WHOLE GRAINS & POTATOES

Daily Physical Activity

Alkalizing Food Pyramid

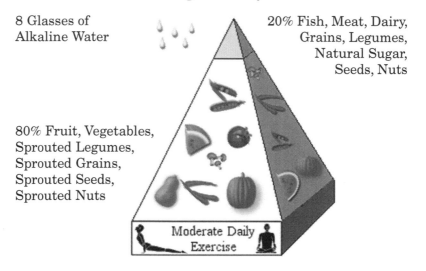

8 Glasses of
Alkaline Water

20% Fish, Meat, Dairy,
Grains, Legumes,
Natural Sugar,
Seeds, Nuts

80% Fruit, Vegetables,
Sprouted Legumes,
Sprouted Grains,
Sprouted Seeds,
Sprouted Nuts

Moderate Daily
Exercise

* Fats & oils are considered neutral

Stress and the Adrenal Glands

"Any stressor that the mind or body interprets and internalizes as too much to deal with, leaves an acid residue. Even a mild stressor can cause a partial or total acid-forming reaction."

— Dr. Theodore A. Baroody

Most Americans spend more time producing acid waste products, especially related to stress than processing it. *Stress is acid-forming.* Two adrenal glands situated, one on top of each kidney, produce hormones in response to stress. The adrenal glands are triangular-shaped organs. Each gland normally weighs about five grams. The adrenal glands produce hormones such as estrogen, progesterone, cortisol, and chemicals such as adrenalin. When the glands produce more or less hormones than required by the body, disease conditions may occur.

The adrenal glands produces cortisol and this helps to maintain salt and water balance in the body and help you cope with stress. Cortisol production has a normal circadian rhythm with peak levels in the morning and low levels in the evening. Your body needs proper cortisol balance to help you meet the daily challenges of life. Eventually, chronic stress creates weak adrenal glands.

Specifically for IC, it is the cortisol produced by our adrenal glands that will help block the histamine response to allergens. We know that it is the degranulation of the mast cells in the IC bladder and the release of histamines that can cause the pain and other symptoms of IC. Mast cells are a part of allergic reactions. Weak adrenal glands mean they have a decreased ability to produce cortisol. Decreased cortisol means we lose our ability to block the release of histamines from mast cells in the bladder.

Progesterone is a precursor or building block to all the corticosteroids. Progesterone is required by the adrenal glands in the manufacture of cortisol. Stress, vitamin C deficiency, vitamin B deficiency, and progesterone deficiency all contribute to adrenal exhaustion and cortisol imbalances. Reduced adrenal function may be indicated by the following: weakness, lethargy, dizziness, headaches, memory problems, food craving, allergies, and blood sugar disorders.

In a stressful situation, adrenal hormones:

֍ Transfer blood from the intestines to the extremities

֍ Increase blood pressure

֍ Increase your heart rate

֍ Suppress the immune system

֍ Increase the blood's clotting ability

There are different types of stress:

֍ Emotional ֍ Thermal
֍ Physical ֍ Chemical

Emotional stress can be positive or negative. For example, a promotion at work might be a positive one, and an IRS audit a negative one. In either case, the excitement elicited from these changes still affects the adrenal glands. *Thermal stress* comes from being exposed to extreme temperatures. Examples of *physical stress* are heavy physical work, lack of sleep, living a sedentary life style, and being overweight. *Chemical stress* comes from exposure to caffeine, toxins, and rapid changes in blood sugar, especially low blood sugar.

Sustained stress from worry, caffeine, and low blood sugar increases cortisol levels. Stress can diminish the immune system, causing a person to be sick often or develop allergies. Adrenal hormones cause an increase in blood clotting, which can lead to arterial plaquing and heart disease. Continued stress decreases blood flow to the bowel and creates digestive problems such as LGS or irritable bowel. Chronic stress reduces the blood flow to the kidneys and bladder, reducing vital alkalizing oxygen and nutrients to these organ systems.

The adrenal glands do not know the difference between the stress produced by a cup of coffee or from being laid off at work. Eventually, accumulated stress wears out the adrenal glands, they fail to meet demands, and varieties of symptoms include fatigue, digestive problems, obesity, depression, allergies, and overacidity of the body.

Food Substitutions

No	Yes
Wheat Crackers or Bread	Rice, Corn, Millet , Amaranth, Quinoa
Chocolate Chip Cookie	Fig or Raisin Cookie
Peanut Butter Crackers	Nut Butter on Rice Cracker
Salted Nuts	Dry Roasted Almonds, Nuts, or Seeds
Salted Chips	Salt-Free/Low Salt Chips or Vegetable Sticks
Sour Cream Dip	Hummus, Guacamole, Salsa
Milk Shake	Fruit Smoothie
Ice Cream	Yogurt Topped with Fruit, Rice/Almond Frozen Desserts
Spaghetti Meat Sauce	Italian Meatless Sauce
Wheat Pasta	Vegetable Pastas, Rice or Lentil Pastas
Sausage Pizza	Spinach or Vegetable Pizza
Beef Stew	Vegetable Minestrone Soup
Burger Fast Food	Vegetable Chow Mein, Vegetable Burrito
Coffee	Coffee Substitutes, Ginger Tea
Carbonated Water	Alkaline Water
Soda	Fruit Juice, Alkaline Water
Pretels	Reduced Salt Popcorn (Air Pop)
Candy	Dried Fruit
French Fries	Sweet or Baked Potato
Sugar	Honey, Molasses, Maple Syrup
Salt	Low Salt or Salt Substitute, Sea Vegetables, or Herbs
Black Tea	Herbal Teas, Ginger Tea, or Green Tea

Solving the Interstitial Cystitis Puzzle

People with weak adrenal glands crave caffeine and sugar because these substances stimulate the failing adrenal glands. What you need is rest, relaxation, and proper nourishment. Minimizing *emotional, physical, thermal* and *chemical* stress wherever possible will go a long way to helping heal the adrenal glands and alkalize the body. To reduce emotional stress in your life, here are some suggestions: mild to moderate aerobic exercise, biofeedback, yoga, Tai Chi, Qi Gong, meditation, progressive muscle relaxation, Pilates exercise, visualization, guided imagery, psychotherapy and counseling, music therapy, and touch therapy (massage, reflexology, Reiki, Rolfing, Feldenkrais, therapeutic touch).

A hypoallergenic alkalizing diet which distributes adequate fats, nuts, and moderate protein throughout the day will stabilize blood sugar and help balance cortisol levels. It is very important as a base of this IC recovery program, to address stress factors in one's life. Being more aware of stress and exploring ways to eliminate or cope with stress is a good starting point. Please consider the list of alkalizing versus acid-forming lifestyle choices in appendix B as a starting point for some life changes.

Adrenal Gland Function Blood Pressure Self-Test (Ragland's Test)

Ragland's test involves comparing your systolic blood pressure readings (BP) while lying down with those taken immediately after standing up. Blood pressure is shown as systolic/diastolic, such as 120/80, which is a normal blood pressure. In this test, you are comparing the systolic (top number) BP between the supine (lying down) and standing positions. Normally, if your adrenal glands are healthy, systolic BP will increase approximately 10 points when changing from a supine position to standing.

Here is how you perform the test to determine if you *might* have an adrenal deficit. Rest for five minutes in a supine position. While remaining supine, take your first BP. Remember this BP. Then stand up, and immediately take the second BP. If the standing systolic reading is lower than the supine systolic reading, suspect reduced adrenal gland function. The degree to which the systolic BP drops while standing is often proportionate to the degree of hypoadrenalism. So, if your stand-up BP is 10 points lower than the BP lying down, you more than likely have an adrenal deficit

Pantothenic Acid

The body relies on pantothenic acid to help the adrenal glands produce stress hormones during times of both psychological and physical strain. This property makes pantothenic acid potentially useful for dealing with emotional upset, depression, anxiety, migraines, chronic fatigue, and withdrawal from alcohol or tobacco. It is commonly taken as part of a vitamin B complex supplement.

Allergy sufferers may find pantothenic acid beneficial for controlling the nasal congestion that can develop during an allergic reaction. An asthmatic response initiated by seasonal allergies may similarly improve with pantothenic acid. There is no RDA for pantothenic acid. There are no known drug or nutrient interactions associated with pantothenic acid.

For psychological or physical stress: Take a daily vitamin B complex supplement that includes 100 mg of pantothenic acid. Many adrenal support combinations designed to help the body cope with stress contain approximately this amount of pantothenic acid. *I strongly encourage the reader to take a good B complex vitamin to help you cope with stress as well as healing the liver and adrenal glands.* Three companies I have discovered that make a good B complex *without vitamin C* are Solaray (50 B complex), Allergy Research Group, and Thorne. Clients I have coached generally tolerate one or the other of these B complex. Make sure you test either brand carefully. Explore other brands if these do not agree with you. You might need to open a B complex capsule and only take ¼ dose at a time once in the morning and afternoon in order to obtain adequate B vitamins. It I best to take your B complex with breakfast and not too late in the day since B vitamins are invigorating.

Adrenocortex Stress Profile

The Adrenocortex Stress Profile is a saliva test offered by Great Smokies Lab, which evaluates bioactive levels of the body's important stress hormones, cortisol and DHEA. It accurately measures unbound levels of cortisol and DHEA and provides a complete circadian analysis of cortisol activity. Controlled collection times allow for accurate testing. Saliva samples can be collected easily at home or at work. Diagnos-Techs is a lab in Kent, Washington that I use for accurate saliva testing of cortisol levels.

Yeast Infections (Candida albicans)

If you have a systemic yeast infection, I encourage you to read *The Yeast Connection* by Dr. William G. Crook, MD. Remember that any infection, including yeast is acid-forming. *The Yeast Connection* is an excellent resource to help you overcome yeast infection. I would caution you to eat only your daily protein requirements. The yeast connection diet consists of a majority of vegetables, so if you are careful with your protein intake, you can resolve your yeast problem as well as alkalizing.

Tea Tree Oil

Tea tree oil has natural antiseptic and fungicidal (anti-yeast) properties. Tea tree oil is found in toothpaste, hand lotions, creams, soaps, household cleansers, and shampoo. It has been used to treat yeast infections, acne, and athlete's foot.

Precautions:

Never take tea tree oil internally by drinking it. Avoid contact with eyes. Do not store it in plastic, as it will dissolve the container. Keep out of reach of children. Store it in a cool place in a glass container. Always test a drop of pure tea tree oil on a small area of the underside of your forearm to check for sensitivity. Wait a few hours to see if you react. If you develop a rash or redness, do not use tea tree oil.

Tea tree oil can be used as a mouth wash for a sore throat, thrush, and canker sores. Add five drops to a small glass of warm water. Three times a day, swish, and spit. Vaginal yeast treatments may contain tea tree oil. You can apply pure tea tree oil to the feet for athlete's foot or add five drops to warm water and soak you feet.

To reduce your exposure to harsh chemicals, tea tree oil cleaning products for the home have natural antiseptic properties. Tea tree oil is a natural insect repellant, too. Apply pure oil to exposed areas of skin to repel insects.

Vulvodynia

Some women at the IC Puzzle support group have reported using a few drops of pure tea tree oil in a warm sitz bath and find this very soothing. You need to test tea tree oil on your inner arm first to make sure you're not allergic to it. Fill a basin with warm water about an inch or two from the top and add 3 to 5 drops of 100% tea tree oil. In the bath, balance over the basin, soak, and wash the perineum gently for 5 to 15 minutes. Use this warm sitz bath twice a day for 3 or 4 days to notice effect, and then only do it once a day. It is very soothing. You may notice a little tingling at the urethra, but this goes away within minutes after soaking.

Anti-fungal Remedies

It has been suggested to rotate anti-fungals in order to help eradicate yeast. The rationale is that the yeast does not adapt or become resistant to a certain herb or medicine if these anti-fungals are rotated every few weeks.

- Tea tree oil (Don't take internally)
- Grapefruit seed extract
- Oregano extract
- Pau D'arco extract
- Garlic
- Propolis
- Golden Seal
- Echinacea
- Caprilic acid
- Clove
- Olive leaf extract
- Diflucan, Nystatin, Nizoral

Protein—What is Protein?

Protein is constructed of amino acids. Amino acids are essential to the production of proteins for enzymes, hormones, and collagen. Of the 20 amino acids found in the human body, 9 are termed *essential* amino acids since they cannot be made by the body and therefore must be provided in the diet. The other 11 amino acids are termed *non-essential* as they can be produced by the body from other components of the diet.

Essential protein in our diets comes from both animal and plant sources. Most animal sources (meat, fish, milk, eggs) provide what's called *complete* protein, meaning that they contain all 9 of the essential amino acids.

Plant sources of *incomplete* protein include legumes (beans), grains, fruits, vegetables, nuts, sprouts, and seeds are missing certain essential amino acids. For example, rice is low in isoleucine and lysine. By combining different plant foods you can get all of the essential amino acids throughout the course of the day. Some plant sources contain quite a bit of protein, like nuts and legumes. An example of plant protein combination to obtain a complete protein would be combining beans with rice. As a rule, grains with legumes or grains with nuts provide you with complete protein. Soy is a legume and a *complete* plant protein.

Non-essential Amino Acids

﹩ Alanine	﹩ Glutamine
﹩ Arginine	﹩ Glycine
﹩ Asparagine	﹩ Proline
﹩ Aspartic Acid	﹩ Serine
﹩ Cysteine	﹩ Tryosine
﹩ Glutamic Acid	

Essential Amino Acids

﹩ Histidine	﹩ Phenylalanine
﹩ Isoleucine	﹩ Threonine
﹩ Leucine	﹩ Tryptophan
﹩ Lysine	﹩ Valine
﹩ Methionine	

How Much Protein Do We Need?

Dietary protein requirements have been contested throughout the brief history of modern nutritional science. The World Health Organization recommendation is that 10-15% of your calories come from protein. Scientific evidence indicates adults require no more than 10-15% of their daily caloric intake from protein. Regular consumption of protein in the U.S. exceeds the recommended daily amount for regular needs, so most people do not need to add more protein-rich foods to their daily intake. We need protein to meet our growth, repair, and reproductive needs, not our energy needs.

Ron Brown, author of *The Body Fat Guide,* takes this approach in determining our daily protein requirements. He claims Nature's answer to the question of how much protein we need lies within a woman's breast. "Human breast milk contains approximately 10% of calories from protein. This supplies all the protein needs during infancy, the time of a human's life when protein needs are the highest. On a diet of 10% protein, an infant will double its weight in 6 months; an infant will triple its weight in a year. How can an adult who is not building new tissue at the same rate possibly need a higher percentage of protein than this?"

Getting Started

"All cure starts from within out and from the head down and in reverse order as the symptoms have appeared."

— Hering's Law of Cure

The Plan

Ideally, for the first few weeks, 80% of your diet will be alkalizing foods, which will be vegetables preferably green vegetables to which you are not allergic. The other 20% of your diet will be eaten from this acid-forming food category: organic meat, poultry, or fish. A basic rule of thumb in the beginning: vegetables for breakfast, vegetables for lunch, vegetables for dinner with small portions of protein, fats, or nuts to stabilize blood sugar. For some individuals they might need to start this program more slowly, selecting 50% of their diet from the alkaline food list and the other 50% from the acid-forming food list. The reason for this approach is that a highly alkalizing diet is detoxing. A 50:50 ratio will create fewer detox symptoms, however your progress will be much slower. Take alkalizing supplements in between breakfast and lunch and between lunch and dinner. Grains, dairy, nuts, seeds, eggs, and legumes are best avoided in the very beginning since they are acid-forming, but most importantly they can cause hidden food allergies, food sensitivities, and gluten intolerance contributing to bladder symptoms. Most fruits and fruit juices will not be consumed for the first few months because they contain citric, malic, or tannic acids which persons with IC do not tolerate at this point. All your food selections should be as fresh as possible. Frozen is OK if you must. No canned or processed foods, please. No additives, food colorings, or preservatives. Organic is the best but not absolutely necessary. Choose natural free-range meat and poultry, organic eggs, and fresh seafood. When you are better alkalized, you can add one food at a time from the food lists in this Getting Started chapter. This diet is somewhat strict in the beginning, but you can lighten up a bit in a few months when your metabolic acidosis improves. Your allergies, fibro, and irritable bowel should start to fade away the longer you are on this diet.

Stress and Exercise

You must learn to relax because stress is very acid-forming. In the beginning of alkalizing, *do not overexercise* since this causes an increase in lactic acid, which adds to the body's acid load. Exercise moderately for the first few months until you understand your body's pH. If you resume a more vigorous exercise program after a few months, monitor your urine pH after exercising so you can see how much it drops after activity. Drinking fresh vegetable juices will help raise the pH after exercising as well as green drinks and green supplements. Some individuals take an extra dose of sodium and potassium bicarbonate to help neutralize acids after vigorous exercise. Drink adequate alkaline water when exercising to stay hydrated.

Eliminate Allergens

Allergies or food intolerances can be a big problem for persons with IC, which is explained in the Allergies chapter. The reason we avoid grains, dairy, eggs, nuts, seeds, legumes in the beginning is these foods tend to be common allergens and are acid-forming. Allergens can be from food, cosmetics, inhalants, et cetera. However, allergies or sensitivities can show up as bladder symptoms. You should have minimal bladder symptoms if you avoid all your allergens. This could take about 72 hours, although it might take several weeks to detect and eliminate your allergens. It is a good idea in the beginning of this program to be tested for food allergies and environmental allergens either with a blood test or MRT. When you detect your food and environmental allergens, eliminate them when you start this diet. By avoiding food allergens for three months to six months, you should be able to add IgG allergen foods back after avoiding them and carefully evaluate their effect. You must always avoid your IgE allergens. Studies have proven that by avoiding allergens for three to six months, the body readjusts, and you should be able to reintroduce IgG food allergens and rotate these foods, eventually eating them once or twice a week without causing bladder symptoms. While avoiding these allergens in the beginning, we are working on alkalizing the body, healing the leaky gut, liver, and adrenals as described in other chapters of this book.

Persons wonder why if their urine pH is 7 or above they can still have IC symptoms. Here is the reason. Histamine is a chemical released by mast cells in the body when the body encounters something to which it is allergic. **Histamine's main effects are to make smooth muscles (in the bronchi, gut, and bladder) contract, to make small blood vessels enlarge and make the capillaries (tiny blood vessels) becomes leakier causing inflammation and discomfort.** Many doctors prescribe antihistamines like Atarax, Zyrtec, and Vistaril for persons with IC. Claritin and Benadryl are also effective over the counter antihistamines. Antihistamines help decrease allergic reactions anywhere in the body, including the bladder, by blocking the effects of histamine. Alkalizing over time will help decrease the tendency to release histamine. Please do not underestimate the impact of allergies or food intolerances on IC. Be a good detective. In the first couple of weeks by consuming a diet of 80% green vegetables and 20% lean meats, poultry, or fish, we will be consuming an alkalizing and hypoallergenic diet.

Stop Supplements

I strongly suggest stopping all supplements, vitamins, or herbs. Supplements, herbs, and vitamins cause IC irritation. Even one supplement can make you miserable. This seems to be a big hurdle for many persons with IC. This is a critical recommendation. Supplements, vitamins, and herbs might contain allergens, irritants, or they might contribute to your acid load. When you are stable on the diet and free from symptoms, you can add each supplement carefully one at a time to test for reactions. Test different brands if one brand disagrees with you. Take all prescribed medications as ordered by your medical doctor. It is possible that a prescribed medicine can be a bladder irritant, but you must work this out with your doctor to determine this for yourself.

Probiotics and Essential Fatty Acid

Test a good hypoallergenic and dairy-free probiotic, and take it every day. HLC Intensive and HLC High Potency probiotics by Pharmax is an excellent probiotic. It must be refrigerated.

Test essential fatty acids. You can usually find these in health food stores in the refrigerated section. If you can't find one that says Total Essential Fatty Acid (Udo's Oil is a good one), then buy flaxseed oil and use one tablespoon a day. (Note: flax seeds and flaxseed oil does seem to be bothersome to many persons with IC.) Another excellent essential fatty acid is fish oil such as salmon oil capsules. These oils need to be refrigerated. I use a pure and tasteless fish oil supplement by Pharmax, Udo's Oil, canola oil and olive oil. Do not cook with your total essential fatty acids. You need to use them raw. Make a salad dressing using these oils, or drizzle them over your cooked vegetables, salads, and soups right before serving.

Be careful when adding probiotics and flaxseed oil, and make sure they do not cause a bladder reaction. Add only one at a time when you are comfortable. Consider testing various essential fatty acids and probiotics for tolerance. If you find you cannot tolerate the probiotics or the flaxseed oil for now, test them again in another few weeks. Keep retesting periodically. When your metabolic acidosis improves, you should be more tolerant of foods and supplements. Organic canola oil, Pharmax fish oil, salmon oil capsules, and olive oil are usually well tolerated by persons with IC. These oils are useful for calories and healthy fats in case you do not tolerate Udo's oil or flaxseed oil in the beginning.

Seafood

Eat two to three servings of fish per week instead of your usual meat or poultry—just not shellfish. Fish provides another important source of essential fatty acid (DHA) that is critical for the brain and all our cells.

pH Testing

Purchase a roll of Hydrion pH paper with the color code for testing your urine. You can dip the pH paper in the urine stream if you wish. I recommend a Hydrion Lo-Ion test kit to accurately evaluate drinking water pH. Start an IC diary that includes your urine pH readings, food intake, supplements, and symptoms. 0 indicates no bladder symptoms, and 10 indicates the worst discomfort. We want to keep the urine pH around 7 to 7.4. The pH paper will be a teal blue color or dark blue. This will indicate that we are consuming an alkalizing diet and creating an alkalizing life style.

Green Supplements

Once you are stable on the hypoallergenic alkalizing diet, test a green supplement such as pure organic barley or wheatgrass. Add liberal amounts of dark green vegetables and grasses from a wide variety of sources. Veggie Magma or Green Magma supplements are a way of adding more greens to your diet fast. However, *fresh* vegetables and grasses are the best and are an excellent source of alkaline salts. The chlorophyll (or blood of the plant) contained in green plants and grasses is identical to the blood of humans, except for only one atom. That atom difference is magnesium in green plants and grasses and iron in human blood! Eating lots of green foods is like giving yourself a blood transfusion. You will feel energized. Green foods, such as wheat grass and barley grass, are some of the lowest-calorie, lowest-sugar, and most nutrient-rich foods on the planet.

Of course, do be careful when taking *any* new supplement to observe for allergies or intolerances. If you feel like you have bladder symptoms from any green supplement, stop the supplement and try it again in another month. Because the wheat and barley are in the developing stages or grass stage of growth, there is *no gluten* in these products. If you have an allergy to wheat or barley, the fact that it is a sprout without the gluten means these supplements should not cause an allergic reaction. Some individuals with allergies to grass might not tolerate wheat or barley grass.

Fresh barley green juice or fresh wheatgrass juice are excellent for IC. Shots of fresh wheatgrass juice can be purchased at Robeks and Jamba Juice. I would not recommend more than one ounce of fresh wheatgrass or barley grass when you start. It will detoxify the body, which can cause nausea, so start with no more than one ounce a day. You can take the green supplements or fresh wheatgrass or barley grass a couple of times a day as you progress. Be careful, these green supplements are invigorating. Do not take these green supplements after dinner. You can grow your own flat of wheatgrass/barley grass or purchase a flat of fresh wheatgrass from Jamba Juice or Robeks. You *must* have a juicer that states it will juice fresh wheatgrass or barley grass. I recommend the Omega 8001 juicer as it will juice fresh vegetables, fruits, sprouts, and grasses. It also makes fresh nut butters and pasta! A web site to purchase fresh wheatgrass or barley grass trays to grow in your own home is http://www.wheatgrasskits.com. An excellent reference on the healing benefits of barley or wheatgrass is *Wheatgrass: Nature's Finest Medicine* by Steve Meyerowitz.

Juicing

Juiced green vegetables are very cleansing. If you have irritable bowel you can juice your vegetables. Green juices are alkalizing and help to replace lost minerals.

Solving the Interstitial Cystitis Puzzle

Fruits

While fruits are a good source of fiber and alkalizing, most persons with IC do not tolerate fruit in the beginning due to the level of *acids* found in most fruits. It is best to avoid fruit for at least the first three to six months. When you are ready to test fruit, add one fruit at a time and evaluate your tolerance. Eventually, fruit should be part of your alkalizing diet—just not at the start. Good fruits to test are low acid yellow or red delicious apples, watermelon, pears, blueberries, dates, avocados, tomatoes, and fresh figs.

Note: When a person is in balanced health, small portions of fresh seasonal fruit may be added as a snack apart from meals. Fruits can be added in about three months and tested for tolerance. I suggest testing tomatoes after about three to six months of alkalizing since tomatoes are low in sugar and high in potassium.

Low Carbohydrate Vegetables

Good low carbohydrate vegetables include broccoli, Brussels sprouts, cabbage, cauliflower, watercress, collards, chard, Swiss chard, celery, cucumbers, lettuce, green beans, spinach, kale, turnip greens, okra, parsley, or zucchini squash. Focus on *green* vegetables for the first few months. If you feel you must have potatoes, in food list *two* try red new potatoes; they might be less prone to cause food allergies. Asparagus is very healing for the kidneys and bladder but has diuretic properties.

Sprouts

Some of the best foods to eat are sprouts. When seeds, legumes, grains, and nuts are sprouted they become alkaline. Sprouts are *live* plant foods that are biogenic, which means they transfer their life energy to us. Sprouts can easily be grown in your kitchen during any season. Make sure to eat a *variety* of sprouts every day. If you are a vegetarian, sprouts are an excellent source of protein.

Heel Homeopathics

When starting your alkalizing program, consider using two BHI homeopathics made by Heel, a Swiss company—one for allergy and one for inflammation. When you encounter a food allergen, you should take one or two allergy and one or two inflammation tablets and let them dissolve in your mouth. Take one or two of each every 5 to 10 minutes until symptoms subside. You might need several doses. These homeopathics are a natural alternative to antihistamines. There are no side effects and no drug interactions. They are completely safe and nontoxic. Even children can take these safely.

Alkalizing Foods

Green juices from all green vegetables are highly alkalizing. In addition, fresh vegetable broths are extremely alkalizing to the body. These need to be yeast-free and preservative free.

Eliminate

Acid-forming drinks and foods you should avoid are coffee, tea, soda, or *any* carbonated beverage, vinegar, sugar, artificial sweeteners, and of course, no candy, cakes, donuts, and fried foods. Citric acid or citrate might be troublesome. Avoid wines of all kinds, beer, and hard liquor. Avoid smoking or chewing tobacco. No *over*-exercising. Diminish stress levels, as stress is very acid-forming. Avoid foods with additives, artificial ingredients, or preservatives. Do not eat shellfish since they are high in toxins. Initially, avoid foods from the *nightshade family*: red or green bell peppers, cayenne pepper, tobacco, tomatoes, potatoes, and eggplant.

Protein

What about protein? Too much animal food provides more protein than is required by the human body. In addition, meats and poultry contain a fatty acid called arachidonic acid that contributes to inflammatory conditions, which is something we don't want. Our bodies are only about 7% protein. Many holistic health care professionals evaluate the amount of protein "Mother Nature" recommends by analyzing the protein content in human mother's milk. Mother's milk is only about 10% protein; i.e. better suited to the human body's protein requirement. Infants whose bodies are growing the fastest they will ever grow thrive on this amount of protein!

If you are *vegetarian*, you can try some of the protein drinks such as soy complete protein drinks. Soy (if tolerated) is an excellent plant source of *complete* protein without adding to the body's acid load. However, grains, nuts, dairy, eggs, and legumes (soy) cause many allergic bladder reactions in the first several months. Sprouts are a good source of protein for vegetarians. If you don't consider yourself a strict vegetarian consider small portions of fresh fish or eggs for a protein source in the first several months until you can carefully test grains, nuts, seeds, and legumes. Feature proteins such as sprouts, garbanzo beans, tofu, or fresh fish with scales and fins. Vegetables carry the subcellular units of amino acids to make proteins in amounts that are congruent with the body's needs.

In a few months after you have eliminated your allergens you will have a nice selection of foods to consume. Your diet should look like this: 80% alkalizing foods: vegetables, fruits, and sprouts. 20% acid-forming foods: meats, poultry, fish, legumes, grains, eggs, dairy, nuts, seeds, and natural sugars. Let approximately 10% of your daily calories be from protein. Instead of the usual American protein intake of 90 to 120 grams of protein a day a more ideal intake would be about 20 to 40 grams per day. For example, if you eat 2,000 calories a day, you would need about 200 of those calories for your protein intake. This will decrease your daily acid load tremendously. In addition, animal protein foods often contribute factors to the body, which are unneeded and then represent a challenge to dispose of (e.g., saturated fats). Avoid organ meats as they are higher in toxins.

Solving the Interstitial Cystitis Puzzle

Alkaline Water

Ideally, drink one to two quarts of alkaline water each day. You might want to explore Evian or other bottled alkaline spring water. Test bottled spring water carefully. Drink only bottled spring water or ionized water with a tested pH of 7 or above. Use your Hydrion Lo-Ion test kit to test your water. Do not drink distilled water unless you add alkalizing minerals or a coral calcium sachet.

Yeast

If you have a yeast infection or have been taking antibiotics off and on for a while due to your IC, eliminate bakers or brewers yeast and all yeast-containing foods. You should especially avoid baked goods such as bread, muffins, pies, cakes, and pastries that contain yeast. Having a yeast condition will add to your acid load, so test for yeast and follow an anti-yeast program.

Limit Milk Products

Some alternatives to dairy are calcium fortified soy, almond or rice milk, or cheese. Soyco makes very good soy, rice, and almond cheeses that are high in calcium. Soy products (if tolerated) are an excellent plant source of *complete* protein without adding to the body's acid load.

What about Calcium?

If milk products are limited, where should one turn for their calcium needs? Many worry that eating an alkaline diet would seriously deplete one's calcium intake, which is vital for so many functions of the body. All leafy green vegetables and grasses are inherently high in calcium. We also need to understand that calcium can be pulled from the bones to help neutralize an over-acid condition caused by incorrect diet, stress and other acid-forming conditions. Thus we see that people are suffering from a *calcium-robbing* problem along with a calcium deficiency problem. As long as we are eating an alkalizing diet that is rich in green foods, green drinks, and other sources of calcium such as fortified soy, rice or almond products, we do not need to worry about getting enough calcium.

Shopping Suggestions:

Produce Section: A fruit to test and eat freely in the beginning is avocado. Do try to include avocados in the beginning since they are alkalizing, increase calories, and usually do not cause bladder symptoms. Persons with IC cannot tolerate fruits in the beginning due to the level of citric acids. In a few months, tomatoes and other fruits can be added one at a time to test for tolerance. Your tolerance will improve with alkalization. See food lists in this chapter for fruit and vegetable suggestions.

Health Food Section: Explore your local health food store and purchase fresh bulk foods from the bins (they contain less mold) such as brown rice, soy beans, garbanzo beans, lentils, and other legumes; raw sunflower, sesame, flax seeds, raw almonds, pumpkin seeds, and walnuts. Look for liquid, no yeast low salt vegetable, chicken, and beef broth, calcium-fortified soy, almond, or rice milks and cheeses, almond butter and sesame tahini, unsalted brown rice cakes. If you find you are gluten intolerant, explore alternative pastas and cereals made from millet, amaranth, quinoa, buckwheat, corn, soy, or brown rice. Use organic virgin, cold pressed olive oil for cooking. Refrigerate nuts and oils to prevent rancidity. Some individuals tolerate sprouted grain products such as Ezekiel or Essene bread.

Refrigerated Section: Consider non-genetically engineered tofu, sprouted wheat tortillas (no yeast), Udo's Oil blend—a good *total* essential fatty acid supplement found in health food stores—, flaxseed oil, and fresh humus. You might tolerate pesto.

Seafood/Meat Section: Small to moderate portions of fresh fish with fins and scales (like trout and salmon), fresh, free-range turkey, chicken, or beef. Eating more than three ounces of animal protein per day starts calcium loss from the body, so do not over eat animal protein. Try to eat two to three servings of fish a week instead of meat and poultry. Buy eggs that say high in DHA or chicken that has been raised free-range and fed high omega-3 fatty acid feed. Do not overcook the eggs since this will destroy much of the DHA in the yolk. DHA is a good omega-3 essential fatty acid that most Americans are deficient in—a deficiency that contributes to inflammatory conditions. One to two eggs a week if you are not allergic to them is reasonable. Have small portions of protein at each meal to help stabilize blood sugar. Fats such as nuts, seeds, and nut butters help stabilize blood sugar as well.

Water: Drink only alkaline bottled spring water or ionized water in the beginning.

Seasonings: Good salt choices are sea vegetable seasoning granules by Maine Coast: dulse, kelp, and nori sea seasoning granules. These are excellent because they are high in potassium and trace minerals yet low in sodium. I summarize the taste of these three sea seasonings as follows: Maine Coast kelp sea seasoning is salty tasting and is good on vegetables, soups, and salads. Maine Coast nori sea seasoning is mild tasting also use on vegetables, soups, and salads. Maine Coast dulse sea seasoning is salty and more "fishy." I would use this last sea seasoning on fish and seafood salads. Strips of dried seaweed added to soups or soaked in water briefly and added to salads add good doses of trace minerals.

Celtic sea salt and Bragg Liquid Aminos are also good salt seasoning choices. Bragg Liquid Aminos, made from soy, is a good way to obtain a salt flavoring and complete protein. If you are intolerant of soy, you need to avoid Bragg's. Be careful not to overdo the Celtic salt or Bragg's, as they are still high in sodium. Onions, garlic, turmeric and ginger are good foods and spices to consider as long as they do not cause IC symptoms in *you*.

Solving the Interstitial Cystitis Puzzle

Remember, we are all unique and can react differently so there are no hard and fast rules for everyone with IC. Onions and apples contain quercetin, which is a natural antihistamine and anti-inflammatory. Garlic is anti-parasitic, anti-fungal and adds nice flavor to use with your vegetables. Ginger and turmeric are anti-inflammatory. Try slicing up some fresh organic ginger and boil in alkaline water for tea. Add a drizzle of honey to taste. As with all food, spices, and supplements test carefully to make sure it does not cause symptoms. In addition, what you cannot tolerate in the first several months, you may tolerate after 6 to 12 months of alkalizing. Remember to read your labels. Watch for ingredients such as MSG, citric acid, yeast (if you have a yeast infection or yeast allergy), vinegar, wheat or gluten, corn syrup, sugar, additives, or preservatives. The easiest way to start is to eat a diet of *whole* foods and keep your recipes simple. This will help you avoid additives and detect allergies.

The First Week Getting Started

First, read this entire book. **Second,** find an open-minded healthcare professional to work with you on this program so that you can determine that the alkalizing hypoallergenic diet, supplements and suggestions are safe for *you*. **Third**, consider food/environmental allergy testing by blood test or MRT to determine your allergens or sensitivities and eliminate them.

Go to Holisticnurse.com for copies of an IC diary. Document all your IC symptoms including other complaints such as fibro, irritable bowel, headaches, etc., ranking them the worst to the least bothersome. Give your bladder discomfort a scale of 0 is no symptom to 10 is the worst. Observe yourself before starting on this program and keep an accurate records. Document the times you void (urinate) and your levels of discomfort. We need to have a record before starting this hypoallergenic alkalizing program to watch for improvements. Some of you may notice that when you awaken in the morning you may have minimal or no bladder symptoms. This is because you have been fasting for about 12 hours. Your bladder is not being subjected to food allergens, irritating supplements, medicines, or vitamins.

Now that you know where you are coming from, let's move on to the food choices for the first several weeks. The first few weeks is the allergy elimination diet. *You must stop all vitamins, herbs, and supplements. Take all medications and supplements your doctor prescribes*. You will choose only foods from list *one*. Although the foods listed are generally well tolerated, you might be sensitive to some. Please use your diary to evaluate *your* individual differences. There is no *perfect* food or supplement list for *everyone* with IC. But there are safer ones.

Start by selecting foods from list *one* that you rarely if ever eat. If you eat a food more than twice a week, exclude that food. The rationale is if you don't eat a food very often, the body does not generally react to that food. For example, if you eat chicken more than twice week, choose turkey or fish you rarely eat. If you eat broccoli more than two times a week choose other vegetables you rarely eat.

When you test foods, understand that you can be *not reactive, slightly reactive, moderately reactive,* or *highly reactive* to a certain food or *quantity* of food. What this means is that you might tolerate a certain *quantity* of a food. For example, you might tolerate soy products a few times a week, but cannot tolerate soy *every* day.

Keep your protein servings small to moderate portions if possible (three to fours ounces per day). A cup or two of vegetables (raw or lightly steamed) per meal would be good. Focus especially on green vegetables. The only seasonings you may use from food list *one* are Celtic sea salt, sea seasonings, seaweed, and vanilla. Only when you are *symptom free,* start to add in foods from list *two.* It might take some of you a few days to be symptom free when eating foods from list *one,* or it might take up to several weeks. Everyone is different. Don't get discouraged!

NOTE: *Green vegetables and foods high in chlorophyll such as wheatgrass are high in vitamin K. Vitamin K is essential to facilitate proper blood clotting. However, if you are on blood thinners such as aspirin, Coumadin or heparin to thin your blood or decrease blood clots you need to review this diet carefully with your health care practitioner and / or a dietician.*

Food and Supplement List One
Meat, Poultry, and Fish

Bass (striped)	Beef (lean)	Bluefish
Bison	Buffalo	Chicken
Cod (Pacific)	Cornish Hens	Duck
Flounder (Pacific)	Goose	Halibut (Alaskan)
Lamb	Ostrich	Perch
Pheasant	Pike	Rabbit
Salmon (Alaskan)	Sole (Pacific)	Trout (rainbow)
Turkey	Venison	Whitefish

Vegetables

Bok Choy	Beans (string)	Broccoli
Brussels Sprouts	Cabbage	Cabbage (Chinese)
Cauliflower*	Celery	Chard
Collards	Cucumbers (peeled)*	Dandelion Greens
Endive	Escarole	Jicama
Kale	Kelp	Kohlrabi
Leeks	Lettuce (Boston)	Lettuce (iceberg)*
Lettuce (Romaine)	Mustard Greens	Okra
Parsley	Parsnips	Peas (green)*
Peas (snow)	Pumpkin	Rutabaga
Seaweed	Spinach	Sprouts*

Squash (acorn)*	Squash (butternut)*	Swiss Chard
Taro	Turnips*	Watercress
Water Chestnuts	White cabbage*	Zucchini*

Legumes, Nuts, Grains and Seeds

Coconut*	Lentils*	Pumpkin seeds

(*studies show pumpkin seeds lower calcium oxalate levels in the urine*)
Rice (white, wild, or brown)*

Fruits

Avocado*

Beverages

Alkaline Water (spring or ionized water with pH of 7 or above)
Broth (Low salt, yeast-free vegetable, chicken, or beef)
Coconut milk*   No Carbonated Drinks.

Seasonings

Celtic sea salt	Maine Coast Sea Seasonings (kelp, nori, dulse)
Seaweed	Vanilla*

Oils

Avocado oil*	Canola oil (Organic)	Olive oil

(Organic virgin cold-pressed. You can cook with olive oil.)

Pharmax fish oil	Pumpkin oil	Salmon oil capsules

Supplements

Calcium/Magnesium with vitamin D   Sodium Bicarbonate (baking soda)
Potassium Bicarbonate

1. Test Healthy Life Harvest Aloe Vera Coral Calcium. 1,000 mg of calcium, 500mg to 1,000mg of magnesium, and 400 to 800 IU of vitamin D daily. Divide calcium/magnesium/vitamin D in two to three divided doses over the day with meals. If you do not tolerate Healthy Life Harvest Aloe Vera Coral Calcium, then test a calcium/ magnesium/vitamin D supplement you do tolerate.

2. Sodium/potassium bicarbonate mix 4:1 [four parts sodium bicarbonate (baking soda) to one part potassium bicarbonate]. Take one eighth to one quarter teaspoon two to three times a day *in between meals on an empty stomach.* If you are on a sodium restricted diet, consider potassium bicarbonate without the sodium bicarbonate.

Food and Supplement List Two

NOTE: Before starting list two do liver flush (See Gallbladder/ Liver Flush chapter.) Now, if you are *symptom free,* you can choose foods from list *two,* which add more calories and variety. However, many persons with IC report more symptoms when adding foods from list *two.* Many food *Low oxalate foods in food list one. Most meats are low oxalate.*

in list *two* and *three* have a higher glycemic food index, some are more acid-forming and are known to cause allergies or hidden food intolerances. There is no "perfect" food list for all persons with IC, but the foods from list *one* are *generally* "safe" hypoallergenic and have a low glycemic index.

Along with list *one*, you can now add and test one new food or supplement at a time from list *two*. When you add the new food you will eat this new food for three days consecutively. For example you may now be comfortable and eating the following foods from list *one*: trout, salmon, turkey, chicken, lean beef, alfalfa sprouts, mung bean sprouts, yellow and green zucchini, romaine lettuce, celery, cucumbers, avocado, pumpkin, string beans, snow peas, Chinese cabbage, acorn and butternut squash, cauliflower, green peas, water chestnuts, pumpkin seeds, brown and wild rice, rice milk, rice cheese, seaweed, Maine Coast sea vegetable seasoning, Celtic sea salt, olive oil, canola oil, pumpkin oil, avocado oil, fresh coconut and coconut milk, low fat, low salt yeast-free vegetable, chicken or beef broths. This would be considered your *base diet* and the diet you know you can return to if you get into a flare.

Moving on to food list *two*, you decide to test millet for the next three days. *Keeping your food diary* you will observe yourself to see if this new food causes any bladder symptoms. For the next three mornings you will eat millet cereal every morning for breakfast. A *small* drizzle of maple syrup or honey is OK provided you do not have a problem with yeast.

I have seen many persons initially react to a certain foods or supplements in the first 6 to 12 months of this alkalizing hypoallergenic diet. These same foods and supplements are temporarily eliminated and are eventually reintroduced and tolerated after 6 to 12 months. *Do not get discouraged or lose hope.*

Categories of Food Reactions
1. First day of testing millet cereal for breakfast and your bladder symptoms appear or increase. Put millet on your *no* list. You are *highly* reactive to millet. Take your homeopathics (allergy and inflammation by Heel) as directed to diminish bladder symptoms and select a new food to test. It should only take about an hour after the homeopathic doses to feel comfortable. *Wait* until the next morning to begin testing a different food from list *two*. You can retest millet in another month or two.

2. First day no reaction after eating millet for breakfast, but on the second day after eating millet, you start to have bladder symptoms you are *moderately* reactive. Take your homeopathics to stop the bladder reactions as directed. Put millet on your *maybe* list. You can probably eat millet once maybe twice a week only. You can test a new food from list *two* the next day.

3. You eat millet cereal for breakfast for three days in a row and by the end of the third day; you develop some slight bladder symptoms. Put millet on your *yes* list. You are *slightly* reactive to millet and you could safely eat millet one to two times a week. Take your homeopathics to stop the bladder symptoms. You can test a new food from list *two* the next day.

4. You eat millet cereal for breakfast for three consecutive days and notice you do *not* develop any bladder symptoms. You are not reactive to millet. You can safely eat millet and put millet on your *yes* list.

Here is food and supplement list *two*. When you have tested all the foods and supplements you want to test on list *two* you can move on to the foods and supplements in list *three*. Testing foods and supplements on list *two* should take a few months. Test only one new food or supplement every three days. If you choose to test dried fruit, make sure to eat only small amounts. Make certain dried fruits are unsulfured and unsweetened. Dried fruits may contain the preservative sulfur dioxide which many persons are allergic to.

Food and Supplement List Two
Vegetables

Artichoke	Asparagus	Beets
Carrots	Garlic	Ginger
Onions	Potato (Fingerling)	Potato (Red)
Sweet Potatoes	Yams	Yukon Gold Potato

Snacks, Nuts, Nut Butters, and Seeds—Unsalted

Almonds*	Brazil Nuts	Cashews
Hazel Nuts	Macadamia Nuts	Pine Nuts (Pignolias)
Pistachio Nuts	Sesame Seeds*	Sunflower Seeds
Walnuts*		

* Nuts in general can cause food allergies and food intolerances. However the nuts and seeds listed and highlighted are very healthy for IC and add calories. I encourage you to test and explore unsalted seeds and nuts. Almonds, walnuts, and pumpkin seeds are especially good for us.

Non-Gluten Grains and Cereal Alternatives

Amaranth	Buckwheat	Corn
Ezekiel or Essene Bread	Quinoa	Millet

Fruits

Apples (dried)	Apples (Gala)	Apples (low acid, yellow)
Apples (Red Delicious)	Apricots (fresh or dried)	
Blueberries	Dates	Figs (fresh or dried)
Olives	Pears	Watermelon

Sugar and Spice

Braggs Amino Acids (use as salt)   Maple syrup (Organic)
Honey   Sugar (Raw organic)   Turmeric

Oils

Flaxseed Oil† (do not heat) Safflower Oil   Sunflower Oil
Total Essential Fatty Acid† supplement or Udo's oil (do not heat)
Flaxseed Oil† (do not heat)

† It is very important to include at least one tablespoon of essential fatty acids in our diet every day. Flaxseed oil, total essential fatty acid supplement, Pharmax fish oil, or salmon oil capsules help to decrease inflammation and build healthy cell walls that are not prone to breakdown.

Supplement Testing

1. Test B complex vitamin (Thorne, Solaray 50, or Allergy Research Group; *No vitamin C* added) Take in the morning with breakfast, as it is invigorating. Take 1/4 to 1/2 capsule if you react to a B complex vitamin. Start slowly.

2. Stool test for parasites and food allergens with Diagnos-Techs. Treat LGS with compounded antimicrobial(s). (See Clark Compounding Pharmacy and Diagnos-Techs in appendix D.) Add loading doses of HLC Intensive probiotics and then follow up with daily HLC High Potency probiotic capsules *after* stool testing. You might need to take HLC probiotics *during* LGS treatment as well as after.

3. Test other essential fatty acids (Udo's oil, flaxseed oil, walnut oil). Take one to two tablespoons daily. Consider fatty acid red blood cell testing to determine fatty acid status.

4. Female or male hormone testing with Diagnos-Techs and supplementation to balance hormones

5. Consider adding leaky gut supplement, Perm A Vite, or L-glutamine powder by Allergy Research.

Food and Supplement List Three

The following is a list of foods and supplements that are known to cause some allergic or hidden food intolerances. You can test these foods and add them carefully and cautiously after you are finished with lists *one* and *two*. Again, take your time with testing. Test each new food one at a time by eating it for three days in a row. For example, if you want to test soy, test soy by consuming plain tofu or drink plain soy milk for three consecutive days. Make sure the food you test is the pure food with no other flavorings or other ingredients.

Meat, Fish, and Poultry
The following *fish* might be high in histamines and might cause bladder symptoms:

Herring   Mackerel   Mahi Mahi*
Sardines
Tuna*   Swordfish* is high in mercury

Lean pork and any other lean meat, fish (except shellfish), and poultry

Legumes
All legumes including soy and peanuts

Fruits
Berries (most)   Cherries   Grapes
Golden Raisins   Mangoes   Melon
Nectarines   Papaya   Peaches
Tomato (sun-dried and fresh, plus juice and mild salsa)

Nuts
Any nuts not previously listed

Supplements
1. Test green supplements such as Veggie Magma or Green Magma, fresh wheatgrass and/or fresh barley grass. Fresh wheatgrass or barley grass one ounce once or twice a day as tolerated. Green supplements between meals. Do not take late in the day as they are invigorating. If not tolerated, test at later dates.

2. Test small dose of buffered vitamin C—consider Thorne or Allergy Research Group.

Food List Four
Here are some foods that I suggest you test in six to twelve months when you are stable.

Fruits and Vegetables
Bananas (fresh or dried banana chips)   Dried Fruits
Grapefruit   Kiwis   Lemon
Lime   Orange   Passion Fruit
Peaches (fresh or dried) Persimmon   Pineapple (fresh or dried)
Pomegranate   Raisins   Tangerine
Night Shade Plants (potatoes, eggplant, red, green, cayenne pepper)
Any other fruits or vegetables not previously mentioned

---

* *These are over-fished.*

Gluten Grains (Caution: May aggravate LGS)

Barley	Kamut	Oatmeal	Pumpernickel
Rye	Spelt	Triticale	Wheat

Dairy and Eggs

Eggs   Kefir or Yogurt (vanilla or plain; good natural probiotics)

To summarize, you should have a healthy group of hypoallergenic foods from a wide range of food groups from lists *one, two, three,* and list *four* to eat and be free of IC symptoms or minimal discomfort. If there are foods not listed in this book, feel free to test them carefully. Your diet should consist of 80% alkalizing foods (vegetables, fruits, and sprouts as tolerated), alkaline water, and the other 20% from the acid-forming foods (meats, poultry, fish, eggs, dairy, legumes, nuts, seeds, natural sugars, and grains). Your urine pH should read 7 or above most of the time when you are better alkalized. You may check your urine pH throughout the day to understand your body's pH trend. Starting with food list *one* should provide a good base.

Do a liver flush before starting list two. Use one to two tablespoons of essential fatty acids every day. Most fats and oils form a neutral ash in the body. Other supplements have been suggested that are useful to hasten recovery: sodium bicarbonate/potassium bicarbonate, buffered vitamin C as tolerated, aloe vera with coral calcium (or any calcium/magnesium/vitamin D supplement *you* tolerate), L-glutamine or Perm A Vite, B complex *without* vitamin C, green supplements, or green drinks such as fresh wheatgrass and barley grass. Use generous amounts of sea seasonings and seaweed for your trace minerals.

Once you are stable on your hypoallergenic, alkalizing diet and supplements, refer to the list of supplements in appendix E to test and explore natural antihistamines or mast cell stabilizers. Slowly test and add liver tonic(s) over time to help support liver function. I have attempted to keep the number of supplements to a minimum. I feel the steps I list in this Getting Started chapter to heal IC and the supplements I have listed are important for long term healing.

If you run into problems and get confused, you can always go back to the foods on list *one.* Foods and supplements on list *one* should cause fewer problems (unless you find medium to high oxalate foods bother you). Our first goal is to alkalize and eliminate your allergens or food intolerances with the elimination diet from food list *one.* **Test your stool for parasites and food allergies, then treat LGS when using food list two.** Take daily HLC probiotics *during and after* treating LGS. Test female or male hormones with Diagnos-Techs, and supplement as needed with food list *two.*

Remember to test supplements and perform food challenges by choosing foods and supplements to test for three consecutive days while using your

Solving the Interstitial Cystitis Puzzle

food diary. Once you have a nice group of healthy foods and supplements, in a few months you can then challenge yourself with other foods and supplements. Work on liver cleansing after the first month or two on this program (coffee enemas, tonics, yoga, et cetera).

Coffee and Tea: If after several months—don't try this in the first six months—you are stable and just can't live without your morning cup of coffee or tea, you can "cheat" a little by using the product Coffee Tamer in your coffee. Coffee Tamer neutralizes the acids in the coffee or tea *before* you drink it. With Coffee Tamer, you are not using all your hard-earned alkalizing elements you are obtaining through this alkalizing diet plan. You can purchase Coffee Tamer at *http://www.tamer.com*.

I suggest adding Coffee Tamer to a *low acid* organic coffee or tea. I make my coffee with low acid organic coffee; one half regular and one half water processed decaffeinated. *Only one cup, please. Caffeine starts the loss of alkalizing elements from our bodies, weakens the adrenal glands and contributes to LGS. In addition, caffeinated drinks are diuretics which will increase urination even if you do not have IC!* Coffee Tamer will neutralize the acid in a cup of coffee or tea, but it does not eliminate caffeine. Puroast and Coffee Bean are two companies that make very flavorful *low acid* coffee, both caffeinated and water processed decaffeinated. Green tea is high in antioxidants and a better choice than coffee. Use Coffee Tamer in the green tea.

As far as your own choice of supplements, it is important to stabilize yourself on this hypoallergenic alkalizing diet first. *Please* add your supplements in a thoughtful careful manner so you will know if any cause discomfort. Test one supplement every three days just like your foods. This is a healthy natural diet high in vitamins, minerals, essential proteins, and fatty acids, and you are not in danger of malnutrition. Some persons have referred to this hypoallergenic alkalizing menu as a "limited diet." I say yes, it is "limited." It is "limited" to *healthy* foods!

I know the food allergy elimination and diet challenge I have suggested in this chapter is time consuming, but it is worth it to get your life back. I do recommend food/environmental testing with Immuno Labs initially if possible. However, the allergy elimination diet and food challenges are the *most* effective ways to determine *your* bladder triggers.

Along with this alkalizing diet and supplements, continue to work with your holistic health care provider to cleanse, heal and support the leaky gut, liver, adrenals, reduce stress and support any other system that is weak for *you*. Remember, healing IC is a total body process. The kidneys and bladder are just the end result of an overly acidic and "sick" body. It has taken years to develop IC; it will take time to completely heal. Stay optimistic and take note of even small shifts in feeling better. The individuals I have seen recover from IC are the ones that stay positive and keep with the program. Even if they "fall off the wagon" occasionally, they persist. It seems healing IC is sometimes two steps forward, one step back, but there is slow and steady healing with time.

Oxalic Acid (Oxalate)

"In the small amounts normally present in food, the only importance of oxalic acid is that it combines with calcium in the diet and so reduces the amount of this mineral element that can be absorbed. Large quantities may cause poisoning by damaging the lining of the mouth and stomach, and interfering with the action of the nerves and muscles.

"A few foods, notably unripe tomatoes and some varieties of strawberries, may have small amounts. However, beetroot has about 100 milligrams per 100 grams, parsley about 150 milligrams, and rhubarb and spinach between 300 and 600 milligrams. As well as deriving oxalate from the diet, the body can synthesize it from citric acid." [1]

Oxalate Food List

The following oxalate food list was adapted from *The Low Oxalate Cookbook* published by the Vulvar Pain Foundation. Some individuals when starting the elimination diet need to follow a low oxalate diet plan for a while. *This is because oxalates bind with our minerals especially calcium and decrease our ability to alkalize.* Not everyone is bothered by high oxalate foods. Use this list as a reference to choosing your foods in the first 6 to 12 months if you feel you are sensitive to oxalates. Start with low oxalate foods and consider adding medium to high oxalate foods as tolerated.

LEGUMES, NUTS, AND SEEDS

Low	Medium	High
Coconut	Cashews	Baked beans
Lentils	Garbanzo beans	Nuts
Water chestnuts	Lima beans	Peanuts
	Split peas	Pecans
	Sunflower seeds (1 oz)	Peanut butter
	Walnuts	Sesame seeds
		Soy Products

CONDIMENTS

Low	Medium	High
Chives	Basil, fresh (1 tbsp)	Pepper (1 tsp)
Mustard, Dijon (1 tbsp)	Cinnamon (1 tsp)	Soy sauce
Nutmeg, dry (1 tsp)	Dill (1 tbsp)	
Oregano, dried (1 tsp)	Ginger, raw (1 tsp)	
Salt		
Vanilla		
Vinegar (apple cider)		

MEATS

Low	Medium	High
Beef	Kidney, beef	*none listed*
Poultry	Liver	
Eggs	Sardines	
Fish		
Lamb		
Pork		

DAIRY

Low	Medium	High
Butter	*none listed*	*none listed*
Buttermilk		
Cheese		
Milk		
Yogurt, nonfat, plain		
Yogurt, fruit		

FATS

Low	Medium	High
Butter	*none listed*	*none listed*
Mayonnaise		
Salad dressing		
Vegetable oils		

VEGETABLES

Low	Medium	High
Acorn squash	Asparagus	Beet tops, roots, greens
Alfalfa sprouts	Artichokes	Celery
Butternut Squash	Brussel sprouts	Collards
Cabbage, white	Broccoli	Dandelion greens
Cauliflower	Carrots	Eggplant
Cucumbers, peeled	Corn	Escarole
Green peas	Cucumber	Kale
Lettuce, iceberg	Garlic	Leeks
Sprouts	Green beans, snap, pod	Okra
Turnips, roots	Kohlrabi	Parsley
Zucchini squash	Lettuce (Butter)	Parsnips
	Lettuce (Romaine)	Peppers, green
	Mushrooms	Potatoes
	Mustard greens	Potatoes, sweet
	Onions	Pumpkin
	Radishes	Rhubarb
	Snow peas	Rutabagas
	Tomato, fresh	Sorrel
	Tomato sauce	Spinach
	Vegetable beef soup	Swiss chard
	Watercress	Turnip greens
		Watercress
		Yams

SWEETS

Low	Medium	High
Honey (1 tbsp)		Fig Newtons
Jellies, jams, or preserves made with low oxalate fruits (1 tbsp)	Jellies, jams, or preserves made with medium oxalate fruits (1 tbsp)	Fruitcake (1 slice)
		Marmalade
Maple syrup (1 tbsp)		
Sugar		

FRUITS

Low	Medium	High
Apples, peeled	Apples with peel	Currants, red
Avocado	Apricots	Dewberries
Cantaloupe	Blackberries	Figs, dried
Casaba	Blueberries	Gooseberries
Cherries, bing and sour	Dewberries	Grapes (Concord)
Cranberries, canned	Currants	Kiwi
Grapes (Thompson)	Cranberries, dried	Lemon peel
Honeydew	Grapefruit	Lime peel
Lemons	Oranges	Orange peel
Lemon juice	Peaches	Rhubarb
Lime juice	Pears	Strawberries
Mangoes	Pineapple	Tangerines
Melons	Plums	
Nectarines	Prunes	
Papaya	Red raspberries	
Raisins (golden)		
Watermelon		

GRAINS

Low	Medium	High
Cornflakes	Bagel (1 medium)	Bread, whole wheat
Cornstarch (1 tbsp)	Barley	Flour
Egg noodles	Corn tortilla (1 medium)	Graham crackers
Rice, white or wild	Cornbread	Grits, white corn
	Cornmeal	Kamut
	English muffin	Oatmeal
	Pasta	Popcorn
	Rice, brown	Spelt
		Wheat bran
		Wheat germ

A Guide to Natural Healing   245

BEVERAGES

Low	Medium	High
Barley water	Coffee	Chocolate milk
Cider	Fruit juices (4 oz)	Cocoa
Fruit juices (4 oz)	Cranberry	Tea, black, Indian
Apple	Grape	Herbal teas (Bigelow)
Grapefruit	Orange	*hot, brew 4 min*
Lemon	Tomato	Apple Orchard
Lime	Herbal teas (Bigelow)	Fruit & Almond
Herbal teas (Bigelow)	*hot, brew 4 min*	I Love Lemon
hot, brew 4 min	Lemon & C	Mint Medley
Apple & Spice	Spearmint	Orange & C
Chamomile Mint	V-8 Juice	Orange Spice
Cinnamon Orange		Perfect Peach
Cozy Chamomile		Red Raspberry
Cranberry Apple		Strawberry
Hibiscus - Rose Hip		Sweet Dreams
Purely Peppermint		Take-A-Break
iced, brew 10 min		
Perfect Peach		
Raspberry Royale		
Red Raspberry		
Tahitian Breeze		
Lemonade/Limeade		
Milk		
Water		

OTHER FOODS

Low	Medium	High
Carob	*none listed*	Chocolate, plain
Gelatin, unflavored		Cocoa, dry powder

Pregnancy and Safe Seafood Guidelines

The federal government has warned pregnant women about eating fish because of mercury contamination, but its recommendations still allow eating up to 12 ounces a week of a variety of species. The federal 12-ounce-a-week advisory would allow for two servings of mixed species and federal data shows very little mercury in salmon, catfish and scallops. Fish-oil supplements are supposed to be free of mercury.

Researchers found that the more omega-3 fatty acids a woman consumed in seafood during the third trimester, the *less* likely she was to show signs of major depression at that time and for up to eight months after the birth.

In fact, the rate of depression in the women with the highest intakes was only about half that of women with the lowest intakes, says senior author and psychiatrist Dr. Joseph R. Hibbeln.

The federal government has warned pregnant women to avoid eating *shark, swordfish, king mackerel, and tilefish* because they can contain high levels of mercury, which might harm the developing nervous system of the fetus. The National Academy of Sciences (NAS) suggests that tuna be added to the FDA list of fish to avoid during pregnancy. NAS states that tuna steaks have higher levels of mercury than canned tuna. Fish in some areas pose other risks of contamination, and women should follow local recommendations about eating them.

Choices for Healthy Oceans
You Have the Power!
Your consumer choices make a difference.
Choose seafood from the Best Choices list
to support those fisheries and fish farms
that are healthier for ocean wildlife and
the environment.

BEST CHOICES	CAUTION
Abalone (farmed)	Clams (wild-caught)
Catfish (U.S. farmed)	Cod, Pacific
Caviar (farmed)	Crab, Imitation/Surimi
Clams (farmed)	Crab, King (AK)
Crab, Dungeness	Crab, Snow
Halibut (Pacific)	Lobster, American
Lobster, Rock/Spiny (CA, Australia)	Mahi-Mahi
Mussels (farmed)	Mussels (wild-caught)
Oysters (farmed)	Oysters (wild-caught)
Sablefish/Black cod (AK, BC)	Pollock
Salmon (CA, AK; wild-caught)	Sablefish/Black Cod (CA,WA,OR)
Salmon, canned	Salmon (OR, WA; wild-caught)
Sardines	Sanddabs, Pacific
Sea Bass, White	Scallops, Bay/Sea
Shrimp/Prawns (trap-caught)	Shark, Thresher (U.S. West Coast)
Squid (CA market squid)	Shrimp (U.S. farmed or wild-caught)
Striped Bass (farmed)	Sole, English/Dover/Petrale/Rex
Sturgeon (farmed)	Swordfish (U.S. West Coast)
Tilapia (farmed)	Tuna, Albacore/Bigeye/Yellowfin
Trout, Rainbow (farmed)	(longline or purse seine-caught)
Tuna, Albacore/Bigeye/Yellowfin	Tuna, canned
(troll/pole-caught)	

Legend
AK = Alaska
BC = British Columbia
CA = California
OR = Oregon
U.S. = United States
WA = Washington

Solving the Interstitial Cystitis Puzzle

How to Use This Guide

It's OK to ask questions when shopping or eating out. Ask staff where their seafood is from. Is it farmed or wild-caught? How is it caught? If they're not sure, choose something else.

This seafood guide is updated at least twice a year. Visit www.montereybayaquarium.org to obtain the latest version and learn more about seafood.

AVOID

Caviar, Beluga/Osetra/Sevruga
Chilean Sea Bass
Cod, Atlantic/Icelandic
Crab, King (imported)
Lingcod
Monkfish
Orange Roughy
Rockfish/Rock Cod/Pacific Snapper
Salmon (farmed/Atlantic)
Sharks (except U.S. West Coast Thresher)
Shrimp (imported)
Sturgeon (wild-caught)
Swordfish (Atlantic)
Tuna, Bluefin

MEAL SUGGESTIONS

"If man made it, don't eat it."

— Fitness Guru, Jack LaLanne

Meal Suggestions for the First Three to Six Months

You should have a fairly high success rate with these meal suggestions. For the first three to six months, I encourage you to choose your foods and supplements from food list *one* and *two*. For best results, consider testing for food allergies with MRT, blood testing, or pursuing an allergy elimination diet and food challenge. Some of you might need to concentrate on low oxalate foods. See the oxalate food list in the Getting Started chapter.

Breakfast

Purée green vegetable soup. Use a low salt, low fat yeast free vegetable, chicken, or beef broth; simmer vegetables such as green zucchini, green peas, and cauliflower with sea seasoning salt substitute. Purée soup. Right before serving, drizzle a small amount of organic canola oil over soup. If tolerated, sprinkle soup with pumpkin seeds as a garnish. Serve with unsalted rice cake or unsalted yeast free rice crackers and sliced avocado and/or rice cheese. Freeze leftover purée soup in individual containers for quick alkalizing breakfast.

Purée acorn squash soup. To make soup use a low salt, low fat yeast free vegetable, chicken, or beef broth with sea seasoning salt substitute, and simmer acorn squash until soft. Then purée. You might like to add a touch of plain rice milk for creamier soup. Drizzle a small amount of organic pumpkin oil over soup before serving. Serve with unsalted rice cake and rice cheese. Freeze leftover soup in individual containers for a quick filling breakfast.

Fresh green vegetable juice. Juice a fresh green vegetable juice made with several celery stalks, peeled cucumber, romaine lettuce, and one low acid red or yellow apple (no seeds). Gala or Delicious apples are usually low acid. Serve with unsalted pumpkin seeds. Add an unsalted rice cake with unsalted pumpkin butter. Add some ripe sliced avocado.

Cooked, non-gluten, whole grain or rice cereal. Serve with plain or vanilla rice milk. Before serving, add some unsweetened shredded coconut to cereal.

Avocado slices and rice cheese with rice cake. Alternatively, unsalted pumpkin butter on unsalted rice cake.

Toasted yeast free rice bread with avocado slices, rice cheese, or nut butter.

NOTE: *Pumpkin oil, pumpkin seeds, and pumpkin squash are very healing for the bladder if you tolerate pumpkin.*

Lunch

Salads are nice. Keep a variety of leafy green lettuce and vegetables ready. Use a salad spinner to remove excess water and place in a covered container with a paper towel in the bottom in the refrigerator. This way it feels like a salad is always ready to serve. Then build a salad of your choice with the following: fresh avocado, sprouts, cucumber, celery, lettuce, etc.

Vegetable sushi made with cucumber, avocado, rice, and seaweed. *Never use raw fish.*

Vegetable soups with rice cake, rice cheese, or nut butter.

You might tolerate low oxalate lentils or brown, white, or wild rice in vegetable soup. Use an unsalted low fat yeast free vegetable, chicken or beef broth with your choice of vegetables with sea seasoning salt substitute. Drizzle organic canola oil over soup just before serving. Serve soup with unsalted rice cake and rice cheese. You might need to use low oxalate vegetables if you are sensitive to oxalates at first. (See oxalate food list in the Getting Started chapter.)

Purée creamy pumpkin soup made with vegetable broth and rice milk. Drizzle soup with organic canola or pumpkin oil. Serve with rice cake.

Large tossed vegetable salad with avocado, softened seaweed strips, one to three ounces of chicken, turkey or salmon, and rice cheese. Avocado dressing: one ripe avocado mixed until creamy with olive oil. Dash of Celtic sea salt and *plenty* of sea seasoning salt substitute sprinkled over greens. Pumpkin or sesame seeds sprinkled over salad as tolerated. Rice cake.

One to three ounces of grilled chicken, turkey, salmon, or trout. Serve with green salad sprinkled with sea seasoning salt substitute and olive oil. Serve with roasted mixed vegetables and/or acorn or butternut squash.

Grilled rice cheese or plain rice cheese sandwich made with yeast free rice bread. Large green tossed salad and mixed vegetables with avocado dressing, and sea seasoning salt substitute on salad.

Dinner

One to three ounces of chicken, turkey, salmon, trout, very lean beef, or lamb. Grilled low oxalate vegetables brushed with olive oil, a dash of Celtic sea salt, and plenty of sea seasoning salt substitute; baked acorn squash. Small portion of brown/wild rice.

Pasta salad made with rice pasta, cooked chicken, chopped, mixed vegetables, and avocado with olive oil dressing. Dash of sea salt.

Beverages

Alkaline water, coconut milk, plain or vanilla rice milk, green vegetable juice, vegetable, chicken, or beef broth. Low oxalate herbal teas.

See supplements and seasonings from list *one* and low oxalate food list in Getting Started chapter.

Juicing Is Highly Recommended

When you are comfortable and are eating a nice variety of foods from list *one* and *two,* use some of your fruit and vegetable choices to start *juicing.* It is a fantastic way to incorporate extra fruits and vegetables in your diet without feeling like a "rabbit" nibbling on greens. It is especially useful for persons with irritable bowel who feel the extra fiber of fruits and vegetables is too irritating. Because no fresh fruits or vegetables have been heated there is no loss of alkalizing elements or enzymes. In addition, the natural enzymes in fruits and vegetables are anti-inflammatory. If you can drink one to two glasses of fresh green vegetable juices a day, your recovery will be hastened.

You might want to start with this combination of vegetables and fruits, and then experiment on your own. Wash the produce thoroughly and juice the following together:

- Romaine lettuce (half a bunch)
- Celery (two or three stalks including the leaves)
- Cucumber (remove the peel)
- One low acid yellow or red delicious apple (no seeds)
- You can add a carrot or small beet for sweetness if you so desire with or without the apple. Care should be taken to avoid apples, beets, and carrots if you feel you have a yeast problem. Beets and carrots are higher in oxalates.

A juicer that I used initially is the Continental CE22311 Juice Extractor, 120V, 250W Motor. This juicer is only about $30.

Its base is 9 x 6 inches and the motor is only 250 watts, but it does the trick. The best juice extractors to buy if you feel you will be juicing for many years is one with a larger more powerful motor of 500 watts or more. Consider disposable filters for easier clean-up. Juicers with a larger motor and disposable filter will cost more, however.

Currently, I use an Omega 8001 because it will juice fresh wheatgrass and barley grass as well as hard and soft fruits and vegetables. It also makes nut butters and fresh pasta (vegetable and wheatgrass pasta)! This juicer is very quiet, does not heat the juice and is versatile. It costs around $200.

Meal Suggestions for Months Six through Twelve
Breakfast

Cooked millet is satisfying as a hot cereal. Millet is an ancient non-gluten, more alkaline grain; serve with rice milk or vanilla rice milk. For each serving, bring ¼ cup millet and 1 cup ionized or alkaline water to a boil. Cover; turn to simmer for 25 minutes.

Cooked non-gluten amaranth cereal with rice milk.

A salt-free brown rice cracker with almond butter.

Fresh green vegetable juice made in a juice extractor (add a low acid yellow or red delicious apple and/or carrots for taste as tolerated). Drink juice with raw unsalted almonds, pumpkin seeds, or nuts as tolerated.

Ezekiel toast with fig jam, nut butter, and/or apple butter.

Organic corn flakes with blueberries and rice milk. Diluted apple juice.

Dates, figs, raw pumpkins seeds, almonds, cashews

Fresh apple or blueberries with ginger tea.

Fruits (fresh or dried) and nuts from lists *one* through *four* as tolerated

Fruit smoothie made with fresh fruits and frozen non-dairy rice, almond, or soy frozen dessert

Lunch

Sprouted wheat yeast-free tortilla wrap, sliced ripe avocado, shredded lettuce, sprouts, sea seasoning salt substitute, chopped vegetables, rice or alternative non-dairy cheese and one to three ounces of lean chicken or turkey. Drizzle Udo's oil, flaxseed oil, or organic canola oil over sandwich.

Soup, salad, sandwiches, vegetables, fruits, and sprouts from food lists *one* through *four*, testing carefully each new food and supplement from each list.

Dinner

Dinner entrées, soup, salad, sandwiches, vegetables, fruits, and sprouts from food lists *one* through *four*, testing carefully each new food and supplement from each list.

Suggested Beverages

Many IC patients report fruit juices and coffee might be bothersome to their IC symptoms. You may dilute juices with alkaline water. Some persons add Tamer or Prelief products to further reduce acids in juices and coffee. If you crave orange juice and coffee in the mornings, consider the reduced acid products and coffee substitutes. I suggest waiting to test these following low acid beverages and substitutes until you are comfortable on the hypoallergenic alkalizing diet, typically 3 to 6 months.

Reduced Acid Orange Juices

Minute Maid® Acid-Reduced Frozen Orange Juice Concentrate: www.minutemaid.com

Tropicana Pure Premium ® Low Acid Orange Juice: www.tropicana.com

Reduced Acid Caffeinated and Decaffeinated Coffees

The Coffee Bean & Tea Leaf®: www.coffeebean.com 1-800-TEA-LEAF

Euromild®: www.euromild.com

Puroast®: www.puroast.com 1-877-LOW-ACID.

Grain Beverages (Coffee Substitutes)

Grain beverage coffee substitutes are not always tolerated by persons with IC, so you must test carefully.

Teeccino® a caffeine-free herbal coffee that helps restore alkaline balance. One tablespoon contains 65 mg of potassium. Teeccino products come in a variety of flavors; Java, Mocha, Almond, etc. The great thing about this new product is you can brew it in your coffee maker like real ground coffee. www.teeccino.com 1-800-498-3434

Cafix®: Used primarily as a coffee substitute, Cafix is a freeze-dried grain beverage made from barley and chicory. 1-201-909-0808.

Natural Touch Roma®: Roma is a multi-grain beverage with chicory www.wfds.com

Postum®: Postum was one of the first of the grain beverage coffee substitutes.

Other Beverages

Golden Milk (See Recipe chapter.)

ALKALIZING RECIPES AND FOOD PREPARATION

Recipes by Mary Sparacino, "The Chef"

"Take the 'die' out of diet—Alkalize!"

—Unknown

Mary Sparacino and I "met" through email in 2001 and began corresponding about alkalizing and healing IC. My luck was to find a very special lady who was interested in healing heath conditions with diet as well as being a great chef! Mary's following recipes are alkalizing as well as tasty. In addition, they are *generally* well tolerated by persons with IC. Mary tried to keep the ingredients simple and the recipes not too time consuming. Many of the ingredients in these recipes such as garlic, onions, and ginger are antiparasitic and anti-inflammatory. Even though garlic, onions, and ginger are not generally tolerated in the first three to six months, as time passes, tolerance improves. Many persons at the IC Puzzle group tolerate tomatoes, lemons, and more fresh fruits after six to twelve months of alkalizing.

Hints: Do not use aluminum or Teflon-coated cookware, and try to avoid microwaves. *Never* microwave in plastic.

You may use any natural, safe sugar substitute in place of natural sugar or honey in these recipes. Wax Orchard Fruit Sweeteners are natural foods and are concentrated fruit juices that Mary and I liked in certain recipes. Wax Orchard Fruit Sweeteners taste sweeter than honey or sugar, so less is needed. With only 280 calories per 100 grams, they beat sugar's 385 calories for the same amount. For conversions, substitute 2/3 cup fruit sweetener per cup of sugar. When using Fruit Sweet, reduce the liquid in the recipe by 1/3 of the Fruit Sweet® used. Some people prefer 1/2 cup Fruit Sweet per cup of sugar.

When changing to an alkalizing diet, consider experimenting with a variety of sea vegetables in the form of flakes, granules, and seaweed. I especially like kelp and nori granules for seasoning and softened seaweed in soups and salads. Using sea vegetable granules or flakes as a salt substitute will increase potassium and trace mineral levels in your alkalizing diet. Celtic sea salt should be used sparingly as it contains inorganic sodium. Bragg Liquid Aminos is used as a salt substitute but is a soy product. So if you are allergic to soy, don't use Bragg Liquid Aminos in the recipes. Always consider your allergies and food tolerances when preparing these recipes. Some recipes or ingredients might not be appropriate for *you*. Certain foods and spices might not be tolerated by everyone, so test each recipe carefully. I have suggested a time schedule for each recipe when it *might be tolerated* in this alkalizing program. Currently, Mary and I are working on alkalizing

IC-friendly recipes and plan to publish an IC Puzzle cookbook. We hope you enjoy the recipes in this second edition.

Dressings and Alternative Mayonnaise

Simple Avocado Dressing (0 - 3 months)

1 whole ripe avocado without peel and pit
1 clove fresh garlic (or 1 tsp garlic powder)
Bragg Liquid Aminos or dash sea salt (to taste)
1 tsp olive oil
Kelp granules (to taste)

Mix together in a blender and serve. Use as salad dressing or as a vegetable dip.

Sesame Salad Dressing (0 - 3 months)

2 Tbsp Bragg Liquid Aminos
1 Tbsp sesame oil
1/2 tsp unprocessed raw sugar

Blend ingredients together. Toss with vegetable salad. This dressing would be nice for a Chinese chicken salad.

Avocado Mayo (3 - 6 months)

1 cup pine nuts (may substitute almonds or nut of your choice)
1 whole ripe avocado without peel and pit
1 Tbsp lemon juice (optional)
2 Tbsp apple cider or apple juice
1/2 tsp Celtic sea salt (optional)
6 medium pitted dates (3 Tbsp packed)
1/2 clove fresh garlic (or 1/2 tsp garlic powder)

Blend until creamy. This makes a sweet mayo for fruit salad. Can be refrigerated for approximately 2 to 3 days.

Tofu Mayonnaise (3 - 6 months)

1 lb firm tofu, drained
1 - 6 cloves fresh garlic, minced (or 1 - 6 tsp garlic powder)
6 Tbsp Bragg Liquid Aminos
4 Tbsp fresh lemon juice (optional)
2 tsp kelp granules
2 tsp curry

Combine all ingredients in a blender. More garlic and curry powder can be added to make the mayo even livelier, as tolerated.

Mock Almond Mayonnaise (3 - 6 months)

1 cup soaked almonds
1/2 cup alkaline water or vegetable broth
1 Tbsp dried onion (or 3 Tbsp chopped onion (optional)
1 clove garlic (or 1 tsp garlic powder)
1/2 fresh lemon, peeled and chopped (optional)
1 Tbsp oil of choice (olive, canola, or Udo's Oil)
1 tsp dried oregano (or 1 Tbsp fresh oregano)
1 tsp nori granules
2 tsp Bragg Liquid Aminos
Pinch each of cumin and curry

In a food processor or blender combine the almonds with water or broth and process until smooth. Add lemon, onion, garlic, oil, oregano, Bragg Liquid Aminos, and spices. Blend until smooth, using additional water if necessary to achieve the desired consistency. This can be a great dressing for salad or dip for vegetables.

Green Mayo (3 - 6 months)

1 lb tofu drained
2 ripe avocados without peel and pit
1/2 Tbsp Curry Powder
3 Tbsp lemon juice (optional)
Dash Celtic sea salt (to taste)

Blend all ingredients in a processor until mayonnaise consistency.

Nature's Delight Almond Dressing (6 - 12 months)

1/2 cup raw almonds
Juice 1/2 lemon (optional)
1/2 cup alkaline water
1 Tbsp raw honey (or natural sweetener substitute)
1/2 tsp lemon pepper (optional)
1 Tbsp chives
1/2 tsp sweet basil
1 slice fresh ginger

1/2 clove fresh garlic (or 1/2 tsp garlic powder)

Blend all ingredients at high speed for 4 minutes.

Green Goddess Avocado Dressing (6 - 12 months)

1 whole ripe avocado without peel and pit
2/3 cup of alkaline water
1 tsp fresh grated ginger (or 1/2 tsp ginger powder)
1/2 tsp cumin powder
Juice 1/2 lemon (optional)
2 tsp Veggie Magma
1 clove fresh garlic (or 1 tsp garlic powder)

Mix together in a blender and serve. It's delicious on a freshly prepared tossed green salad.

Salads

Cold Shredded Cucumber w/ Bean Sprouts (0 - 3 months)

1 cup fresh bean sprouts
1 peeled cucumber
1 small fresh carrot
Kelp granules (to taste)

Sesame Dressing

2 Tbsp Bragg Liquid Aminos
1 Tbsp sesame oil
1/2 tsp unprocessed raw sugar
Blend ingredients together.

Shred cucumber and carrot. Rinse bean sprouts in water and drain. In bowl, mix kelp granules, bean sprouts, shredded cucumber, carrot. Toss with Sesame Dressing and serve. (I add a few shreds of dried nori seaweed, which softens with the vegetables and dressing.)

Simple Wakame Salad (6 - 12 months)

1 clove fresh garlic, grated (or 1 tsp garlic powder)
1/2 tsp fresh ginger, grated (or 1/4 tsp ginger powder)
1/2 ripe avocado without peel and pit
Bragg Liquid Aminos (to taste)
3 cups greens (spinach, lettuce, sprouts, etc.)
1 cup soaked wakame seaweed (or substitute other seaweed)
Optional: Add tomatoes, walnuts, pecans, almonds, or pine nuts

Grate the ginger and garlic. In a bowl, mash the avocado, ginger, garlic and Bragg's together. Break greens and wakame up into bite size pieces. Toss all ingredients together thoroughly.

Soups

Alkalizing Soup (0 - 3 months)

To incorporate generous servings of *organic* sodium and potassium in your diet, please use this soup liberally. For those of you who find high oxalate foods troublesome, choose low oxalate vegetables for this soup. See the oxalate food list in the Getting Started chapter.

Use 1 - 2 quarts of low sodium vegetable broth. Refer to appendix C for vegetables high in potassium and organic sodium (suggested vegetables: spinach, kohlrabi, zucchini, crook neck squash, carrots, beet greens, Swiss chard, and celery). However, select high sodium/potassium vegetables *you* tolerate. Wash and chop the vegetables. Season with 1 - 2 teaspoons of sea vegetable granules (nori or kelp). Simmer all ingredients in vegetable broth until vegetables are raw crisp. Consume several cups of this soup daily in the beginning of your program. Some IC Puzzle members like to purée this soup. In addition, you can freeze leftovers in individual containers for a quick alkalizing breakfast.

Cream Style Celery Soup (3 - 6 months)

1/2 small sweet white onion (optional)
1 Tbsp oil of choice (olive, canola, butter)
1 cup milk product of your choice (plain soy milk is a good choice)
1/4 tsp cloves (optional)
1 bay leaf
1/4 tsp thyme
7 stalks celery (include leaves)
1 medium steamed, peeled potato (or 1/2 cup cooked non-gluten grain)
3 cups low sodium vegetable bouillon
Dash Celtic sea salt (optional)
1 clove fresh garlic, crushed (or 1 tsp garlic powder)

Chop onion finely. Heat oil of choice in a soup pot and add the onion. Sauté until the onion is soft. Add milk product of choice, bay leaf, cloves, garlic, and thyme and keep warm on a low flame until the rest of the ingredients are ready. Stir from time to time. This allows the liquid to take on the flavor of the spices. Cut celery into smaller pieces, and place celery and leaves into a food processor or blender and chop until fine. Add the steamed potato and continue chopping. Add the bouillon, a little a time, continuing to work the machine until a soup-like consistency is achieved. Add soup to pot and warm. Do not allow the soup to simmer. Stir frequently. Add a dash of Celtic sea salt to taste.

Cauliflower Soup (3 - 6 months)

2 Tbsp butter
2 cups finely chopped white sweet onion (optional)
4 1/2 cups cauliflower florets (about 1 head)
3 cups diced, peeled baking potato
1/2 cup finely chopped carrot
6 cups fat-free, low-salt chicken broth
1/2 tsp Celtic sea salt (optional)
1/8 tsp freshly ground black pepper (optional)

Melt butter in a Dutch oven (or large pot with lid) over medium high heat, add onion. Cook 4 minutes or until lightly browned, stirring occasionally. Add the cauliflower, potato, and carrot. Cook 6 minutes or until cauliflower begins to brown, stirring frequently. Add broth, bring to a boil. Reduce heat, simmer 20 minutes or until vegetables are crispy tender. Stir in salt and pepper. Hint: Add your favorite sea seasoning or a clove of crushed garlic for taste. For an alternative consider puréeing this soup after it is cooked.

Sprouted Pea Soup (3 - 6 months)

3 cups alkaline water
2 cups pea sprouts
1 Tbsp canola oil or light olive oil
1 small sweet onion, chopped (optional)
1 medium potato cubed
2 small carrots cubed
1 Tbsp kelp granules
1/4 tsp dulse granules
1/2 tsp nori granules

Sauté onion, carrots and potato in oil a few minutes Add water, sprouts and granules, and cook slowly for 30-40 minutes.

For those into sprouting, this soup is unique. You can also substitute 2 cups of regular cooked split peas or 1 cup of green peas instead of pea sprouts.

Stir Fry
Easy Chinese Stir Fry (0 - 3 months)

1 Tbsp light olive oil
Dry seaweed strips
4 carrots, peeled and cut into thin strips or diced
1/2 small cabbage, chopped into thin strips
1 cup bean sprouts
2 Tbsp Bragg Liquid Aminos

In a wok, or a large saucepan, heat the oil. Add the carrots and stir fry for about 2 minutes. Add the remainder of ingredients except seaweed, and stir fry for a further 3 minutes. Toss in dry seaweed strips until softened (a few seconds). Remove from the heat and serve immediately.

Stir fry any vegetable that you tolerate and prefer.

Spring Vegetable Stir-Fry (3 - 6 months)

1 Tbsp sesame oil
1 clove fresh sliced garlic (or 1 tsp garlic powder)
1 inch fresh ginger root, finely chopped
1/2 cup baby carrots
1/2 cup fresh summer squash
1/2 cup fresh green beans
1/2 cup fresh sugar snap peas
1/2 cup fresh young asparagus, cut into 3 inch pieces (optional)
(1/2 cup fresh bean sprouts can be substituted for asparagus)
8 scallions, trimmed and sliced (optional)
1/2 cup cherry tomatoes (cut in half)

Dressing
Juice of 1/2 lime (optional)
1 Tbsp raw honey (or natural sweetener substitute)
1 Tbsp Bragg Liquid Aminos
1 tsp sesame oil

Heat 1 Tbsp sesame oil in wok or large frying pan. Add garlic and ginger, stir-fry over med-high heat for 1 minute. Turn the heat to high. Add the carrots, squash, and green beans, and stir-fry 3-4 min. Add the peas, asparagus (or bean sprouts), scallions, and tomatoes for 2 more min. Add the dressing, and fry 2-3 minutes more or until just crispy tender. Serve with brown rice.

Desserts

Pumpkin Pie (3 - 6 months)

2 eggs
1/2 tsp cinnamon
1/8 tsp ginger
1/8 tsp cloves
2 cups pumpkin
1 cup *Wax Orchards Pear Sweet**
1 cup almond milk or milk of your choice
1 9" natural no preservative pie shell
Pinch of Celtic sea salt

Beat eggs, spices, and salt until well blended. Add pumpkin and stir. Pour in Wax Orchards Pear Sweet and almond milk. Stir until well blended. Pour filling into pie shell and bake at 350 degrees for 35 minutes or until a knife inserted into the center comes clean.

* Wax Orchard Fruit Sweeteners are natural foods and are concentrated fruit juices.

Rice Stuffed Apples (3 - 6 months)

2 Tbsp sweet butter
1 medium sized sweet white onion, chopped (optional)
1/2 cup uncooked rice
1 1/4 cups alkaline water
1/2 tsp ground nutmeg
1/2 tsp ground ginger (optional)
1/2 cup raisins
4 large golden apples
1/4 cup apple juice (no sugar or vitamin C added)

Preheat the over to 350 degrees. Heat the butter in a medium size skillet. Add the onion and sauté for 5 minutes. Stir in the rice, water, allspice, and ginger. Bring to a boil, reduce the heat, and cover the skillet. Simmer for 20 minutes or until the rice is tender, but not soft. Stir in the raisins. Core the apples, leaving about 1/4 inch flesh at each bottom. Scoop out approximately 1/4 flesh from the centers. Chop and add to the rice mixture. Place the cored apples in a baking dish and spoon the rice stuffing into and on top of the apples. Add the apple juice to the pan. Cut the remaining tablespoon of butter into small pieces and dot over the rice mixture. Cover the pan loosely. Bake for 45 minutes.

Golden Milk

Golden milk helps to relieve pain and inflammation all over the body. First, prepare a golden turmeric paste by combining 1/8 cup of turmeric powder with 1/4 cup of alkaline water and boil in a saucepan until a thick paste is formed. (Be careful. The paste can splatter as it heats.) This paste can be stored in the refrigerator for one week.

For each cup of golden milk, combine 1 cup of milk (milk of your choice) and 1/4 to 1/2 teaspoon of the turmeric paste. I like rice or almond milk for this drink. Stir over low heat, bring the milk just to the boiling point. Optionally, add *small* amount of honey or maple syrup to taste. Add one teaspoon of almond oil after removing golden milk from heat. If you are allergic to almonds, try canola oil instead.

If you like, this mixture can then be blended in an electric blender to make a frothy drink served with a sprinkle of nutmeg on top.

Juicing
Juicing Is Highly Recommended

It is a fantastic way to incorporate extra fruits and vegetables in your IC alkalizing diet. It is especially useful for persons with irritable bowel who feel the extra fiber of fruits and vegetables is irritating. Because no fresh fruits or vegetables have been heated, there is no loss of alkalizing elements or enzymes. In addition, the natural enzymes in fruits and vegetables are anti-inflammatory. Care should be taken to avoid fruits, carrots, and beets if you feel you have a yeast problem since these are higher in sugar. Some fruits and vegetables are higher in oxalates (beets and carrots—see low oxalate fruit and vegetable list for juicing in the Getting Started chapter). If you can drink one to two glasses of fresh green vegetable/ fruit juices a day, your recovery will be hastened.

You might want to start with the Puzzle Delight and then experiment on your own. Wash produce thoroughly and juice.

Puzzle Delight (0 - 3 months)

Romaine lettuce (half a bunch)

Celery (3 - 4 stalks including the leaves)

Cucumber (remove the peel)

1 apple (low acid yellow or red delicious with no seeds)

Add a carrot or small beet if you so desire—with or without the apple. In the very beginning, you might only tolerate the romaine, celery, and cucumber. You might not be able to tolerate the apple, carrot, or beets for this juice.

Anti-Inflammatory Juice (3 - 12 months)

1/4 inch slice of fresh ginger root
3 - 4 carrots (greens removed)
1/2 low acid apple (seeds removed)

Allergy Rescue Juice (3 - 12 months)

1/4 inch slice of fresh ginger root
1 small beet (no greens)
1 low acid apple (seeds removed)
2 carrots (greens removed)

Food Preparation for Grains, Legumes, Nuts & Seeds

"Some food preparation techniques such as soaking and sprouting beans, grains, and seeds, can hydrolyze phytate and may improve iron absorption."[1]

"Soaking legumes, sprouting grains, and roasting nuts and seeds...will increase zinc absorption..." [2]

"Phytic acid is a compound of inositol and phosphoric acid. It occurs partly as an acid and partly as salts such as calcium phytate in plant foods, especially in the bran of cereals, and in pulses and nuts.

"It readily combines with minerals including calcium, iron and zinc, and if these are present in only marginally adequate amounts in the diet, phytic acid may reduce their availability sufficiently to cause deficiency. There are, however, a few ways in which this hazard is reduced. Germination, soaking fermentation and cooking all reduce the effect of phytate..." [3]

"Soybeans are high in phytic acid, present in the bran or hulls of all seeds. It's a substance that can block the uptake of essential minerals—calcium, magnesium, copper, iron and especially zinc—in the intestinal tract.

"Although not a household word, phytic acid has been extensively studied; there are literally hundreds of articles on the effects of phytic acid in the current scientific literature. Scientists are in general agreement that grain- and legume-based diets high in phytates contribute to widespread mineral deficiencies in third world countries.

"Analysis shows that calcium, magnesium, iron and zinc are present in the plant foods eaten in these areas, but the high phytate content of soy- and grain-based diets prevents their absorption.

"The soybean has one of the highest phytate levels of any grain or legume that has been studied, and the phytates in soy are highly resistant to normal phytate-reducing techniques such as long, slow cooking. Only a long period

Solving the Interstitial Cystitis Puzzle

of fermentation will significantly reduce the phytate content of soybeans."[4]

Grain Preparation and Cooking

"Most people consume whole grains and flours in a manner that can have harmful effects on health.

"Our ancestors and peoples all over the world soaked or fermented their grains before using them in porridges, breads, pilafs and casseroles. From "ogi" porridge in Africa made from fermented millet, to Mexican "pozol" made from fermented corn, people have taken great care with whole grains. Europeans made slow-rising breads from fermented starters, and our own American Pioneers made buttermilk pancakes and biscuits by soaking flours in sour milk–a practice largely forgotten today. Many older people may recall, though, that cooking instructions on oatmeal boxes used to include an overnight soaking.

"What did our ancestors know that we have forgotten? They knew that grains treated this way were more digestible and "better for you." Modern science understands three big reasons for this.

"The first is that all grains contain phytic acid in the outer layer of the bran. Phytic acid combines with calcium, phosphorous, iron, and especially zinc in the intestinal tract and blocks their absorption. This means that a diet high in whole grains which have not been soaked, fermented or sprouted can lead to bone loss and serious mineral deficiencies.

"The second reason is that there are enzyme inhibitors in all grains, which are neutralized by the soaking process. Enzyme inhibitors literally wear down the body's digestive capabilities, leading to digestive problems ranging from chronic indigestion to irritable bowel syndrome, chronic fatigue, candida overgrowth and food allergies, among others. The people most at risk for these problems are vegetarians and vegans, who base their diets around grains and grain-products.

"The third reason applies only to grains that contain gluten, which is a kind of protein. Different grains have different amounts of gluten. Oats, barley, rye, and especially wheat all contain gluten. Rice, quinoa and millet do not (they do all contain phytates, however). Gluten can be hard to digest, and many people are allergic to it. The good news is that during the process of soaking and fermenting, lactobacilli help break down the gluten, making the grains' nutrients more available to our bodies.

"Different people have different digestive capacities, and there are plenty of people who can consume just about anything with no discomfort. Others are more sensitive and will feel heavy, bloated or in pain after consuming various foods. It often takes a while for the digestive tract to break down, so vegetarian, vegan or macrobiotic diets that work so well at first (and the benefits are well documented) may cause problems later on.

"Many of my clients have reported great results using properly prepared grains. They have more energy and less digestive discomfort, as well as a sense of satisfaction from truly nourishing themselves.

"So what if you want to make a pot of brown rice? Or you want to make quinoa pilaf, rye berry salad, or millet?

"What should you do? It's very simple:

1. Put the grains in the pot you're going to cook them in.

2. Rinse them off, then add ionized or alkaline water to the pot to cover the grains, plus a little.

3. Add a pinch of salt.

4. Add a spoon of something sour such as apple cider vinegar, lemon juice, umeboshi vinegar or whey. The acid in the sour ingredient helps to neutralize the phytic acid in the grains.

5. Soak the grain overnight if you're going to cook it in the morning, or all day if you're going to have it in the evening (7-24 hours).

6. Discard the soaking water. Now you're ready to cook the grains like you usually would.

"The grain will have a little different texture than you may be used to. It's slightly softer and more moist. I've found that most people adjust very quickly and come to prefer the taste of soaked grains.

"If you soak your grains and then change your mind and decide to go out that night or something, don't worry! Just change the water and keep soaking! You need to change this water about every 12 hours or so." [5]

Legume Preparation and Cooking
Preparation

Wash and rinse legumes thoroughly. Sort through and discard dirt and stones.

Soak legumes for 12 hours overnight in 4 parts ionized water to 1 part legume. For beginners, remembering to soak beans is simply a new habit to get into. Put beans out to soak before you go to bed at night, or when you get up in the morning

For best results, change the water once or twice. Lentils and whole dried peas require shorter soaking, while soybeans and garbanzos need to soak longer. Soaking softens skins and begins the sprouting process, which eliminates phytic acid, thereby making more minerals available. Soaking also promotes faster cooking and improves digestibility, because the gas causing enzymes and trisaccharides in legumes are released into the soak water. Be sure to discard the soak water.

For a different flavor and more nutrients, place soaked seaweed in the bottom of the pot. Add 1 part seaweed to 6 or more parts legumes. Use seaweed soak water to cook grains and vegetables.

Cooking

After bringing legumes to the boil, scoop off and discard foam. Continue to boil for 20 minutes without lid at beginning of cooking to let steam rise, which breaks up and disperses indigestible enzymes.

You can flavor beans with garlic, onion, and herbs during cooking, but you must not add salt, sugar, lemon juice, or tomato products until the beans are completely tender, since these toughen the beans.

Herbal Combinations to Consider

❧ Coriander, cumin, or ginger (lentil, mung, black, aduki)

❧ Sage, thyme, or oregano (black, pinto, lentil, kidney)

❧ Dill or basil (lentil, garbanzo, split pea)

❧ Fennel or cumin (pinto, kidney)

❧ Mint or garlic (garbanzo, lentil)

Sprouts

Despite their deceptively inconspicuous appearance sprouts are incredibly nutrient-rich, tasty, and versatile, and can be ready for harvest in just a few days! 1/2 cup of most sprouts contains more vitamin C than five glasses of orange juice! Perhaps more relevant is the fact that sprouts are powerful antioxidants that can help prevent cancer, heart disease, osteoporosis, and menopausal symptoms. Furthermore, sprouts are a good source of protein (particularly soybean and wheat sprouts) and B-complex vitamins. They are also very easy to digest. It is important to eat a variety of sprouts—not just one or two types.

If you are new to eating sprouts, don't make too much at first. Once you get the hang of it, you can start another jar three days after you start the first jar. The next jars will be ready after you finish eating the first batch.

The most important point: when you strain seeds, make sure that they are well strained. Sprouting is easy; all you need are the seeds and alkaline water. But add too much water and the seeds may rot. Nevertheless, it is difficult to make the seeds rot, as long as you follow the steps carefully.

Choose and Measure

Here are the best choices of each type of sprout source.

Best seeds: alfalfa, clover

Best beans: mung, lentil, garbanzo

Best nuts: almonds, filberts (hazelnuts)

Best grain: wheat berries

The next list indicates what amount of sprout source is appropriate.

small seeds: 2-3 tablespoons

medium seeds: 1/4-1/2 cup

large beans and grains: 1 cup

sunflower seeds: 2 cups

A large variety of seeds, beans, nuts, and grains can be sprouted. I will describe alfalfa sprouting.

Measure: Before you go to bed one night, measure the correct amount of seeds—in this case, 2-3 tablespoons of alfalfa seeds.

Any time you cook with seeds or beans, it's a good practice to inspect them. Take the portion of seeds or beans, and pour them out onto a large plate, serving dish, or baking sheet. Inspect the seeds for broken or withered seeds and small stones or lumps of dirt. After they are sorted, pour them into a strainer and give them a good rinse.

Pour the rinsed seeds into a glass mason jar. If you're sprouting large beans, grains, or nuts, use a large bowl.

Cover them with adequate alkaline water—a few inches above the level of the seeds. Let the seeds soak overnight. Medium-sized seeds should be soaked 8-12 hours, and large beans and nuts can soak for 12-24 hours.

Note: Many municipal water supplies around the world have been contaminated with chlorine and other chemicals If you soak the seeds in that water, your sprouts may absorb those pollutants and pass them on to you. Consider using filtered or spring water for sprouting.

Strain

The next morning, cover the mouth of the jar with cheesecloth, and fasten with the rubber band. Turn over the jar in the sink. The cheesecloth acts as a strainer, holding in the seeds and letting out the water. If you are using the bowl method, use the strainer to strain out the soaking water and rinse the seeds.

Note: Some people save this soaking water. It contains valuable nutrients that you can mix into a smoothie with other ingredients like fruit and yogurt. You can also water your plants with this discarded soaking water.

Shake the jar (or strainer) a few times to remove all of the water from last night's soak.

Rinse: Fill the jar with water, and again drain out the water, ending with a few hearty shakes. Hold the jar up to the light; the seeds should be mostly dry. If there's too much water left in the jar, the seeds may rot over the next few days. But if you're even slightly careful to drain the seeds, that probably won't happen.

To ensure complete drainage, some individuals store the jar upside-down in a glass baking dish. Rest the jar on the side of the dish, or up against the wall—any excess water drains out, without any more attention from you.

Repeat

On the evening of the same day, you'll repeat the rinsing process. You'll continue this morning and evening rinsing for 4 or 5 days (in warm climates, figure a day or two less than that). If you're feeling particularly keen on sprouting, you can rinse it a third time at noon.

Watch for the growth: you'll see green leaves sprouting on seeds, and white shoots on beans, nuts, and grains.

Harvest

After four or five days, the sprouts will reach their peak of flavor and nutritional value. Give them a final rinse; drain with a hearty shake. Now they're ready to be prepared and eaten.

Your biggest problem with sprouting is choosing among these serving alternatives:

Add to salads, sandwiches, and as a garnish on soups.

Puree seed and bean sprouts to make a sandwich spread or vegetable dip. For flavors, try adding tahini, lemon, and garlic for a middle Eastern flair; or fresh tomato and basil for a Mediterranean touch. (Garlic, lemon, tomato need to be tested carefully and probably only after three months of the hypoallergenic and alkalizing diet.)

Cook bean sprouts: lightly stir-fry them with other vegetables, or add to other recipes like vegetable burgers. Also they are very good when steamed with shredded carrot and cabbage.

Sprouted grains are a bit trickier to use. They're often ground up and baked at low temperatures (220° F) to make bread or added to recipes like vegetable burgers and casseroles.

AYURVEDA

by Dawn R. Mahowald and Dr. Emmey Ripoll, MD

"The guiding principle of Ayurveda is that the mind experts the deepest influence on the body, and freedom from sickness depends on contacting our own awareness..."

—Dr. Deepak Chopra

What Is Ayurveda?

Ayurveda is a 5,000 year old medical system from India. It is interested in both the prevention of disease as well as curing it. In some ways it is very similar in practice to western medicine. In some ways it is *very* different.

If an Ayurvedic doctor from ancient India and a modern day western doctor were to meet, they could easily discuss and agree upon many things. Both would know about and understand various details of coronary heart disease and its progression, inherited genetic weaknesses in families, and the long-term effect of protein in the bloodstream on the kidneys of a person with diabetes. Both would also understand the concept of prescribing medications (or herbs) to people who were already sick. Both might recommend dietary changes to a patient to help with a certain condition.

However, since Ayurveda is by and large non-technical, the Ayurvedic doctor would never have held a hypodermic syringe or seen an x-ray machine. And, the western doctor would not understand how their Ayurvedic counterpart could tell so much about a patient just from taking their pulse, or why they put so much emphasis on lifestyle choices.

Being reasonable people however, they would both soon recognize that despite their differences in training and skills, their goals of helping people to heal are the same. They would also conclude that they each served important, but different and necessary positions in the world of medicine.

Basics of Ayurveda

Ayurveda is about balance. According to Ayurveda, even human beings have their own individual balance. When a person gets out of balance, their body will try to restore the natural balance through a minor illness. If the body cannot restore the balance, the person will eventually become seriously sick. When the person becomes seriously sick, the Ayurvedic practitioner will work to help restore the person's innate balance and in so doing, also restore their health.

Although this basic concept of balance is very simple, Ayurveda is a complex, deep, powerful, and very detailed medical system. Fortunately, you don't have to understand it to use this guide. It is, however, helpful to get a brief overview to start. If you find you are interested in going deeper into the theory and science of Ayurveda we have included the names of three books others have found helpful at the end of this section for you to explore.

Ayurveda & the Universe

At its very core Ayurveda looks at the universe in different way from modern, western science. The ancient thinkers—or *rishis*—of India who developed Ayurveda looked at the universe in a way more similar to that of the ancient Greek philosophers.

Elements & Forces

The rishis saw the universe as a system containing five elements and three forces. The five elements are *ether, air, fire, water,* and *earth.* The three forces (also called *doshas)* are *vata, pitta,* and *kapha.*

According to the rishis the three doshas move the elements around and combine them in different ways to form all the individual pieces of the universe. Everything from the tiniest sub-atomic particle to the most complicated life-form is made up of the five elements moved into place and combined by the three doshas, even human beings.

Doshas & the Human Body

The three doshas, vata, pitta, and kapha, each have different qualities and affect the elements in different ways.

Vata is dry, light, cold, irregular, mobile, rough, quick, and subtle.

Pitta is hot, oily, light, fluid, intense, liquid, and sour-smelling.

Kapha is heavy, stable, oily, dense, smooth, sticky, dull, slow, soft, sweet, and cold.

Because of the qualities of each of the doshas, they are associated with specific organs and process in your body.

Vata is associated with your brain, nervous system, heart, colon, bones, lungs, urinary bladder, and bone marrow.

Pitta is associated with your skin, small intestine, eyes, spleen, endocrine system, liver, brain, and blood.

Kapha is associated with your brain, joints, pericardium (the protective tissue around the heart), pleurium (the protective tissue around the lungs), mucous linings of the organs and sinuses, lymph system, mouth, and stomach.

You are born with a balance of doshas in your body and during the course of your life more of each of the doshas enters your body through the food you eat and from other parts of your environment. Your body uses them up as it needs them throughout the day. If the doshas are not used up they will begin to accumulate and affect your body in unhealthy ways. Eventually you will get sick.

People

Because of its emphasis on elements and forces, Ayurveda looks at people somewhat differently than the way western medicine looks at them. A western doctor is interested in a few of your physical characteristics (height, weight, etc.), your symptoms, medical history, and a little bit about your lifestyle. A practitioner of Ayurveda will not only be interested in those things but, also how the doshas are working in your body.

How Ayurveda Looks at People

When you go to a practitioner of Ayurveda they will examine your hair, your skin, your mouth, eyes, face, and tongue, your hands and finger nails, and your build. They will ask you about your symptoms and then ask about your sleeping and eating patterns and habits, your emotional life, your work situation, exercise habits, bowel as well as urinary habits, if you gain weight easily or not, and many other things about you and your body. Many of them will take your pulse for several minutes and maybe at a couple of different places on your body.

The doctor will also be very interested in how any of these things have changed over time. The progression of any disorders, from the first symptoms to their current stage of development will also be of great interest to them.

All of this information will help the doctor determine the balance of the doshas in your body (also called "your individual body-type") and what type of treatment is appropriate for you.

Your Body-Type

Western medicine typically pays little attention to body-type. In Ayurveda, body-type is a critical component of diagnosis and treatment. Ayurveda defines the body terms of the three doshas and has characterized seven basic body-types. They are: Vata, Pitta, Kapha, Vata-Pitta, Vata-Kapha, Pitta-Kapha and Sama (all three equally).

Each body-type expresses the characteristics of the dosha or doshas it is named after. Without going in to too much detail the various body-types have the following characteristics:

Vata Body-Type – very tall, or very short, thin to underweight, joints large or very noticeable, uncoordinated movements, irregular and uneven features, hair is dark, dry, and dull, skin is dry, dark, and rough with more moles than average, eyes are dark and narrow or protruding, mind is quick and eager, but memory is poor, sleep is light with chaotic dreams and wakes easily, constipates easily and is subject to nervous disorders, emotionally perceptive, but sensitive and easily hurt, sensitive to pain, loves heat and sun.

Pitta Body-Type – medium frame with good muscle tone, athletic, rarely overweight or underweight, regular, even features, hair is oily with light to dark blond or black with reddish highlights, skin is ruddy or reddish and subject to freckles, eyes are blue, green or light brown, mind is sharp and retentive, sleep is moderate with intense or violent dreams, prone to anger and has a quick temper, good health but subject to ulcers and other stomach problems, personality is competitive and driven to success and loves cool, green, wet environments.

Kapha Body-Type – lush to heavy or overweight body on a large, solid frame, with graceful movements, even round features, hair is lustrous, wavy, and thick, skin is soft and oily, eyes are round and dark, the mind is slow, steady and once information is learned it is rarely forgotten, sleep is deep with beautiful dreams, excellent health, personality is calm, collected and loving, loves warmth and sun.

The other four body-types are mixtures, in varying degrees, of Vata, Pita, and Kapha body-types.

Changes in Body Type
Everyone is born with a specific body-type. It does not change during their lifetime. However, stress, damaging lifestyle choices, toxins and other things can change the appearance and responses of the body. If the changes are large enough, a person becomes ill. To get well again, people must make the right changes in their lifestyle to bring their body back into balance.

Environment
A western medical doctor rarely puts too much consideration into evaluating your environment when diagnosing you. The only exceptions would be if you had been exposed to an extreme or highly toxic environment or if you were in a highly stressful environment for a long period of time. A practitioner of Ayurveda, on the other hand, is *very* interested in your environment and how it affects you.

How Ayurveda Looks at Your Environment
In Ayurveda no one is separate from their environment. Everything you hear, see, smell, taste, touch, absorb, and eat contains the three forces and affects you and your health, for better or for worse. Everything you do, how you do it, and even when you do it also has an effect on your body-type and its balance. Time of day, the seasons, and even the weather can also have an effect. And, on top of all that, the effect of each of the three forces (vata, pitta, and kapha) in all of these things is different for each of the seven body-types.

Because your environment is such a powerful force on your body and health, Ayurveda not only looks at it as one potential cause of disease, it also looks at environment as a potential cure.

Healing & Ayurveda
How Ayurveda Helps You Heal
Because a practitioner Ayurveda works with both your body-type and your environment, they have a very large number of alternatives to offer

their patients in their journey towards restored health. They also have different tools for each stage of a disease from the first symptoms to its more serious stages. When you go to an Ayurvedic practitioner for a consultation you may be offered solutions similar to those from a western medical doctor including dietary recommendations and medicines (herbs in the case of Ayurveda). You may also get recommendations of aromatherapy, essential oil application, music therapy, cleanses, changes to your immediate environment, yoga, meditation, visualizations, color therapy, and others.

What are the Limits of Healing in Ayurveda?

In the proper hands, with a good practitioner and a patient who is willing to work with it, Ayurveda is a powerful, effective tool for healing. However, like all forms of medicine, it does have limits.

If you are in need of Emergency Medicine, broken bones, severe trauma, etc., Ayurveda is not the answer, the hospital emergency room is. After the emergency or trauma has been addressed Ayurveda can offer ideas on making you more comfortable and herbal nutritional supplements to help your body heal.

In the United States, Ayurveda also defers completely to western medicine in the cases of cancer, terminal illnesses, and treatment of other very serious diseases. If you have a serious, life threatening disorder and want to use supplemental Ayurvedic nutritional herbs or any other Ayurvedic techniques, seek a practitioner who is also trained in western medicine. They often have a deeper understanding of herb/drug interactions and will be better able to help you find herbs and techniques that will work for you.

Ayurveda also depends on you to help heal yourself. Much of Ayurveda is concerned with individual lifestyle choices. Typically, people who are willing to make more choices that support their body-type will have the most success with Ayurveda.

Ayurveda & Interstitial Cystitis

Both IC and Urethral Syndrome have been recognized as legitimate disorders by Ayurveda for over 5,000 years. Ayurveda lists the same symptoms for these disorders as western medicine. However, Ayurveda has defined specific causes for them as well as specific solutions to help cure or control them.

What is Interstitial Cystitis?

In Ayurveda, both IC and Urethral Syndrome are part of a continuum of a vata based bladder disorders. The classic explanation of the disorder is:

1. The patient has a genetic weakness in the bladder and/or urethra or the urinary system has been damaged in some way.

2. The patient has accumulated excess vata and pitta as a result of poor lifestyle choices. Because the bladder is weaker than other parts of the body, vata is able to move the excess pitta into the bladder and or

urethra where it attacks the mucous producing cells and nerve cells of the bladder.

3. Pitta causes pain and creates more vata. The excess vata moves more and more pitta into the bladder and the disorder becomes self-perpetuating.

4. When pitta has caused enough damage, kapha becomes provoked, and the ability of the bladder to heal itself is compromised.

Pulse Diagnosis

When a person has IC an Ayurvedic pulse diagnosis will show both kapha and pitta spikes in the bladder pulse.[1]

Who Gets It?

IC and Urethral Syndrome most often occur in people with vata-pitta body-types. People with vata and pitta body-types can get it occasionally and people with the other body-types get it only in very rare circumstances. Women are more susceptible than men.

How is it Treated & Can it be Cured?

Ayurveda has many treatments available for IC. The effectiveness of the treatments depends on how advanced the disease is and how long it has been left untreated. Effectiveness is also dependent on how willing the patient is to begin making lifestyle choices more appropriate to their body-type.

The treatments prescribed can include aromatherapy, carefully organized dietary plans, herbs (taken orally), environmental and lifestyle changes, various types of massages with specific medicinal oils, enemas, carefully selected yoga exercises, cleanses, stress reducing programs, and other treatments.

Other Disorders

There is a very clear link in Ayurveda between IC and muscle and joint pain, migraines, allergic reactions, and gastrointestinal problems. If left untreated, Ayurveda believes that IC patients are at risk of developing certain other chronic diseases and pain syndromes such as vulvar vestibulitis, fibromyalgia, endometriosis, irritable bowel syndrome, and others.

Resources

If you are interested in learning more about the specifics of Ayurveda we recommend the three books listed in this section. All three can easily be ordered by your local bookstore or through one of the on-line book sellers.

Perfect Health, by Dr. Deepak Chopra, MD, ISBN 0-51-58421-2. This is an excellent book for someone who is new to Ayurveda. It is written in a clear, simple style and covers the basics of Ayurveda theory and treatment very well.

Ayurveda A Life of Balance, by Maya Tiwari, ISBN 0-89281-490-X. This book gets into more depth both with regard to Ayurveda theory and covers the subject of Ayurveda, food, and nutrition. It contains in-depth discussions on foods for the various body-types and has many wonderful recipes for each.

Prakruti Your Ayurvedic Constitution, by Dr. Robert E. Svoboda, ISBN 0-945669-00-3. This book is very good for the more serious student of Ayurveda. It delves deeper into the theory of Ayurveda than the previous two and even discusses some the medicinal Ayurvedic herbs.

ACUPUNCTURE & ACUPRESSURE

by Dawn R. Mahowald and Dr. Emmey Ripoll, MD

"There are three categories of drugs; the lowest one of which is poison, the second one is a little poisonous, the highest one is no poison. The lowest drug cures six out of ten sicknesses, leaving poisons in the patient. The middle one cures seven out of ten sicknesses, leaving a small amount of poison. Even the highest medicine can only cure eight or nine out of ten sicknesses. The sicknesses that medicine cannot cure can be cured only by foods."

— The Nei Ching

What are Acupuncture & Acupressure?

Acupuncture and acupressure originated in China over 5,000 years ago and are key elements of traditional Oriental medical practice. The theory behind acupuncture and acupressure is that the human body has "Meridians" or pathways through which energy or "chi" travels. Chi is believed to be a key component of the body and necessary for life and health. If the flow of chi is interrupted or even slowed in the meridians, ill health (mental, physical, or emotional) can result. The meridians have certain points along their path where the chi can be manipulated to flow faster, slower, or more effectively; these are the acupuncture or acupressure points.

Types

Several different schools of acupuncture have been found to be useful. These include Traditional Chinese, Meridian or Japanese, Five Element, Korean Hand, Auricular (performed on the ear), Medical, and Scalp Acupuncture.

Meridians

The human body has over 20 interconnected meridians. Some meridians travel just beneath the skin; others are located much deeper in the body. Some of the meridians are named after a major body function, e.g. the Great Regulator Meridian or organ, e.g. the Bladder Meridian.

Points

Over 350 points are distributed among the various meridians. Some of the points on the meridians are associated with diseases related to that function or organ. For example, many points on the Bladder Meridian are used to treat bladder disorders. However, not all points are limited to treating that organ. Some points can be used to harmonize and regulate body functions, while others are associated with diseases or disorders involving other parts of the body.

Tools for Treatment

The most common tools for administering acupuncture are very thin needles. Because the needles are so thin, patients usually report they feel no pain when the needles are inserted. Some patients say they feel a slight tingling or sometimes heat or cold sensations when the needles are inserted. Rarely are any of these sensations unpleasant.

The needles can be any length from less than ¼" to over 2"; the shorter needles are often used in places like the ears, while the medium and longer are used in the limbs and trunk of the body. The needles often have handles on one end to make it easier for the doctor to hold. They can be made of different metals, including gold, silver, and stainless steel. The different types of metals are used to treat different types of diseases. If you have an allergy to any particular metal, it is important to let the doctor know ahead of time, so an alternate type of needle can be selected.

Individual needles are not the only tools used in acupuncture treatments. Other traditional methods involve finger pressure or massage on the individual points, as well as applying suction or heat to the points (also called "cupping" and "moxa"). Patients can also be taught many different physical exercises to stimulate both meridians and individual points; these are called "Meridian Exercises." Hatha Yoga exercises may also be prescribed.

More recent innovations in the acupuncture field include using needles attached to electrodes and using very low-power cold lasers. When electricity is used, the doctor attaches an electrical source to two or more of the needles and sends a very small electrical charge through them while they are in the body. A slight "tingling" sensation is often associated with this type of treatment, but it is not unpleasant or painful. The lasers are use to stimulate a specific point.

Tips for People with Frequency, Urgency, Bladder Pain or Pelvic Pain

A typical acupuncture treatment session lasts from 30 minutes to one hour. During much of this time, you are lying down on your back or stomach with all or some of your clothes off and with acupuncture needles in your body. It may be difficult or even painful to move around. For people with frequency or urgency problems, it may be difficult, if not impossible, to go to the bathroom. For those with pelvic or bladder pain, lying flat on your stomach may become uncomfortable.

To help with frequency and/or urgency issues, try going to the bathroom immediately before the needles are inserted. You may also want to bring an adult diaper or request an absorbent pad. You can use them only if you need to and the doctor and medical staff will certainly understand.

To help with bladder and pelvic pain, request that the doctor use pillows or folded blankets to help keep the weight off your bladder. Also, ask that someone come in halfway through your treatment time and help you adjust your position on the table to make you more comfortable. Some doctors even have intra-office pagers or buzzers you can use to call one of the staff members to help you. Again, the medical staff knows what you are up against and should be very willing to help. If the doctor or medical staff is not willing to help you with these adjustments, get another doctor.

An opinion from Dr. Ripoll, MD, CYI, Board Certified in Urology and Holistic Medicine, Medical Acupuncturist on Acupuncture for Cystitis and IC

"After several years of experience of using Acupuncture on people with Chronic Cystitis and IC, my opinion is that it can be very effective. The degree of effectiveness, however, does depend on the individual and how long they work with it. People who try Acupuncture for several treatments (10-12) usually have more success than people who try it only once or twice. Some people are helped a lot; they experience a large reduction in both pain and symptoms. Some even appear to be in remission. Others have experienced moderate success in pain reduction or symptom control. Still others feel they do not get relief for either.

"Before you let this dampen your enthusiasm for trying Acupuncture, remember that the situation in Western Medicine is not significantly different. For example, in the case of Chronic Infectious Cystitis, many people respond to antibiotics and they respond in varying degrees. Unfortunately, some people do not respond at all or they cannot tolerate the antibiotics long enough to get rid of the infection. In the case of IC, the situation is similar; some respond to available treatments, some do not. In the case of long-term control of chronic pain resulting from these incurable forms of Cystitis, most drug treatment programs become ineffective after a time or include serious drug dependence issues.

"Another important point for people with IC to remember is to very carefully explain to your acupuncturist that IC is *not* an infectious cystitis. Even though IC is now widely accepted by urologists and other western medical practitioners, it is a relatively rare disorder. Many excellent and experienced Acupuncturists have never heard of it. For your first visit to an acupuncturist it may be helpful to take along a list of reference materials so the acupuncturist can get up to speed quickly. Or you could mail your list or drop it off ahead of time. Armed with good information they will be more able to help you."

YOGA

by Dawn R. Mahowald and Dr. Emmey Ripoll, MD

"There is no disease that yoga cannot heal."

—Amma Karunamayi

What is Hatha Yoga?

Hatha Yoga (often referred to as "yoga") is a 7,000-year-old fitness science developed in India. Hatha Yoga is a complete fitness art and is often used as a medical tool to prevent illness, aid healing, induce relaxation, and reduce stress and its effects. Students of it gain physical strength, muscle tone, flexibility, stamina and endurance, plus relaxation and inner calm.

Yoga aims for balance in the mind, body and spirit. The word yoga is Sanskrit for union or joining (like our word "yoke"). The word ha means sun; tha means moon. Thus Hatha Yoga joins and balances different emotional, mental and physical elements in a human being as symbolized by the sun and moon

There's nothing magical, mystical, or religious about Hatha Yoga. You don't have to believe a thing to experience its benefits. All you have to do is use your mind, body, and breathing to bring you into a state of balance and peacefulness coupled with physical strength and vitality.

The exercises in Hatha Yoga are called asanas—sometimes they are called poses, or postures. There are about 84 basic poses and over 800,000 variations and combinations. Asanas are believed by the people who have worked with them to affect the muscles, nerves, and glands in the body; bathing them with fresh blood, massaging them, stretching them, and toning them.

Hatha Yoga differs from other exercise systems in these ways:

♦ It's noncompetitive.

♦ It's non-judging. You observe yourself in asanas, without criticism.

♦ It's nonviolent. You never bounce, force, or allow pain.

♦ It's mentally stimulating and fascinating as you explore stretching and your mind-body response to it.

♦ It's fun.

♦ You can start it at any age.

♦ You can practice it for the rest of your life.

The essence of doing Hatha Yoga is for you to be aware of how your body feels and responds as you are doing the asana. The degree of physical flexibility achieved doesn't determine your success in yoga, nor does the number of times you do an exercise or how long you hold a pose. Success is measured by your inward attention to the body and mind in the poses. Only by not straining or forcing does true progress in physical flexibility and strength come.

Not straining or forcing is good advice for anyone who wants to do Hatha Yoga, but it is especially good advice for people who have interstitial cystitis (IC), or urethral syndrome. Many of us who have dealt with these disorders know that jumping into a new type of exercise program and pursuing it vigorously at the start can bring on an attack of the disorder. We may exercise strenuously and enthusiastically one day only to wake up the next day in severe pain. The best way, with any new program, including yoga, is to start gently and build up gradually, take it easy. In addition, never exercise beyond your means.

Hatha Yoga works by using the static stretch. This means that you enter a pose with a slow, steady motion and then you hold it for as long as you are comfortable and breathing comfortably. This doesn't mean you can be lazy. You learn to "play your edge" between comfort and discomfort, always reaching as far as you can within our own comfort zone and *never* allowing pain. Always, you are responsible for deciding how much you can or should do in yoga.

Hatha Yoga has recently come to the attention of western medical practitioners because of the vast array and range of exercises and its ability to help reduce feelings and effects of stress. It also appears to be very helpful for people with IC and urethral syndrome. Hatha Yoga can help you to learn how to relax tense muscles, both pelvic floor and other muscles. Feelings of stress, which often accompany chronic disorders, can greatly be reduced with regular Hatha Yoga practice. Muscles can be toned and strengthened without sweating, bouncing, or running[1]. Hatha Yoga also helps to cleanse the body of accumulated toxins. As you gently stretch and move tense muscles, blood circulation in those muscles increases and slowly, but surely toxins are washed away.

What Can You Expect from Hatha Yoga?

An opinion from Dr. Ripoll, MD, CYI, Board Certified in Urology and Holistic Medicine, and Medical Acupuncturist and Dawn R. Mahowald, MIM, CYI

During the more than five years we have been teaching yoga to people with cystitis and IC, we have had a number of common questions come up and some interesting responses to the exercises from our students. We would like to share them with you. Before we do, we would like to caution you that this information is a combination of our opinions and observations as a doctor and as yoga teachers as well as feedback in the form of questionnaires from our yoga students. It is not based on formal, long-term, double blind studies backed up by secondary and tertiary research and therefore cannot yet be considered scientific or medical fact.

Solving the Interstitial Cystitis Puzzle

The first and most common question we get is "Will yoga help cure cystitis or IC"? The answer from both of us and from our students is no, yoga will likely *not* cure either. However, over 90% of the students who answered said that yoga was helpful in reducing their symptoms, including: pelvic and abdominal pain, burning, pelvic floor spasticity, frequency, urgency, difficulty starting the flow of urine, and feelings of physical exhaustion and mental or emotional stress. Many felt they could sleep better when they did yoga.

The degree to which students thought yoga helped, varied from "some what" to "very much". And, when looking at specific symptoms, the students felt they were helped more in certain areas than in others. For example, some had a large reduction in frequency, but only a moderate decrease in urgency, and so on.

So, the second part of our answer to the question is that even if it won't cure cystitis and IC, it might help you work with and/or control some or all of your symptoms.

Another question we get is, "If yoga is going to help me, how quickly will I see results"? The answer seems to be, "It depends." A few students reported they saw some results after only a week's worth of practice. Most students, however, said that over a period of several weeks, they noticed a slow, gradual improvement or a "hills and valleys" pattern of improvement. Some days are better, some worse, but the general trend was towards better.

Some Tips on Starting a Hatha Yoga Program

Is Hatha Yoga for You?
As with all other new exercise programs, check with your physician or other personal health care provider who is familiar with your situation before beginning a Hatha Yoga program. Most people with light to moderately severe cases of IC or urethral syndrome can handle a gentle yoga program. For people with very severe to extremely severe symptoms, private lessons with a certified yoga instructor or one with several years experience teaching would be better. They can help you adapt this material to your specific needs.

What to Wear
Most Hatha Yoga books suggest that people doing yoga exercises wear leotards and tights. Because people with IC and urethral syndrome often find tight clothing uncomfortable and since women wearing tight clothing are more prone to bladder infections, it is better to wear loose comfortable clothing. You might want to try loose knit pants or sweat pants and a t-shirt. Also, women may even want to consider wearing cotton or no underwear as they exercise. *Bare feet* are essential for good traction on the floor, but you can always wear socks when you are not doing the standing exercises if your feet get cold.

Equipment to Have On Hand

Have 2 thick blankets available. Cotton thermal blankets are best. Wool blankets are a good second choice. Be certain to avoid slick, shiny, or satin finish blankets or bedspreads. These can cause you to slip and hurt yourself.

The extra padding blankets can provide can be especially important for people who also have fibromyalgia. Doing the exercises on the floor or the carpet without that extra padding can cause extreme pain either while you're doing exercises or the next day. Occasionally, an exercise will use a strap. Any strong, long belt, rope or even old necktie will suffice for most people.

If you really like yoga and have some money to spend there are all kinds of equipment, bolsters, pillows, sticky mats, straps, blocks, cushions, and wooden and metal contraptions. You don't need them. Get them only if you want to try something a little different. You can find out about them and where to get them from ads in the bi-monthly yoga magazines available at most well stocked newsstands.

Keeping your Energy Up

Like most forms of exercise, eating a heavy meal before doing yoga can cause you indigestion or nausea. Eat a light snack if you want before you start your exercise session, but don't eat a heavy meal for at least two to three hours before your session. Also, if you need a small snack after you exercise, have it. But, wait an hour or so after you finish exercising to eat a large meal.

Where to Do your Yoga

If you have an exercise room in your house, you can do your yoga there. If you have an extra room or large, airy space, you can do it there. In truth, however, most of us live in a limited space; a small apartment, a house with three kids, a dog, a spouse, and a home office, or we live in a condo with a roommate. Don't worry, you can do your yoga anywhere you have the space to do it. With this set of exercises you need a space no larger than 3' x 6', at most. Even the space between your bed and the wall will often be enough. You may have to roll over carefully or turn around often, but you can still get your yoga done. You may want to keep any blankets you use tucked away in the spot where you do your yoga. Never mind the mess. If the blankets are readily available, you'll be more likely to exercise.

How Much? How Often? And When?

It would be nice if you could do your yoga three to six days a week, for 30-60 minutes a session, and at the same time everyday. However, most of us not only have limited space, we have limited time and varying schedules. The recommendation of three to six times a week, for 30-60 minutes a session, and at the same time, everyday is the ideal, but not a requirement. Do what you can, when you can, as often as you can (but, no more than six times a week). Give it a sincere effort and concentrate on enjoying the process.

People often want to know what time of day is best. What ever fits into your schedule is best. You will probably notice that when you do yoga in the morning you will have more energy and less flexibility. When you do it in the evening you will have more flexibility and less energy. If you remember that and pace yourself accordingly, any time of day should be fine.

One note, if you do yoga late in the evening, you should go to bed right away. Usually people feel very relaxed for 15-30 minutes after they have done yoga and later feel very energetic. If you wait too long to go to bed, you may find yourself staring at the ceiling in the dark for longer than usual. On the other hand, some students with frequency issues report that they get up fewer times per night if they do their yoga just before they go to bed.

Some Extra Tips

♦ Some of the exercises in a class may be too difficult for you. That's okay. Skip them and rest until the other students are done.

♦ Some exercises may seem too easy for you. That's okay too. You might want to try them anyway. Sometimes the simplest exercises can provide the most dramatic relief.

♦ A whole class may be too much at first for someone with IC or urethral syndrome. Stop when you are tired.

♦ Don't try to work up a sweat. Keep your movements slow and gentle, and rest when you need to.

♦ Women should not do inversions (exercises where the hips are higher than the head) during their menstrual period.

♦ Do the breathing exercises! They can be very helpful in dealing with stress and can give you a temporary focus away from pain.

♦ Remember to *always* rest for a few minutes at the beginning and end of each session. A little rest can do wonders for the mind and body.

Yoga Poses to Avoid

There are some poses and types of Hatha Yoga a person with IC or urethral syndrome should avoid, either because they may irritate the bladder or because they stimulate the meridians incorrectly for a person with these disorders. However, if you are in remission the poses are fine. These include:

♦ Headstand and Headstand variations, which put the entire weight of the body on the top of the head or require the tightening of the pelvic floor muscles.

♦ Full Shoulder Stand and variations which cause tightening of the pelvic floor muscles.

♦ Breathing exercises where the stomach muscles are forcefully pulled in (i.e., Kapalbhati and Bhastrika).

♦ Breathing Exercises done lying on back with weights on the abdomen.

♦ Nauli or Stomach Churning.

- Lower body muscular contractions, locks, or bhandhas (i.e., Uddiyana, Asphenia, and Moola) if they cause pain.

- Standing or Sitting Forward Bends that put pressure on the abdomen or parts of the abdomen (i.e., Forward Bends with legs or one leg in the lotus position, etc.).

- Twists that put pressure on the abdomen.

- Triangle Poses (some people find these helpful; try to see).

- Yoga done in very warm or hot rooms.

- Intense Ashtanga or Aerobic Yoga (if you like moving yoga, try a more gentle Vinyasa style Yoga).

- Water Yoga (if chlorine irritates your bladder).

- *Any pose* which makes your symptoms worse.

Finding a Yoga Teacher & Classes

Yoga has become very popular lately, teachers abound, and classes are offered almost everywhere. The real key is finding a class and a teacher that work for you.

Getting Started

Places to start looking for both teachers and classes can include: the yellow pages of your phone book under yoga, local health clubs, universities, colleges, continuing education centers, recreation centers, hospitals, doctor's offices, HMO's, bulletin boards at work, at church, or in health food stores, newspaper ads, the Internet, yoga magazines, professional yoga teachers associations (Yoga Teachers of Colorado, California Yoga Teachers Association, etc.), and any other places you can think of. You can also ask friends, health care providers, or local physical education teachers.

Questions to Ask a Teacher

Remember, as in other professions, there are many types of yoga teachers: specialists, generalists, those with many years of experience, new ones, some with a religious approach, and some with a secular approach. So, set your preferences and questions up beforehand and don't feel discouraged if you don't find a match right away.

Once you find a teacher, try to contact them by phone or go to their class and arrange a time to talk with them later. When you get a chance to talk with them here are some questions you can ask them.

- What kind of classes do they teach, beginning or more difficult, gentle or more strenuous? Beginning and very gentle classes are usually better to start with.

- What is their background in yoga? Do they have training? How long have they been teaching? For people with chronic disorders, it is usually better to pick a teacher who has over 5 years or more of direct teaching experience and some form of training. There are even some teachers trained specifically in yoga therapy.

♦ Do they know what your needs are, or since many forms of chronic cystitis are not very well known, are they willing to learn what your needs are? Some teachers may not be able to accommodate you. They may have contractual obligations to the organization they work with, or the needs of the other students they teach may conflict with your needs.

♦ How large are their classes or do they teach privately? Smaller classes, 10 or less, are usually better for people with chronic disorders. You may also want to consider a couple of private classes to get you started, and then later join a group class.

♦ Are they willing to give references or can you talk to some of their students?

Most teachers will gladly talk with you and, if they are not the right person, will give you leads to other teachers. Again, don't feel discouraged if you don't find what you want on the first try. Take your time, find a teacher, and class that works for you. It will pay off in the end.

Dr. Emmey Ripoll, MD

Dr. Emmey Ripoll, MD is board certified in Urology and Holistic Medicine. She has been practicing Medical Acupuncture for 8 years and is certified in Structural Yoga. She also works with Osteopathic manipulation and rehabilitation and has authored over 25 scientific publications. She practices Urology with the Fergus Falls Medical Group in Fergus Falls, MN.

Dawn R. Mahowald

Dawn R. Mahowald, CYI, certified in Structural Yoga, has been working with yoga for over 40 years. She has co-authored two books and also incorporates Ayurveda into her practice. Dawn currently practices and teaches privately in Boulder, Colorado.

See the Resources appendix D for more information about *Cystitis A Time to Heal with Yoga & Acupressure—An Eight Week Course with Special Information for People with Interstitial Cystitis & Urethral Syndrome.*

Solving the Interstitial Cystitis Puzzle

PELVIC FLOOR THERAPY: AN ANECDOTE OF ONE

by Wm. Zeckhausen, D. Min.
Pastoral Psychotherapist, Laconia, NH

For 3 years I have struggled with IC. I have been helped by Amrit's program, but as she often says, we are all different, respond to similar as well as different things, and need to continue learning from each other. Though her research and testing has led to a remission of her own symptoms, her commitment and compassion to helping other IC patients has her responding individually to many of us, as well as exploring new hopeful treatment possibilities in figuring out and overcoming the suffering produced by IC. In that spirit, she has invited me to share my recent experience of pelvic floor treatment with Dr. Jerome Weiss and his team based in San Francisco.

A physician friend in California, Jeff Kane, author of *The Healing Companion*, sent me an article by Dr. Jerome Weiss on pelvic floor muscles and myofascial release techniques. Dr. Kane had met a member of Dr. Weiss's team, Janice Gigliuto at a conference, and learned from her about their success in treating IC patients with these techniques. Although it can typically take several months of weekly treatment for major progress, I learned from calling the Pacific Center for Pelvic Pain and Dysfunction in San Francisco that it should prove helpful to come for one week's treatment. I was assured that was the experience of numerous IC patients living far from San Francisco who could only come for a week. So I signed up, expecting to gain some understanding of what was happening inside of me and that I would learn some things that I could follow up on in Boston or NYC, as a regular commute to San Francisco was not in my plans. It's now a week since I returned. Though I went with hope for some help, I felt even without help, I would err by deciding to go rather than err the other way.

I knew the concept of trigger points, but I wasn't clear what they were or how they are found. And I thought, what if they don't find any. I will have wasted time and money, but worse, repeat a common experience of being disappointed in my sometimes—desperate hopes for relief from my symptoms (pain and frequency, with the usual qualitative restructuring of one's days). I didn't need to worry about that. I had trigger points, and it was clear where they were!

In the internal exam by Dr. Weiss, who is described as a brilliant diagnostician, he found at least 3 trigger points internally. When he touched on those muscles, it was uncomfortable enough to not be subtle or easy to miss! He did whatever he does inside to stretch and relax those muscles. His treatment the first day was perhaps 30 minutes. The second day a couple of the trigger point spots were somewhat "relaxed" and less painful, but an important central trigger point (layman's description, with apologies to Dr. Weiss) remained tight and painful, so he injected it with an anesthetic agent. It felt like a slight pinprick. I thought that was preparation for a more painful injection, but discovered, no, that first one was it. It was more than tolerable. On Wednesday, I had more internal treatment. Thursday, Dr. Weiss said that the muscles were stretched and relaxed...and in fact I felt no pain with what he was doing. After 15 minutes of treatment, he said he wouldn't continue for another 15 minutes, as it would be a waste of time, the muscles were in a normal condition, which was the goal. Friday, my last day there, he again examined the muscles and indicated there was no need for him to continue.

I would find after the treatments that for several hours I was completely pain free. I felt normal temporarily, the way I had been before IC. I found that later stressful situations during the day, or eating something that I reacted to, would bring discomfort, but that discomfort lasted shorter periods than usual. Real hope was being born! I was excited that I was getting results so soon, as well as receiving convincing evidence that this process is effective.

Dr. Weiss has created a holistic approach, and utilizes a staff of several disciplines. After my treatment sessions with Dr. Weiss, Stephanie Prendergast, MPT, would have an hour to massage or manipulate connective tissues, muscles, and reduce adverse neural tension. As she pointed out, research has demonstrated the involvement and significance of connective tissue restrictions when dealing with the bladder and IC. The fifth and last day, she had sheets and instructions on the kind of exercises I should follow up with to strengthen the relevant pelvic floor muscles. Stephanie suggested running was not a smart exercise to be doing, because of its impact on certain muscles, though swimming was an excellent form of exercise. I would recommend not swimming in chlorinated pools as the chlorine increases IC symptoms for most persons with IC. She cautioned against doing crunches for abs, but that Pilates would be excellent. Pilates works on several sets of muscles simultaneous with pelvic floor muscles, thereby providing needed support to pelvic floor muscles while strengthening them. That extra support was absent with crunches, and could make the condition worse. Since my return, I took a Pilates class at our health club, and it went well.

Janice Gigliuto, biofeedback therapist with a background and practice as a urological nurse, teaches patients how to do Kegel exercises correctly. It's common for other muscles to become engaged when doing Kegel. Janice teaches conscious isolation of the pelvic muscle to build strength and endurance. She also teaches diaphragmatic breathing and other relaxation techniques, to release some of the hypertonicity seen in the pelvic floor. In addition, she is helpful in trying to obtain resources for when one leaves.

Georgina Ritchie is a counselor/consultant who may be seen at Dr. Weiss's clinic for support facing emotional and psychological health challenges.

All of the members of the team have great credibility and integrity in their work, which comes through as being a calling or a commitment on their part to relieving patient suffering through their competent contributions. Moreover, the respect, sensitivity, and support each of them embodied is an important component of the program.

There are others who do this kind of work. After three tough years with IC, I'm most grateful to have learned about and benefited from their care. In my experience, the work with Amrit and with Dr. Weiss and his team, were a right and a left hand for the treatment of my IC.

You may wish to read an informative article by Dr. Weiss titled: *Pelvic Floor Myofascial Trigger Points: Manual Therapy For Interstitial Cystitis and the Urgency-Frequency Syndrome in the Journal of Urology*, Vol.166, 2226-2231, December 2001.

SUCCESS STORIES

"The food you eat can either be the safest and most powerful form of medicine, or the slowest form of poison."

— Ann Wigmore

Julie R.

In July of 2001, I was on Imipramine and Elmiron and still having breakthrough symptoms of urgency, frequency and irritation. I had had two major flares that took a month or more to get under control. I had recently met with a dietician who said that it sounded like the foods I was able to eat were more alkaline based. I left her office with a one-page handout on acid and alkali foods. Then, one day at work, I was desperately surfing the Web for information on bladder treatments when I saw Amrit's site with the yin/yang and acid/alkali on the book cover. Since it sounded similar to what the dietician was talking about, I wrote to Amrit for her book and to ask her some questions. This book and the diet in it have really changed my life.

I began the diet on the last day in July and was a bit saddened to think I wouldn't be able to have chocolate chip cookies, iced coffee, bread and all the things I used to eat. I remember driving to the health food store with a twenty item list and coming home with 4 bags of food. I cleared out a kitchen cabinet that was then called "Mom's special diet food." It was hard those first few weeks, as I realized I had been eating way too much sugar. It was amazing though as I began to feel so much better after only 3 days! As I felt better, I started to really eat tons of green vegetables and limit how much carbohydrates I was getting. I haven't lost more than 7 pounds because I eat a lot of almond butter, almonds, Brazil nuts and avocado along with vegetables, rice, and soy products. I tried to keep at least 80% of the diet alkaline, and the other 20% acid. I was very careful to read the labels on items and would buy only the purest products. When I look back, I think I was very strict and only ate alkaline foods for several months. I even cut out dairy for about a year, only now I will occasionally eat cottage cheese.

I also met with a homeopathic physician who had me take some supplements along with the alkaline diet. The supplements were glutamine powder, kyodophilus, calcium, lax seed oil, and vitamin E. I wanted to make sure I was getting all the nutrients and vitamins to keep me healthy as I couldn't take vitamins or vitamin C. I am not able to eat fruit, but I have started on figs and dates and do OK with them. I drink 2 glasses of Barley grass juice a day. It's the powdered kind, but I've gotten used to it and it picks me up the same way coffee used to, but without the headaches and withdrawal symptoms. I had allergy testing, but nothing really stood out except apples, which I had been eating all my life! I also use Alkalife drops to put in filtered water or bottled water.

Katie S.

My name is Katie. I am aged fifty, live in UK, have been happily married for over thirty years and have two grown up sons. I work as an accountant.

I cannot recall a time when I could say that I felt "well" or enjoyed what I would think of as normal good health. As a child I suffered from frequent headaches, often severe, and chronic catarrh/sinus problems. In my late teens I began to get bouts of tonsillitis for which I was always prescribed antibiotics and my period pains would incapacitate me for at least two days each month. At nineteen I had the first of my many early miscarriages. My first successful pregnancy, at twenty, was uneventful, but with all my health issues I found it difficult to cope with caring for my husband and baby.

During my twenties my headaches became worse and I continued to suffer from miscarriages. I was therefore delighted at twenty six to carry my second baby to term. By now, my headaches were daily and the period pains never really went away. I was diagnosed with advanced endometriosis and at twenty nine underwent a total hysterectomy and removal of ovaries. I was put on HRT (Premarin). After the operation I had what was to become the first of many bouts of cystitis. I don't recall ever getting a positive urine test for bacteria, I would just be given antibiotics at the first symptoms and it would seem to go away.

I discovered that certain things I was eating and drinking (red wine, cheese, cured meats, citrus, and chocolate) were causing the worst of my headaches so I cut these from my diet. With no more period pains and less headaches I felt better for a while. However I was putting on weight, craving sweet foods and getting more frequent bouts of tonsillitis and cystitis. I also developed IBS. I seemed to be on antibiotics as often as I was off them. I wish I had taken the trouble to research at that point and discover why I was so sick all the time. I just trusted my doctor who said I was simply an unlucky woman and I took all the medicines he prescribed for me.

At forty two I had the first attack of cystitis which didn't respond to antibiotics. It was worse than the previous ones with visible blood in my urine. After three courses of antibiotics and a bucket load of painkillers I was referred to a urologist who said I just had an irritable bladder from so many infections and put me on Ditropan (oxybutynin hydrochloride). He also told me to drink cranberry juice! This didn't help much and the treatments I received at the hands of the urologist (more antibiotics, hydrodistension, and DMSO) made things worse. It took two years to diagnose IC. Finally the urologist suggested that I should consider surgery. I got out of that hospital as fast as I could and decided to do some research on my newly acquired computer. I was unable to work at this time and spent most of my time lying on the couch clutching a hot water bottle. It was difficult for me to sit up for long but I was fascinated with the information that was available on the internet, yet my urologist had been able to give me no hope.

I discovered that I was not the only woman in the world who suffered like this and that my story was alarmingly all too common. I joined support groups and read up all the information I could get my hands on. I had to order books from America as very little is known about IC in England. From what I read, I decided that all my illnesses were linked and that my body was crying out to say it wasn't happy with the way it was being treated. I realised that my health had been slowly breaking down for years and that all the medicines I took were just masking the symptoms.

About a year ago, I finally heard about Amrit's book, Solving the Interstitial Cystitis Puzzle. It took weeks for my copy to arrive from America. As soon as I started to read it I knew I had hit upon the answer. I had tried various herbal remedies before and knew that they all blew my bladder up, so I decided that my first step was to STOP doing what was adding to my problem and to clean up my diet completely. I had been eating lots of fruit so I cut that out and drank just plain water.

I had the York IgG blood test and tested positive to dairy, ALL grains, eggs, pork and nuts. I knew that I was also intolerant to red wine, raisins, chocolate and citrus, but as I don't ever eat them, they didn't show up in the test. I was by now in a state of panic. Whatever could I eat? I didn't want to eat too much protein to add to my over acidity, so that really left just vegetables.

The only supplement I could tolerate in the beginning was a mixture of sodium bicarbonate and potassium bicarbonate which I added to my drinking water between meals. Slowly I began to see an improvement. The first thing that improved was my IBS, then I noticed I was getting fewer headaches, and finally the burning in my bladder calmed down to a dull ache. After several attempts I was able to introduce a daily probiotic capsule. I felt this was important after all the years of antibiotics. Then I started to take flaxseed oil and after several tries I can now tolerate MSM. However I still react adversely to wheatgrass and barleygrass. I know this is holding back my progress as they are very alkalising, but I presume it because I am so allergic to grains.

After many years of being incapacitated with my various ailments and in particular, IC, I am slowly getting my life back piece by piece. I have returned to work on a part-time basis and can now go walking with my husband. My diet is the biggest hurdle I have to cope with. I manage fairly well at home and am still enjoying the challenge of a whole new way of eating, but on trips and holidays it can be difficult to obtain things that I can safely eat.

For breakfast I either have some home-made vegetable soup, that I make in quantity at the weekends and freeze in individual portions or some avocado. Lunch is normally a large salad with new or baked potato. For evening meal I have a small portion of fish, chicken or lamb with a huge selection of vegetables.

I have recently been able to take a small amount of fruit with no consequences, so feel hopeful that things are still improving. Yes, at times I feel hungry and I still crave sweet things. When I am at work and the girls go and buy sticky cakes to eat with their coffee my tummy will rumble and I find it best to go to the bathroom and wait until they have finished. Then I remove their plates to the kitchen as fast as I can! Whenever I long for something that I know it is better not to eat I tell myself that it is the yeast asking to be fed. If I give in to them and satisfy their request for something sweet, they will enjoy it more than me and then jump up and bite me in the bladder.

My story isn't complete as I am not yet as well as I would like to be. I expect I will experience some more ups and downs on the road to recovery as I don't always get things right at the first attempt. However I am out of pain now for the most part and slowly regaining my energy and enthusiasm. I sleep all night and only need to go to the bathroom every three hours during the day, despite drinking a lot of water. It is helpful to understand what was happening with me over the years and why I kept getting one problem after another.

It is now one year since I received the book and 11 months since I received my blood test results. I started the diet and the potassium and sodium bicarbonate at that stage. I felt better in myself almost straight away, but it took two months before my bladder symptoms really died down. If I try a new supplement that I am not ready for, or if I make a mistake with my diet....and I have made quite a few!.....it is always my bladder that suffers first. I was 3 months into my diet when I was able to resume work. I saw that as a giant stepping stone as I regained most of my self worth.

I will be eternally grateful to Amrit for writing her book and sharing her experience with other IC sufferers to give hope where there seemed to be none.

Solving the Interstitial Cystitis Puzzle

Solving the Interstitial Cystitis Puzzle

Conclusion

"That which is above is the same as that which is below."

— Hermes Trismegistus

In solving the IC puzzle, I was reminded that the body is a microcosm of our natural external environment. It is important to view one's health holistically. By this, I mean exploring and altering ones diet is vital in resolving IC. As such, while my emphasis has been on maintaining an alkalizing diet/lifestyle, it is important to remember that we all exist within a macrocosm. While researching information for my recovery from IC, I discovered the parallels of the acidification of our bodies and that of our world. We eat acid-forming food, drink water, and breathe air that has been exposed to acid deposition. To understand IC and acidity more thoroughly, we need to explore the world in which we live.

Parallels

While searching for information about "acid water" on the Internet, I came across myriad websites regarding the effects of acid rain. I was saddened by the devastating acidic conditions of the world's fresh-water lakes, rivers, streams, and wetlands. The devastation is particularly prevalent in Norway, Sweden, and Canada. However, the lakes and rivers of the United States have not been spared. "In the United States acid-sensitive areas are found in Minnesota, Wisconsin, upper Michigan, several Southeastern states, the mountainous areas of the West, as well as the Northeastern states.

"Other acid-sensitive parts of the world include the Netherlands, Belgium, Denmark, Switzerland, Italy, West Germany, Ireland, the United Kingdom, Scandinavia, and in the Precambrian and Cambrian geology in Asia, Africa, and South America." [1]

Acid Rain

"When fossil fuels such as coal, gasoline, and fuel oils are burned, they emit oxides of sulfur, carbon, and nitrogen into the air. These oxides combine with moisture in the air to form sulfuric acid, carbonic acid, and nitric acid. When it rains or snows, these acids are brought to Earth in what is called acid rain.

"During the course of the 20th century, the acidity of the air and acid rain has come to be recognized as a leading threat to the stability and quality of the Earth's environment. Most of this acidity is produced in the industrialized nations of the Northern Hemisphere—the United States, Canada, Japan, and most of the countries of Eastern and Western Europe.

"The effects of acid rain can be devastating to many forms of life, including human life. Its effects can be most vividly seen, however, in lakes, rivers, and streams and on vegetation. Acidity in water kills virtually all life forms. By the early 1990s, tens of thousands of lakes had been destroyed by acid rain. The problem has been most severe in Norway, Sweden, and Canada.

"The threat posed by acid rain is not limited by geographic boundaries, for prevailing winds carry the pollutants around the globe. For example, much research supports the conclusion that pollution from coal-powered electric generating stations in the Midwestern United States is the ultimate cause of the severe acid-rain problem in eastern Canada and the northeastern United States. Nor are the destructive effects of acid rain limited to the natural environment. Structures made of stone, metal, and cement have also been damaged or destroyed. Some of the world's great monuments, including the cathedrals of Europe and the Coliseum in Rome, have shown signs of deterioration caused by acid rain.

"Scientists use what is called the pH factor to measure the acidity or alkalinity of liquid solutions. On a scale from 0 to 14, the number 0 represents the highest level of acid and 14 the most basic or alkaline. A solution of distilled water containing neither acids nor alkalies, or bases, is designated 7, or neutral. If the pH level of rain falls below 5.5, the rain is considered acidic. Rainfalls in the eastern United States and in Western Europe often range from 4.5 to 4.0.

"Although the cost of such antipollution equipment as burners, filters, and chemical and washing devices is great, the cost in damage to the environment and human life is estimated to be much greater because the damage may be irreversible. Although preventative measures are being taken, up to 500,000 lakes in North America and more than 4 billion cubic feet (118 million cubic meters) of timber in Europe may be destroyed before the end of the 20th century." [2]

Experts note that forestry is another cause for acidification. In the natural cycle, bases once taken up from the soil by trees eventually return once the trees decompose. The removal of large trees from the forest also removes large amounts of the bases that are needed for the acid-base balance of the forest. This slowly leads to acidification.

Human health is not spared either. We eat food, drink water, and breathe air that has been exposed to acids. This acidic air pollution can cause respiratory problems among children and asthmatics.

Although the primary focus of this book has been to change to an alkalizing diet with pure alkaline water to heal IC, let us not forget the air we breathe. This air contains sulfuric acid, nitric acid, and hydrochloric acid that needs to be neutralized. In solving the IC puzzle, we cannot afford to ignore the big picture, for we are all a part of the world. In solving the IC puzzle, doctors, and researchers have been busy looking through a microscope when what we might need to do is view this problem with a "macroscope."

The macroscope can be considered the symbol of a new way of seeing, understanding, and acting. We need to view our health holistically.

"Many urologists have come to the conclusion that we are dealing with a multifactorial disease entity that needs to be reclassified." [3]

"While much of the effort to treat interstitial cystitis has focused on identifying specific causes and markers for the disease, pain researchers at Johns Hopkins University in Baltimore have concluded that multi-faceted strategies are apparently needed to effectively treat the variety of underlying pain mechanisms that may exist in the same patient… A spectrum of different insults likely leads to chronic visceral pain in IC." [4]

Acid Air, Acid Rain

What I discovered to my amazement was that Norway and Sweden spend an equivalence of $40 to $50 million US dollars each year "liming" their lakes. What does liming entail? They are doing exactly what I have been discussing in this book. They add alkaline elements to an acidic environment to attain a neutralizing effect. They administer 300,000 tons of fine-grained limestone yearly into lakes, streams, and wetlands to raise the pH in surface water. Limestone, also known as calcium carbonate, an alkalizing element, is used to raise the water's pH level from a low 4 or 5 to a higher and life-sustaining pH of 6 to 8.

The liming solution is a shortsighted intervention rather than a long-term "cure." I feel taking a simple alkaline supplement instead of a balanced alkalizing diet/lifestyle change is not recommended for IC. People and environments are too complex to be governed by one or two molecules.

Viewing IC Holistically

"We no longer feel responsible for our illnesses. Microbes, germs, the weather, communism, or the wrath of an unfair God is blamed for the imbalance—and a miracle cure in the form of a pill is recommended as the cure. Rarely does the physician ask the patient to look at his entire lifestyle in order to find the source of stress, dietary or otherwise, that has created the problem" [5]

Traditionally, most Americans have been led to believe that one remedy could solve their health problems, that a visit to a doctor's office could cure what ails them or that one type of treatment or a pill could improve their condition. In my healing process, I went to numerous medical doctors as well as holistic health care providers where I received pieces of the puzzle over many years.

When evaluating any disease it is vital that one examines the "big picture" and assesses all aspects of the person's life and environment. I doubt if very many IC sufferers have had a complete history and examination of their lives including their intake of foods, water and air quality, physical activity, vitamin, mineral and essential fatty acid sufficiency, stress levels and coping, allergies and system reviews.

What I have discovered with IC is there are many pieces to this puzzle—, that ones health needs to be viewed macroscopically. In solving the IC puzzle, I needed to consider the following: diet, including supplements and medications, water quality, air quality, allergies, stress, and lifestyle choices. These considerations needed to be evaluated from the perspective of pH and their correlation with each other. In addition, the systems that needed to be addressed for myself were the bladder, the gastrointestinal system, the liver, and the adrenal glands. These systems, too, needed to be evaluated with respect to pH and my body's balance.

All systems of the body affect ones pH. If a child has asthma, he would tend to be more acidic, since more carbon dioxide would be retained. If the kidneys were weak, one would see signs of acidosis as well. Each person with IC needs to evaluate the systems in their body, their external environment, diet, and lifestyle in order to resolve IC. My point is you will need to do your own self-inventory to determine what is causing your body's acid state.

I am of the belief that most persons with IC, if not all, have been treated with multiple courses of antibiotics. This history creates the LGS, allergies, and malnutrition that in turn tax the liver. These problems are acid-forming and need to be addressed. It has been documented that the majority of Americans eat an acid-forming diet, are deficient in their nutrition, and lead stressful lives. Converting to a nutritious alkalizing diet with pure alkaline water and adequate supplementation plus finding ways to reduce stress and heal other body systems is mandatory for persons with IC.

With respect to inhaling acidic air, I did not cover oxygen therapy. Remember that oxygen is an alkalizing element. There are oxygen therapies and ozone therapies that purify the air we breathe at home and in the office and provide the body with supplemental oxygen. Actually, ozone is simply pure, activated oxygen. I encourage the reader who wants not only relief from IC, but would like to live a *vigorous* life, to explore holistic applications of oxygen therapy.

I would also like to emphasize that consuming an acid-forming diet, drinking acid-forming beverages, and choosing an acid-forming lifestyle cannot merely be "treated" with an antacid or a supplement or two. I have witnessed after twenty years of nursing practice that this is a common history of persons who develop chronic disease.

Over the years I suffered from IC, when I was not diagnosed accurately and wondered what was wrong with me, I was very discouraged. Now that I am healed, I can see that for me IC was truly a blessing. Having IC has been a humbling experience and has helped me to remember that in life there is suffering. It has made me more conscious of others who are hurting in this world. It motivated me to search for answers to my healing. In doing so, IC has helped me to heal in body, mind, and Spirit.

In nursing school, we studied nutrition, and it has always been an interest of mine. Although I thought my diet was healthy, I learned I was making some wrong choices and had many deficiencies, and so did my family.

Even though I do not have a crystal ball to see into the future, I am sure learning about the pH factor and its effect on my health will help to contribute to my continued well-being. I know the healing journey I describe might not be easy. However, for myself, because I endured such pain, I was highly motivated to make these changes. I consider myself a spiritual person, but I found IC had renewed my sense of awe when I was reminded how the mystery of life is so beautifully interwoven. We really are one.

My wish in offering you this book about my discovery and healing IC is that it offers you a safe alternative option for dealing with IC. Choosing an alkalizing diet/lifestyle, healing the LGS, allergies, liver, and the adrenal glands has eliminated my suffering. I wish those of you who have endured so much pain for so long from IC have been given new hope. I welcome further exploration and study from persons with IC as well as caregivers and researchers who work with us regarding the effect of the pH factor and IC. Hopeful, I remain.

May you be well,

Amrit

APPENDIX A — FOODS

In appendix A, I have compiled a table of foods and categorized them according to their level of acidity or alkalinity. This appendix adapted from Dr. Baroody's *Alkalize or Die*. Attempt to eat a diet that contains 80 percent of your food choice from the alkali-forming categories.

Fruits

Highly Alkaline		
Cantaloupe	Dates (dried)	Figs (dried)
Lemons	Limes	Mangos
Melons (all varieties)	Papaya	Watermelon
Moderately Alkaline		
Apricots	Avocados	Bananas
Berries (except blueberries and cranberries)		Breadfruit
Cactus	Citron	Currants
Dates (fresh)	Figs (fresh)	Grapefruit
Grapes	Guavas	Kiwis
Kumquats	Nectarines	Passion Fruit
Peaches	Pears	Persimmons
Pineapple	Quince	Raisins
Tamarind	Tangerine	Umeboshi Plums
Slightly Alkaline		
Apples	Carob	Cherries
Olives (ripened and sun dried)		Oranges
Pomegranate	Raspberries	Strawberries
Neutral		
None Noted		
Slightly Acidic		
None Noted		
Moderately Acidic		
Blueberries	Cranberries	Plums
Prunes		
Highly Acidic		
None Noted		

(Overcooked fruit becomes acid-forming.)

Vegetables

Highly Alkaline		
Kelp	Parsley	Seaweed
Watercress		
Moderately Alkaline		
Asparagus	Carrots	Celery
Dandelion Greens	Endive	Escarole
Lettuce (all types)	Oyster Plant (Salsify)	Pumpkin
Rutabaga	Spinach	Squash
Slightly Alkaline		
Artichokes	Bamboo Shoots	Beets
Broccoli	Brussels Sprouts	Cabbage
Cauliflower	Chicory	Collards
Corn, sweet	Cucumbers	Daikon
Eggplant	Ginger (fresh)	Kale
Kohlrabi	Leeks	Lettuce, Iceberg
Mushrooms	Mustard greens	Okra
Onions	Parsnips	Peppers, Bell
Pickles	Potatoes	Swiss Chard
Taro (baked)	Tomatoes	Turnips
Radishes	Water Chestnuts	
Neutral		
Horseraddish	Rhubarb	Sauerkraut
Slightly Acidic		
None Noted		
Moderately Acidic		
None Noted		
Highly Acidic		
None Noted		

(Overcooked vegetables become acid-forming.)

Solving the Interstitial Cystitis Puzzle

Grains

Highly Alkaline		
None Noted		
Moderately Alkaline		
None Noted		
Slightly Alkaline		
None Noted		
Neutral		
Amaranth	Millet	Quinoa
Slightly Acidic		
Barley	Corn Meal	Rye
Spelt		
Moderately Acidic		
Basmati Rice	Brown Rice	Buckwheat
Oats	Whole Wheat	
Highly Acidic		
Wheat (bleached)	White Rice	

(All grains become neutral to slightly alkali-forming when sprouted.)

Beans

Highly Alkaline		
None Noted		
Moderately Alkaline		
None Noted		
Slightly Alkaline		
French Bean (fresh)	Green (fresh)	Lima (fresh)
Peas (fresh)	Snap (fresh)	String (fresh)
Neutral		
Soy Beans	Soy Cheese	Soy Milk
Tempeh	Tofu	
Slightly Acidic		
Aduki	Black	Broadbean
Garbanzo	Kidney	Lentils
Mung	Navy	Pinto
Red	White	
Moderately Acidic		
None Noted		
Highly Acidic		
None Noted		

(Acid-forming beans become slightly to moderately alkali-forming when sprouted.)

Other Starches

Highly Alkaline		
None Noted		
Moderately Alkaline		
Arrowroot Flour		
Slightly Alkaline		
Potatoes (all types)		
Neutral		
Essene Bread	Granola	
Slightly Acidic		
Bran	Popcorn (plain)	Popcorn with Butter
Unrefined Cold Cereals		Unrefined Crackers
Whole Grain Pastas		
Moderately Acidic		
Buckwheat Cereal (hot)		Corn Bread
Cream of Wheat (hot)	Popcorn with Butter and Salt	
Oat Bread	Oatmeal Cereal	Rice Bread
Rye Bread	Spelt Bread	Tapioca
Whole Grain Pastries	Popcorn with Salt	
Highly Acidic		
Refined Flours	Refined Pastas	Refined Pastries
Wheat Bread		

Nuts

Highly Alkaline		
None Noted		
Moderately Alkaline		
None Noted		
Slightly Alkaline		
Almonds	Coconut (fresh)	
Neutral		
Chestnuts	Pignolias	
Slightly Acidic		
Brazil	Cashews	Coconut (dried)
Filberts	Macadamia	Pecans
Pistachios	Walnuts	
Moderately Acidic		
Peanuts		
Highly Acidic		
None Noted		

Seeds

Highly Alkaline		
None Noted		
Moderately Alkaline		
Alfalfa (sprouted)	Chia (sprouted)	
Slightly Alkaline		
Radish (sprouted)		
Neutral		
Sesame (unsprouted)		
Slightly Acidic		
Pumpkin	Sunflower	
Moderately Acidic		
Wheat Germ		
Highly Acidic		
None Noted		

Meat

Highly Alkaline		
None Noted		
Moderately Alkaline		
None Noted		
Slightly Alkaline		
None Noted		
Neutral		
None Noted		
Slightly Acidic		
None Noted		
Moderately Acidic		
Crab	Fish (fins and scales)	Lobster
Oysters	Scallops	Shrimp
Highly Acidic		
Beef (organically grown)		
Chicken (organically grown)		Fish (other types)
Lamb	Pheasant	Pork
Rabbit	Turkey (organically grown)	
Turkey (wild)	Venison	

Animal Products

Highly Alkaline		
None Noted		

Moderately Alkaline		
None Noted		

Slightly Alkaline		
None Noted		

Neutral		
Butter (fresh unsalted)	Cow's milk (fresh, raw)	Cream (fresh, raw)
Egg Yolk	Goat's milk (raw)	
Lactobacillus Acidophilus		Lactobacillus Bifidus
Whey (cow's milk)	Whey (goat's milk)	Yogurt plain

Slightly Acidic		
Butter (fresh salted)	Butter (processed)	Cheese (crumbly)
Cheese (mild/medium)	Cottage Cheese	Cream (processed)
Egg Whites	Milk (cow's, homogenized)	
Milk (goat's homogenized)		

Moderately Acidic		
Cheese (sharp)	Custard	Sweetened Yogurt
Whole eggs		

Highly Acidic		
None Noted		

Oils

Highly Alkaline		
None Noted		

Moderately Alkaline		
None Noted		

Slightly Alkaline		
None Noted		

Neutral		
Almond	Avocado	Canola
Castor	Coconut	Corn
Margarine	Olive	Safflower
Sesame	Soy	Sunflower

Slightly Acidic		
None Noted		

Moderately Acidic		
None Noted		

Highly Acidic		
None Noted		

Sugars

Highly Alkaline		
None Noted		
Moderately Alkaline		
None Noted		
Slightly Alkaline		
Brown Rice Syrup	Dr. Bronner's Barley Malt Sweetener	
Honey (unprocessed)	Maguey	
Neutral		
Dried Sugar Cane Juice		
Slightly Acidic		
Barley malt syrup	Fructose	Honey (processed)
Maple syrup (unprocessed)		
Molasses (organic, unsulfured)		Milk sugar
Turbinado		
Moderately Acidic		
Maple syrup (processed)		
Molasses (processed, sulfured)		
Highly Acidic		
Beet sugar (processed, bleached)		
Cane sugar (white processed)		

Beverages

Highly Alkaline		
Alkaline Water	Fruit Juices (fresh)	Vegetable Juices
Moderately Alkaline		
Herbal Teas		
Slightly Alkaline		
None Noted		
Neutral		
None Noted		
Slightly Acidic		
Coffee Substitutes	Fruit Juice (naturally sweetened)	
Moderately Acidic		
Wine	Fruit Juice (sweetened with white sugar)	
Highly Acidic		
Beer	Caffeine Drinks	Carbonated Drinks
Coffee	Liquor	Soft Drinks
Tea (black)		

Condiments

Highly Alkaline		
Agar-Agar	Cayenne Pepper	
Moderately Alkaline		
Bay leaves	Chives	
Dr. Bronner's Mineral Bouillon		Garlic
Gelatin (plain, unsugared with fruit or vegetables)		
Marjoram	Vegetable Salt	
Slightly Alkaline		
Apple Cider Vinegar (raw, unprocessed)		Basil
Caraway Seed	Celery Seed	Cloves
Coriander	Cumin Seed	Curry Powder
Dill Leaves	Fennel Seed	Ginger (powdered)
Ketchup (natural)	Miso	Oregano
Paprika	Potassium (Bio-salt)	Rosemary
Sage	Sea Salt	
Sweet Brown Rice Vinegar		Tamari
Tarragon	Thyme	Vanilla Extract
Neutral		
Anise	Brewer's Yeast	Cinnamon
Distilled Water	Nutritional Yeast	Soy Sauce
Slightly Acidic		
Gelatin (mixed with water)		Mustard (dried spice)
Mustard (stone ground, natural)		Nutmeg
Moderately Acidic		
Gelatin (mixed with sugar)		Ketchup (refined)
Mayonnaise (refined with sugar)		Soy sauce (processed)
Highly Acidic		
Mustard (refined)	Salt (refined, white)	White Vinegar

APPENDIX B — LIFESTYLE CHOICES

Alkali-Forming Lifestyle	
Alkali-forming diet	Laughter
Counseling or therapy can reduce stress	Adequate alkaline water intake 6-8 glasses per day
Yoga improves breathing	Deep breathing
Silence	Chew food thoroughly
Parasite and yeast elimination program (Clear® supplement)	Essential fiber in diet decreases constipation
Adequate nutrition with essential vitamins, minerals and fatty acids	Hobbies that relax the body and mind
Meditation	Mineral baths
Allergy testing and elimination to decrease inflammation	Massage helps clean the lymphatic system
Aromatherapy (lavender essential oil can be added to a bath, handkerchief or a few drops diluted in almond oil for a relaxing massage)	Green foods high in chlorophyll removes toxins from the body and increase magnesium and oxygenation (spirulina, chlorella, alfalfa, barley grass; look for Green Magma™ and/or Kyo-green™ on the market)
Saunas help eliminate toxins, but be sure to replace lost minerals and fluids with juices and alkaline water	Enteric-coated probiotics (lactobacillus bifidus and lactobacillus acidophilus)
Liver/ gallbladder flush (bile: pH 8 from the liver helps to digest food which enhances ones nutritional state and the liver helps to detoxify the body of harmful chemicals)	Detoxification programs (consult a holistic health care provider)

Solving the Interstitial Cystitis Puzzle

Alkali-Forming Lifestyle	
Oxygen therapies	Eat moderately
Reflexology helps to strengthen and rebalance body systems	Biofeedback (learn to modify responses to stress)
Sodium bicarbonate	Potassium bicarbonate
Kidney flushes (consult a holistic health care provider)	Attend to your spiritual needs as well as physical and mental
Relaxing walks in nature	A day at a health spa
Pets have been shown to reduce stress and blood pressures in their owners	Homeopathics and appropriate supplements that support acid-alkali balance
Adequate rest and relaxation every day	Acupuncture to assist in balancing the acid-alkali balance
Colonics and enemas are good for detoxification (consult a holistic health care provider)	Mild to moderate fasting (fruit or vegetable juice fasting) can help rebalance acid-alkali balance
Relaxing environment such as the use of natural-scented candles, incense and flowers (provided they are not allergens) water fountains, wind chimes, pleasant colors, inspiring artwork and music, aquariums etc.	Mild to moderate exercise every day (walking, swimming, or bike riding are a good start, but see a health care provider if you have medical conditions or are over 40 years old before starting such a program)
Sunlight (exposure for 30 minutes to two hours a day benefits the adrenal glands; these glands help us regulate our stress fight or flight response)	Ozone air purifiers (placed in a room they will eliminate fungi, bacteria, molds pollutants and chemicals in the air)

Acid-Forming Lifestyle	
Cosmetics, shampoo, soap, hair dye, makeup not organically based since these are absorbed through the skin and scalp	98% of prescription and over the counter drugs produce acid forming reactions
Stress (situations that cause anxiety, anger, fear, disappointment; even success can still be stressors)	Decreased pancreatic fluids (pancreatic fluids are alkaline with a pH of 8.4 to 8.9 and help to neutralize acids)
Respiratory conditions (carbon dioxide an acid is retained and not enough oxygen is absorbed)	Gallbladder and liver diseases from over-consumption, obesity, alcohol and drugs
Drinking acidic water	Kidney disease
Increased hydrochloric acid in the stomach; increases acid load in the body	Alcohol causes excretion of nutrients in the urine especially calcium and magnesium
Sedentary lifestyle	Over-exercising
Parasites and Infections	Allergies and inflammatory conditions
Toxins/chemicals in food and environment	Salt (too much sodium causes potassium to be excreted)
Sugar	Overcooked foods
Tired adrenal glands from too much stress, caffeine and sugar	Caffeine causes the kidneys to excrete alkaline elements
Thyroid disease	Leaky Gut Syndrome
Refined and processed foods	Tobacco (smoking or chewing)
Antibiotics destroy normal gut flora	Air pollution decreases oxygen, an alkaline element

Solving the Interstitial Cystitis Puzzle

Acid-Forming Lifestyle	
Constipation (toxic acid wastes are reabsorbed into the system instead of eliminated)	Malnutrition and anemia (lack of essential vitamins, minerals and essential fatty acids)
Sluggish lymphatic system related to sedentary life style and decreased water intake	Shallow breathing and holding the breath causes the retention of carbon dioxide, an acid

APPENDIX C — FOOD SOURCES OF MINERALS

Potassium (2,500mg RDA for 150 lb adult)

Avocado, raw, 1 fruit	1,097mg
Papaya, raw, large (6 inch x 3 inch)	977mg
Lima beans, boiled, 1 cup	955mg
Potato, baked with skin, 1 medium	925mg
Yam, boiled or baked, 1 cup, cubed	911mg
Spinach, boiled, 1 cup	839mg
Pinto Beans, boiled, 1 cup	800mg
Lentils, boiled, 1 cup	731mg
Almonds, raw, 3.5 ounces	728mg
Acorn squash, boiled, 1 cup, mashed	644mg
Parsnips, boiled, 1 - 9 inch	587mg
Butternut squash, cooked, 1 cup, cubed	582mg
Pumpkin, boiled, 1 cup, mashed	564mg
Kohlrabi, cooked, 1 cup, sliced	561mg
Coconut meat, dried, 3.5 ounces	543mg
Dates, 10 pieces	540mg
Pumpkin, canned, 1 cup	505mg
Molasses, blackstrap, 1 Tablespoon	498mg
Cantaloupe, raw, 1 cup, diced	482mg
Zucchini, boiled, 1 cup	455mg
Green peas, boiled, 1 cup	434mg
Artichoke, boiled, 1	425mg
Tomato juice, unsalted, canned, 6 ounces	400mg
Sweetpotato, baked with skin, 1 medium	397mg
Carrot, raw, 1 cup	394mg
Snap green beans, cooked, 1 cup	374mg
Carrot, cooked, 1 cup	354mg
Crookneck squash, cooked, 1 cup, sliced	346mg
Celery, raw, 1 cup, diced	344mg
Mango, raw, 1 fruit	323mg
Banana, raw, 1 - 6 inch	321mg
Black beans, cooked, ½ cup	305mg
Grapes, red or green, 1 cup	296mg
Nectarine, raw, 1 fruit	288mg
Strawberries, raw, 1 cup, sliced	276mg
Cherries, sweet, raw with pits, 1 cup	262mg
Okra, boiled, ½ cup, sliced	258mg
Oranges, raw, 1 medium	249mg
Lentils, sprouted, raw, 1 cup	248mg
Brussels sprouts, cooked, ½ cup	247mg

Potassium (continued)

Apple, raw with skin, 1 large	244mg
Raisins, 1 ounce	210mg
Pear, raw, 1 medium	208mg
Corn, sweet white, boiled, ½ cup	204mg
Peach, raw, 1 medium	193mg
Corn, sweet, boiled, 1 ear	192mg
Cashews, raw, 1 ounce	187mg
Watermelon, raw, 1 cup, diced	176mg
Pine nuts, dried, 1 ounce	170mg
Brazilnuts, raw, 6 - 8 nuts	170mg
Spinach, raw, 1 cup	167mg
Romaine lettuce, raw, 1 cup, shredded	162mg
Endive, raw, 1 cup, chopped	158mg
Cabbage, red, raw, 1 cup, shredded	144mg
Tomato, raw, 1 medium	138mg
Figs, dried, 1piece	135mg
Peaches, dried, ½ piece	129mg
Bamboo shoots, canned, 1 cup	105mg
Asparagus, boiled, 4 spears	96mg
Cauliflower, boiled, ½ cup	88mg
Waterchestnuts, chinese, canned, ½ cup	83mg
Apricots, dried, 1 piece	41mg

Calcium (1,000mg RDA for 150 lb adult)

Sheep's milk, 1 cup	474mg
Goat's milk, 1 cup	326mg
Cow's milk, 1 cup	291mg
Sesame seeds, roasted & toasted, 1 ounce	280mg
Soybeans, boiled, 1 cup	261mg
Almonds, raw, 3.5 ounces	248mg
Collard leaves, boiled, 1 cup, chopped	226mg
Turnip greens, boiled, 1 cup, chopped	197mg
Kelp, raw, 3.5 ounces	168mg
Kidney beans, boiled, 1 cup	117mg
Dandelion greens, raw, 1 cup, chopped	103mg
Swiss chard, boiled, 1 cup, chopped	102mg
Kale, boiled, 1 cup, chopped	94mg
Broccoli, boiled, 1 medium stalk	83mg
Pinto Beans, boiled, 1 cup	82mg
Sesame seed, tahini, raw, 1 Tablespoon	63mg
Brazil nuts, raw, 6 - 8 nuts	50mg
Watercress, raw, 1 cup, chopped	41mg
Figs, dried, 1piece	30mg

Magnesium (350mg RDA for 150 lb adult)

Almonds, raw, 3.5 ounces	275mg
Corn, sweet, 1 ear	192mg
Filberts or Hazlenuts, 3.5 ounces	163mg
Pumpkin or squash seeds, raw, 1 ounce	152mg
Swiss chard, boiled, 1 cup, chopped	151mg
Soybeans, cooked, 1 cup	108mg
Navy beans, boiled, 1 cup	108mg
Sunflower seeds, hulled, 1 ounce	100mg
Peanuts, dry-roasted, 2 ounces	100mg
Pinto Beans, boiled, 1 cup	94mg
Coconut meat, dried, 3.5 ounces	90mg
Buckwheat, groats, roasted, 1 cup	86mg
Brown rice, cooked, 1 cup	86mg
Cashews, raw, 1 ounce	83mg
Lima Beans, boiled, 1 cup	81mg
Kidney beans, boiled, 1 cup	80mg
Garbanzo beans, boiled, 1 cup	79mg
Millet, cooked, 1 cup	77mg
Artichoke, boiled, 1	72mg
Avocado, 1 fruit	71mg
Pine nuts, dried, 1 ounce	66mg
Brazilnuts, raw, 6 - 8 nuts	64mg
Molasses, blackstrap, 1 Tablespoon	52mg

Iron (10mg RDA for 150 lb adult)

Spinach, boiled, 1 cup	6.4mg
Lentils, boiled, 1 cup	6.6mg
Liver, beef, cooked, 3.5 ounces	5.9mg
Kidney beans, boiled, 1 cup	5.3mg
Garbanzo beans, boiled, 1 cup	5.0mg
Lima Beans, boiled, 1 cup	4.5mg
Pinto Beans, boiled, 1 cup	4.5mg
Soybeans, boiled, 1 cup	4.5mg
Swiss chard, boiled, 1 cup, chopped	3.9mg
Molasses, blackstrap, 1 Tablespoon	3.5mg
Beet greens, boiled, 1 cup	2.7mg
Pine nuts, dried, 1 ounce	2.6mg
Green peas, boiled, 1 cup	2.5mg
Lentils, raw, sprouted, 1 cup	2.4mg
Prunes, dried, 10 pieces	2.1mg
Cashews, raw, 1 ounce	1.9mg
Dates, 10 pieces	1.0mg
Brazilnuts, raw, 6 - 8 nuts	1.0mg

Sodium (2,000mg RDA for 150 lb adult)

Beet greens, boiled, 1 cup, chopped	347mg
Swiss chard, boiled, 1 cup, chopped	313mg
Kelp, raw, 3.5 ounces	233mg
Goat's whey, dehydrated, extract, 2T	187mg
Artichoke, boiled, 1	114mg
Celery, raw, 1 cup, diced	100mg
Spinach, boiled, 1 cup	126mg
Goat's milk, 1 cup	122mg
Sheep's milk, 1 cup	108mg
Spinach, raw, 3.5 ounces	79mg
Apples, dried, 3.5 ounces	87mg

Solving the Interstitial Cystitis Puzzle

APPENDIX D — RESOURCES & SUPPLIERS

AlkaLife®
A 1.2 oz. bottle lasts about two months and costs about $18.95.

Sang Whang Enterprises, Inc.
8445 SW 148 Dr
Miami, FL 33158
(888) 261-0870
http://www.alkalife.com
sang@alkalife.com

Allergy Research Group
30806 Santana Street
Hayward, CA 94544
(510) 487-8526 or (800) 545-9960
Fax: (510) 487-8682 or (800) 688-7426
http://www.allergyresearchgroup.com
info@allergyresearchgroup.com

American Holistic Nurses Association
PO Box 2130
Flagstaff, AZ 86003-2130
(800) 278-2462
http://www.ahna.org
info@ahna.org

American Holistic Medical Association
12101 Menaul Blvd. NE, Suite C
Albuquerque, NM 87112
(505) 292-7788
Fax: (505) 293-7582
http://www.holisticmedicine.org
info@holisticmedicine.org

Dr. Roger Barnes, DC
10801 National Blvd Ste 250
Los Angeles, CA 90064-4126
(310) 441-9682

BHI Homeopathic Remedies
Manufactured and distributed by:
Heel Incorporated
PO Box 11280
Albuquerque, NM 87192-0280
(800) 621-7644
(505) 293-3843
Fax: (505) 275-1672
http://www.heelbhi.com
info@heelusa.com

The Bluestone Group
Water Ionizer
(412) 833-9640
http://www.bluestonegroup.com

Clark's Compounding Pharmacy (Mark Clark)
15615 Bel-Red Road
Bellevue, WA 98008
(425) 881-0222

Clear® Herbal Formula
(800) 69AWARE or (800) 692-9273
Mention Distributor Number **11157401**
http://www.holisticnurse.com/topics/aware/

Awareness Corporation
25 South Arizona Place
Suite 500
Chandler Corporate Plaza
Chandler, AZ 8522
http://www.awarecorp.com
customerservice@awarecorp.com

Diagnos-Techs
Building J
6620 South 192nd Place
Kent, WA 98032
http://www.diagnostechs.com
(800) 878-3787
Fax: (425) 251-0637
diagnos@diagnostechs.com

Great Smokies Diagnostic Laboratory
63 Zillicoa St
Asheville, NC 28801
(800) 522-4762
Fax: (828) 252-9303

Healthy Life Harvest Aloe Vera Coral Calcium
(877) 444-2563
(208) 938-2789
http://www.icaloe.com

Holistic Life Enterprises
Amrit Willis, RN, BSN
9461 Charleville Blvd Ste 198
Beverly Hills, CA 90212-3017
Fax/voicemail: (877) 682-1634
http://www.holisticnurse.com

Immuno Laboratories, Inc.
1620 West Oakland Park Blvd
Fort Lauderdale, FL 33311
(954) 486-4500 or (800) 231-9197
Fax: (954) 739-6563
http://www.immunolabs.com

Interstitial Cystitis Association
110 N Washington St Ste 340
Rockville, MD 20850
(800) HELP-ICA
(301) 610-5300
http://www.ichelp.org

Interstial Cystitis Network
4983 Sonoma Hwy Ste L
Santa Rosa, CA 95409
(707) 538-9442
http://www.ic-network.com

Shira Lee, MA
Shira Lee, MA, offers intuitive counseling, flower essence therapy and self-healing support. She is available for e mail and telephone consultations. She can be reached at gentlybe00@yahoo.com.

Shira Lee
PO Box 1036
Mendocino, CA 95460

Maine Coast Sea Vegetables Inc.
3 Georges Pond Rd
Franklin ME 04634
(207) 565-2907
Fax: (207) 565-2144
http://www.seaveg.com

Dawn R. Mahowald, CYI
Dawn R. Mahowald, CYI, certified in Structural Yoga, has been working with yoga for over 40 years. Dawn currently practices and teaches privately in Boulder, Colorado. http://www.yogamed.net

The book *Cystitis A Time to Heal with Yoga & Acupressure—An Eight Week Course with Special Information for People with Interstitial Cystitis & Urethral Syndrome*, is available from 1stBooks Library Publishers.

1stBooks Library Publishers
2595 Vernal Pike, Bloomington, IN 47404 USA.
(800) 839-8640 (Toll Free)
(812) 339-6000 (Outside USA and Canada)
(812) 339-6554 (Fax)
http://www.1stbooks.com/
The electronic version is $3.95
The printed and bound version is $17.95 + S&H

Dr. Kinne McCabe, MD
2366 Eastlake Ave East Ste 205
Seattle, WA 98102
(206) 325-4681
KinneMcCabe@earthlink.net

MetaMetrix Medical Laboratory (Red Blood Cell Analysis)
500 Peachtree Ind Blvd Ste 110
Norcross, GA 30071

Monro Medical Laboratory (Red Blood Cell Analysis)
Route 17
PO Box 1
Southfield, NY 10975

Nambudripad Allergy Research Foundation (NAET)
6714 Beach Blvd
Buena Park, CA 90621
(714) 523-0800
(714) 523-8900
Fax: (714) 523-3068
http://www.naet.com

Dr. Shera E. Raisen, MD
1260 15th St Ste 1006
Santa Monica, CA 90404
(310) 458-9200
http://www.DoctorRaisen.com

Dr. MarkRhodes, PhD (Diagnos-Techs Consultant)
500 Willamette Avenue
Umatilla, OR 97882

Mailing Address:
PO Box 1640
Hermiston, OR 97838
(541) 922-4823
Fax: (413) 451-6364
http://www.drmarkrhodes.com
Mark@DrMarkRhodes.com

Dr. Emmey Ripoll, MD
Dr. Emmey Ripoll, MD is board certified in Urology and Holistic Medicine. She practices urology with the Fergus Falls Medical Group in Fergus Falls, MN.

http://www.yogamed.net

Slippery Stuff® Gel
Wallace-O'Farrell
11302 164th Street East
Puyallup, WA 98374
(800) 759-7883 or (253) 845-6633
A web site that sells Slippery Stuff® Gel is http://www.drugstore.com

(800) drugstore

Dr. Jim Smith, DO
11263 Reading Road
Cincinnati, OH 45241
(513) 769-7546
Fax: (513) 769-7547
http://www.DrJimSmith.com
drjim@drjimsmith.com

Tamer pH Laboratories
17230 12th Ave NE
Seattle, Washington 98155
(206) 364-6761
Fax: (206) 364-5369

Tamer pH Sciences
(800) 42-TAMER
(800) 428-2637
http://www.tamer.com
customercare@tamer.com

Thorne Research, Inc.
PO Box 25
Dover, ID 83825
(208) 263-1337
Fax: (208) 265-2488
http://www.thorne.com
sales@thorne.com

Herbal Resources in the United States:

Avena Botanicals
219 Mill St.
Rockport, ME 04865
207-594-0694
http://www.AvenaHerbs.com

Frontier Herbal Coop
Box 299
Norway, IA 52318
800-669-3275
http://www.FrontierHerb.com

The Herb Pharm
POBox 116
Williams, Oregon 97544
800-348-4372
http://www.Herb-Pharm.com

Pacific Botanicals
4350 Fish Hatchery Road
Grants Pass, Oregon 97527
541-479-7777

http://www.PacificBotanicals.com

Herbal Resources in the United Kingdom:

Herbs Hands Healing,
Station Warehouse
Station Rd.
Pulham Market, Norfolk IP214XF
Herbs: 01953-60356
School: 01379-608082

Hambleden Herbs
Court Farm
Milverton, Somerset, TA41WF
01823-401205

Herbal Apothecary
70a High St.
Syston, Leicester
0116-2602690

APPENDIX E — SUPPLEMENTS
See Appendix D for Resources and Suppliers

AlkaLife® is a patented alkaline concentrate. Mix 2 drops of AlkaLife solution in an 8-oz glass of water changes ordinary drinking water to high pH alkaline drinking water.

Aloe Vera: Patients with interstitial cystitis should be cautious about using liquid aloe vera since it must be preserved with high concentrations of citric acid, which is irritating to the bladder. Freeze-dried aloe vera from the whole plant—with no additives, no fillers, and no heat treatment—has been proven to be the most effective type of aloe for treating interstitial cystitis. The aloe plant is also a natural anti-inflammatory, antibiotic, and antifungal agent but only when used in its whole-leaf form. Aloe Vera high in muccopolysaccarides, has been shown to have healing properties for the GI tract and benefits for the immune system. Three capsules two to three times a day is recommended. Take with or without food.

Aloe Vera with Coral Calcium by Healthy Life Harvest: Each capsule contains high grade whole leaf aloe vera powder, and bio-available, ionic coral calcium as well as 72 trace minerals. This special IC formula is prepared to maximize absorbability. Suggested dosage is four capsules one to two times a day thirty minutes before meals. Take with 6 to 8 ounces of water. Four capsules contain 616 mg of calcium, vitamin D3 (cholecalciferol) 120 iu, magnesium (from coral, citrate, oxide) 172 mg, plus whole leaf aloe vera powder. These coral mineral supplements have been tested and are reported to *not* be a source of toxic heavy metals or other organic pollutions.

Antihistamines: Over the counter Benadryl or Claritin (not Claritin D) can help stabilize mast cells. Prescription antihistamines such as Vistaril, Atarax, Zyrtec, Allegra may prove useful for IC flares in the beginning of this alkalizing hypoallergenic program. Seek medical advice before taking over the counter antihistamines as they do have side effects such as drying of mucous membranes and can cause urinary retention. Natural mast cell stabilizers such as HMC Hesperidin, pycnogenol, quercetin, buffered vitamin C, and MSM would have fewer side effects than over the counter or prescription antihistamines.

B Complex without vitamin C: This will contain pantothenic acid. Recommended companies: Solaray, Allergy Research Group, or Thorne.

BHI Homeopathic Remedies for allergy flare-ups: allergy homeopathic and inflammation homeopathic. These two homeopathics worked in eliminating IC flare-ups when I was allergic to foods I consumed.

Bromelain is derived from a natural plant source in the stem of the pineapple. Bromelain is an enzyme that acts as a natural aspirin without any side effects. It reduces inflammation. For inflammation, suggested dosage is 500mg taken two to four times per day apart from meals for inflammation. Bromelain can be purchased at health food stores. Prosta-Q and Cysta-Q both contain bromelain and some persons with IC have found these supplements useful to decrease inflammation. It *should not be taken by pregnant women or persons with bleeding disorders.*

Clear®: herbal formula intestinal cleanse, one capsule each morning on an empty stomach with water only

Coffee Tamer: Sprinkle one all natural flavorless tiny packet into your coffee and it will help neutralize the acid. This product does not alter the flavor of the coffee. *Note*: I prefer to use a low acid coffee from Puroast and still add a packet of Coffee Tamer just to be safe.

Cromolyn sodium (disodium cromoglycate): Gastrocrom® may be useful for IC patients who have leaky gut syndrome or food allergies since it is a mast cell stabilizer for the intestinal tract and may help heal leaky gut. This is a prescription medication.

Ginger is a powerful anti-inflammatory agent and helps to reduce pain and fever in a variety of conditions. Dry, powdered ginger root in dosages of 500mg to 1,000mg per day can help reduce inflammation. 3,000mg to 4,000mg of ginger may provide more rapid relief, however do not use dosages beyond this limit. Try using fresh ginger in recipes if you tolerate it.

HCl and Pepsin is for diagnosed hypochlorhydria (low stomach acid) and aids with protein digestion. I recommend Thorne HCl and Pepsin. Dosage:1-2 capsules with each meal

HMC Hesperidin is a natural mast cell stabilizer. Dosage 250 mg one to two capsules three times a day. The methyl chalcone form of hesperidin is more water-soluble than hesperidin. HMC stabilizes mast cells.

L-Glutamine is the primary treatment for inflamed leaky gut, ulcers, and disorders of the small & large intestine such as Irritable Bowel Syndrome (IBS) which is characterized by either constipation, diarrhea or both. L-glutamine *directly feeds the tissue* of the small intestine enabling the villi to grow and improve absorption of nutrients across the cell membrane. L-glutamine also works inside the liver to produce the super powerful amino acid glutathione, which is one of the main free radical fighters within the body.

Dosage of L-glutamine for healing LGS: Start slowly with 500mg at bedtime on an empty stomach. You may increase the dose to 500 mg three times a day; take this on an empty stomach, with your last dose at bedtime. Take this dose for at least three to six months. (Dosages of 500 mg to 40 grams have been recommended for leaky gut. See a health care professional for doses larger than 2,000 mg a day.} Consider Allergy Research Group powder L-glutamine.

Livatone or Livatone Plus: A liver tonic by Dr. Sandra Cabot, MD, the tonic can be taken in a dose of one teaspoon mixed in fresh juice just before meals, twice daily, or two capsules just before food, twice daily. Take this dosage for eight to twelve weeks. Then go on to a maintenance dose of one teaspoon daily, or two capsules daily, which can be continued for as long as needed.

Milk Thistle as a liver remedy, suggested dosage is 70 - 200 mg up to three times daily.

MSM (methylsulfonylmethane): a safe powerful anti-inflammatory supplement and a pain reliever derived from natural foods. MSM is a natural compound that contains sulfur and helps to build new cells and connective tissue. You can take MSM even if you are allergic to sulfa drugs or sulfites. MSM contains sulfur not to be confused with sulfa drugs or sulfites. MSM has *anti-parasitic* and *antifungal* properties that block the binding sites for parasites in the intestines and the urogenital tract. The suggested starting dosage is 250mg to 1000 mg taken with meals. Do not take MSM at dinner or late in the evening, as it is invigorating. Dr. Jacobs, MD, Author of *The Miracle of MSM: The Natural Solution for Pain* suggests healing doses of 2,000mg to 8,000mg of MSM may be safely taken. Taking too large of a dose for your system might cause minor gastrointestinal upset, increased stool, or abdominal cramping. Most persons with IC need to start with very low doses of MSM, increase your MSM doses very slowly, and find a brand that agrees with you. You may experience die-off symptoms of yeast and parasites when starting MSM or increasing dosages which may increase your IC symptoms. MSM can be purchased at health food stores in capsule form or crystals you mix with water. MSM can also be applied topically in creams for arthritis pain relief. OptiMSM brand is recommended.

Pancreatic enzymes: If your pancreatic enzyme test is low, I recommend testing vegetarian Thorne Plantizyme, one capsule a day with a meal and building up to one to two capsules with each meal. Each capsule contains protease concentrate (47,000 HUT units), lipase concentrate (9,000 lipase units), cellulase concentrate (185 GD units), lactase concentrate (1,400 FCC units), and amylase concentrate (19,000 SKB units).

Papain is derived from papayas. It is an enzyme, and along with bromelain is a useful treatment of inflammatory conditions. For inflammation, suggested dosage is 200mg to 300mg with or immediately following meals, upon rising, and before bedtime. Papain can be purchased at health food stores. Prosta-Q and Cysta-Q both contain papain and some persons with IC have found these supplements useful to decrease inflammation. *It should not be taken by pregnant women or persons with bleeding disorders.*

Perm A Vite is a healing powder by Allergy Research Group for LGS. Ingredients: cellulose, L-glutamine, N-Acetyl-D-Glucosamine, slippery elm bark, MSM, Stevia, bovine intestinal glandular complex with epithelial growth factor. 1 to 3 level tablespoons per day. Best taken one hour before meals. (The source of N-Acetyl-D-Glucosamine is crabshell.)

Potassium bicarbonate, USP*: This should generally not be taken by itself. Recommended to mix with sodium bicarbonate 4:1 or 8:1 (four parts sodium bicarbonate to one part potassium bicarbonate or eight parts sodium bicarbonate to one part potassium bicarbonate) If you are on a sodium-restricted diet, you can take 1/8 to 1/4 teaspoon mixed in water on an empty stomach in between meals.

Pharmax Pure Fish Oil: One teaspoon contains DHA 750 mg, EPA 1050 mg, Total omega-3 2250 mg, tocopherols 25 mg. Dosage: one to four teaspoons daily with meals.

pH Control: pH Control can be helpful for those who suffer from interstitial cystitis and urinary urgency and frequency and or overactive bladder. Reducing the acid in urine promotes a healthier environment in the bladder. pH Control is not a drug. It is a dietary supplement made from 100% GRAS (Generally Regarded as Safe by the U.S. Food and Drug Administration) ingredients and has been tested for effectiveness and demonstrated its ability to significantly reduce urinary acid. Dosage is one tablet with each meal not to exceed 6 tablets a day. *Note*: pH Control is *NOT* an expensive calcium supplement. This is an ingenious scientific formula with special hydroxyl ions (OH-) that binds with acid (H+) to form water! (H2O) Each pH Control tablet contains approximately 200mg of calcium. There is a minimum of magnesium and potassium (less than 1% of DV) per tablet. Therefore, this supplement can cause constipation if not balanced 1:1 with a magnesium supplement. You also need 400 to 800 IU of vitamin D daily to help utilize calcium and magnesium.

Probiotics: Oral dose daily, as recommended by product label. I recommend Pharmax HLC probiotics.

Pycnogenol: This safe natural product is made from the bark of the European coastal pine, pinus maritima. It is a powerful antioxidant which quenches free radicals that are involved in the inflammatory process. Pycnogenol has been highly successful in the treatment of hay fever and allergies and is the first choice of many physicians in European countries. *Pycnogenol inhibits the enzyme histidine decarboxylase, and this lowers histamine levels. It prevents excessive histamine release.* Pycnogenol has anti-inflammatory and antihistamine properties. Because of these properties, it is a good choice for persons with interstitial cystitis.

Note: Pycnogenol may have anticoagulant properties taken in high doses. Persons on Coumadin, heparin, or aspirin should only take Pycnogenol under medical supervision. A recommended dose is one half milligram to one milligram per pound of body weight per day.

Quercetin is a natural substance found in plants that has anti-inflammatory, anti-allergenic and antimicrobial effects. Quercetin acts as a natural antihistamine and can be useful by decreasing mast cell breakdown. Quercetin is not absorbed well by the body unless taken in combination with bromelain. Suggested dosages of quercetin are 300mg to 600mg once or twice a day. Cysta Q and Prosta Q both contain quercetin, bromelain and papain. These supplements have been helpful for some persons with IC. *Quercetin can interfere with estrogen production and reduce menstrual flow. It should be used cautiously with menstruating women.*

Sodium bicarbonate *: For IC symptoms, oral dose ¼ teaspoon to ½ teaspoon mixed in 4 oz of water every hour or two until IC symptoms abate

Sodium citrate, USP: for sustained relief from IC, oral dose ½ to ¾ teaspoon mixed in 4 oz of water twice a day.

Sodium and potassium bicarbonate mixture *: (4:1 or 8:1 depending on your tolerance for potassium) for inflammatory conditions, oral dose ¼ to ½ teaspoon mixed in 4 oz of water three to four times a day preferably ½ hour before a meal or two hours after a meal. *Both sodium and potassium bicarbonate can be stimulating. It is best not to take in the evening.*

Turmeric (Curcumin) is an herb in the ginger family and used widely in India. It reduces inflammation and in one study was as effective as cortisone, a potent anti-inflammatory. Suggested dosage is 400mg to 600mg three times a day. Consider using turmeric in recipes if tolerated for its anti-inflammatory effects. See *Golden Milk* recipe in Recipe chapter.

Vitamin C reduces inflammation by decreasing histamine levels in the blood. *Buffered* vitamin C may be useful to decrease mast cell break down in the bladder and decrease the release of histamines. Vitamin C can have a laxative effect if taken in large quantities. Initial doses of vitamin C should be low 500mg to 1,000mg one to three times a day. Persons with IC must take a buffered vitamin C, which means vitamin C is buffered with calcium, magnesium and potassium. Allergy

Research Group makes a good-buffered vitamin C.

*Warnings and Precautions

You may not be able to take potassium bicarbonate, sodium bicarbonate or sodium citrate if you have kidney or heart disease or high blood pressure; are taking a potassium sparing diuretic; have Addison's disease; have a stomach ulcer or intestinal blockage; or have chronic diarrhea. If you are pregnant or nursing a baby, do not take any supplements without consulting your health care provider. Medications can compound the effects of the supplements and certain medical conditions may contraindicate the use of any supplements so consult your health care provider before starting supplements.

Taking too much sodium or potassium bicarbonate can make you too alkaline. Some signs and symptoms of being too alkaline are these:

Feeling overly energized, unable to sleep, tingling in the arms, hands, legs, and lips as well as feeling anxious.

Severe overdosing can result in muscle spasms or tetany, which can start in the forearms and spread throughout the body. Muscle spasms in the chest that effect breathing can be *fatal*. Bicarbonate can cause bloating or gas in some individuals.

If you experience any of these symptoms, reduce the dosage and frequency of sodium and potassium bicarbonate.

To reduce alkalosis, drinking coffee, black tea, lemonade, or cola drinks will cause the body to become more acidic and restore your pH balance. Vigorous exercise also will increase acidity.

It is important to take sodium and potassium bicarbonate 30 minutes before a meal or two hours after a meal so the supplement does not interfere with digestion. Sodium bicarbonate and potassium bicarbonate will neutralize stomach acids temporarily, which is not helpful for digestion.

When taking sodium and potassium bicarbonate or sodium citrate start with the lowest dose recommended to obtain symptom relief. I encourage maintaining a hypoallergenic alkalizing diet and use alkalizing supplements as needed in the first year or two of alkalizing. It may take as long at one to three years to completely reverse tissue acidosis.

APPENDIX F — ENDNOTES

Preface
1. Dr. Dennis Meyers, MD, *A New Biology*, p. 72
2. Catherine M. Simone. *Along the Healing Path, Recovering from Interstitial Cystitis*, Kearney, NE: Morris Pub, 2000, pp. 6 - 7
3. Dr. Susan Lark, MD, and James A. Richards, MBA, *The Chemistry of Success*, San Fransisco: Bay Books, 2000, p. 55
4. *ibid.*
5. Dr. Theodore A. Baroody, Jr., MA, DC, ND, PhD, *Alkalize or Die*, Waynesville, NC: Eclectic Press, 1993, pp. 21 - 22
6. Linda G. Rector-Page, ND, PhD, *Healthy Healing*, 9th, Carmel Valley: Healthy Healing Publications, 1992, p. 9

Testimonial
1. Burton Goldberg Group, *Alternative Medicine: The Definitive Guide*, Puyallup, WA: Future Medicine Publishing, 1883, p. 669
2. Herman Aihara, *Acid and Alkaline*, 5th Edition, Orovile, CA: George Ohsawa Macrobiotic Foundation, 1986, p. 23
3. *ibid.* p. 36

Defining Interstitial Cystitis
1. Meridith F. Campbell (Editor), *Campbell's Urology*, Update 14, W. B. Saunders, Co., 1995, p. 1
2. *ibid.* p. 5
3. Dr. Robert M. Moldwin, MD, *The Interstitial Cystitis Survival Guide*, Oakland: New Harbinger Publications, 2000, p. 37
4. Dr. Susan Lark, MD, *Op. Cit.*, pp. 84-85
5. *ibid.*, p. 75
6. Dr. Larrian Gillespie, MD, *You Don't Have to Live with Cystitis*, New York: Avon, 1996, p. 58
7. *ibid.*, p. 57
8. *ibid.*, p. 65
9. *ibid.*, p. 67
10. *ibid.*, p. 67
11. OB/Gyn.NET, Article: *Chlamydia pneumoniae May Play Role In Pathogenesis*, June 28, 2001
12. Campbell, *Op. Cit., p. 3*
13. Dr. Dennis Meyers, MD, *Op. Cit.*, p. 88

Foundation of Acid-Alkali Imbalance

1. Keichi Morishita, MD, *The Hidden Truth of Cancer.* San Francisco: George Ohsawa Macrobiotic Foundation, 1972

2. *The Atlantic Monthly*, A New Germ Theory by Judith Hooper, February 1999

3. *ibid,*

4. OB/Gyn.NET, Article: *Chlamydia pneumoniae* May Play Role In Pathogenesis, *June 28, 2001*

Understanding Acid-Alkali Balance and its Effect on Interstitial Cystitis

1. Adapted from Dr. Dennis Myers' *The New Biology*, pp. 75 - 76

2. Dr. M. Ted Morter, Jr, MA, *Your Health Your Choice,* Hollywood, FL: Lifetime Books, p. 26

3. *ibid.*

4. Aihara, *Op. Cit.,* pp. 9 - 10

5. Dr. Shaun Kerry, MD, http://www.cfsdoc.org/biological_terrain.htm

6. Lark, *Op. Cit.*, p. 65

7. *ibid.*

8. Moldwin, *Op. Cit.*, p. 37

9. Dr. William Philpott, MD, *Biomagnetic Handbook*, Enviro-Tech Products, 1989

10. Lark, *Op. Cit.*, p. 75

11. Myers, *Op. Cit.*, p. 75

12. Lark, *Op. Cit.*, p. 75

13. Aihara, *Op. Cit.*, p. 23.

14. Lark, *Op. Cit.*, p. 67

15. *ibid.*, p. 68

16. Aihara, *Op. Cit.*, pp. 9 - 10

17. Adapted from Dr. Theodore Baroody, *Alkalize or Die*, pp. 185 - 187

How to Measure your Body's pH

1. Lark, *Op. Cit.*, pp. 84-85

2. Dr. Shaun Kerry, MD, http://www.cfsdoc.org/biological_terrain.htm

3. Robert R. Barefoot and Carl J. Reich, MD, *The Calcium Factor: The Scientific Secret of Health and Youth*, Arkansas City, Kansas: Gilliland Printing Inc., 1996

Leaky Gut Syndrome
1. Dr. Deborah Metzger PhD, MD, FACOG, Helena Women's Health, 2101 Forest Avenue, Suite 220, San Jose, CA 95128 (408) 999-7900

Allergies
1. Moldwin, *Op. Cit.*, p. 43
2. Devi S. Nambudripad, DC, LAc, RN, PhD, (Acu), *Say Goodbye to Illness*, *2nd Edition*, Buena Park: Delta Publishing Co., 1999, p. 9
3. Metzger, *Op. Cit.*
4. Lark, *Op. Cit.*, p. 75
5. Dr. William G. Crook, MD, *Detecting Your Hidden Allergies*, Jackson, TN: Professional Books, 1988, pp. 35 - 36
6. Nambudripad, *Op. Cit*, p.70

The Liver
1. Dr. Hery Bieler, MD, *Food Is Your Best Medicne*, New York, NY: Ballentine Books, pp. 63-65
2. Lark, *Op Cit.*, p. 325

Hormones
1. Dr. Neal Barnard, MD, *Foods That Fight Pain*, New York, NY: Three Rivers Press, 1998, p. 126
2. ibid., pp. 126-127
3. Steven Foster, "Black Cohosh" article online at:
   http://www.herbphoto.com/education/monograph/bkcohosh.html

Essential Fatty Acids
1. Portions of this chapter have been adapted and quoted from Michael A. Schmidt, *Smart Fats*, Berkeley, CA: Frog Ltd., 1997

Vitamin D
1. Shari Lieberman, PhD, and Nancy Bruning, *The Real Vitamin and Mineral Book*, Garden City Park, NY:Avery, 1997, pp. 74-75
2. Dr. Susan Lark, MD, Women's Health Update (Newsletter), July 23, 2003

Nourishing Ourselves with Herbs
1. See the Herb Pharm webpage: www.herb-pharm.com
2. Peter Holmes, *The Energetics of Western Herbs*, Revised Third Edition, vol.2, Boulder: Snow Lotus Press, 1998, p. 679
3. *ibid.3*

4. Susun Weed, *Healing Wise,* Woodstock, New York: Ash Tree Publishing, 1989, pp.144-145

5. Hong-Yen Hsu, *Oriental Materia Medica; A Concise Guide* (Long Beach, California: Oriental Healing Arts Institute, 1986) p. 238

6. Holmes, *Op Cit.*, p. 679

7. Susun Weed, *HealingWise*, p. 172

8. *ibid.* p.171-173

9. Michael Moore, *Medicinal Plants of the Pacific West*, Santa Fe, New Mexico: Red Crane Books, 1995, p.188

10. *ibid.* p.189

11. *ibid.* p. 188

12. *ibid.* p. 189-190

13. Rosemary Gladstar, *Herbal Healing for Women*, New York: Fireside/ Simon and Schuster, 1993, p.247

14. Michael Moore, *Herbs for the Urinary Tract*, New Canaan, Connecticut: Keats Publishing, Inc. 1998, p. 58

15. Peter Holmes, *Energetics of Western Herbs*, vol.1 p.297-298

16. David Hoffman *The Holistic Herbal,* Dorset, England: Element Books, 1988) p. 205

17. Steven Foster and Yue Chongxi, *Herbal Emissaries*, Vermont: Healing Arts Press, 1992, p. 114

18. Stephen Harrod Buhner, *Herbal Antibiotics,* Pownal, Vermont: Storey Books, 1999, p. 53

19. *ibid.* p.54

20. Peter Holmes, *The Energetics of Western Herbs*, p. 438

21. Thomas Bartram, *Bartram's Encyclopedia of Herbal Medicine*, New York: Marlowe and Company, 1998, p.14

22. Susun S. Weed, *New Menopausal Years; The Wise Woman Way*, Woodstock New York: Ash Tree Publishing, 2002, p.72

23. Steven Foster, *Herbal Renaissance*, Salt Lake City: Peregrine Smith Books, 1993, p. 66

24. Peter Holmes, *The Energetics of Western Herbs, vol. 2*, p. 662

25. *The study described on this web page included 13 participants:* http://www.desertharvest.com/interstitial_cystitis.html

26. Thomas Bartram, *Bartram's Encyclopedia of Herbal Medicine*, p.16

27. *PDR for Herbal Medicines*, First Edition, Montvale, New Jersey: Medical Economics Company, 1998, p. 849

28. Michael Castleman, *The New Healing Herbs*, New York: Bantam Books, 2002, p. 531

29. Peter Holmes, *Energetics of Western Herbs*, vol. 2, page 790

30. Lynn Lawson, *Staying Well in a Toxic World; Understanding Environmental Illness, Multiple Chemical Sensitivities, Chemical Injuries and Sick Building Syndrome*, Chicago: Noble Press, 1993, p.175

31. Michael Murray and Joseph Pizzorno, *Encylopedia of Natural Medicine*, Revised Second Edition, Rocklin, California: Prima Communications, Inc., 1998, p. 311

An Alkalizing Program

1. Lark, *Op. Cit.*, p. 248

2. EarthSave Taste of Health seminar by Brenda Davis, RD (1996, Seattle, WA)

3. Shari Lieberman, CNS, PhD, and Nancy Bruning, *The Real Vitamin and Mineral Book,* Garden City Park, NY: Avery, 1997, p. 139

4. *ibid.*, p. 140

5. These data are current as of 1998

6. Lieberman and Bruning, Op. Cit., p. 147

7. *ibid.*

8. These data are current as of 1998

9. Lieberman and Bruning, Op. Cit., p. 147

10. Bieler, Op. Cit., pp. 163-164

11. Dr. John McDougall, MD, http://www.drmcdougall.com/debate.html

12. Jill Carroll, *The Wall Street Journal*, Health, The Government's Food Pyramid Correlates to Obesity, Critics Say, June 13, 2002

Getting Started

1. The Penguin Encyclopedia of Nutrition, 1985

Alkalizing Recipes and Food Preparation

1. Canadian Journal of Dietetic Practice and Research, Vol. 62, No 2, Summer 2003

2. EarthSave Taste of Health seminar by Brenda Davis, RD (1996, Seattle, WA)

3. The Penguin Encyclopedia of Nutrition, 1985

4. Sally Fallon & Mary G. Enig, Ph.D, Cinderella's Dark Side, (Mercola.com Newsletter)

5. Jennette Turner, Certified Holistic Nutritionist, Wedge Co-op Newslatter, Apr/May 2002, Preparing Whole Grains the Traditional Way for Health

Ayurveda

1. *Secrets of the Pulse. The Ancient Art of Ayurvedic Pulse Diagnosis,* Dr. Vasant Lad

Conclusion

1. D. W. Schindler, *Effects of Acid Rain on Freshwater Ecosystems,* Science, vol. 239, 1988, pp. 149-157

2. Compton's Encyclopedia Online v3.0 © 1998 The Learning Company

3. Dr. Raymond A. Hurm, MD, *Urology Times*, Letter to the Editor, July 1999

4. Dan Emerson, *Urology Times*, Jan, 2001

5. Ann Wigmore, *The Hippocrates Diet and Health Program*, Avery, 1984, p. 10

Index

A

G

H

irritable bowel 87
irritable bowel syndrome 160

J

Jarrow 21
Jewish 165
Juicing 265

K

Kapha 274
kava (piper methysticum) 184
kidney failure 205
kinesiology 92

L

L-glutamine 80, 81
lactic acid and exercise 53
lactobacillos casei 79
lactobacillus acidophilus 79
latent acidosis 56, 58
   endogenous conditions 61
   exogenous conditions 60
   mast cell breakdown 59
latitudes
   vitamin D 139
leaky gut
   healing 78
leaky gut, dysbiosis, allergies, and IC 85
Leaky Gut Syndrome (LGS) 75
lecithin 103
leukotrienes 131
LGS. *See* Leaky Gut Syndrome (LGS)
licorice root (glycyrrhiza glabra, g. uralensis) 174
lifestyle
   health effects on modern man 147
liming 305
linoleic acid 131
   sources of 132
liver
   coffee enemas 107
   enzymes 96
   massage 106
   stress 76

Q

quality of life 33

R

radiation 147
Ragland's test 219
rectum 159
riboflavin 102

S

safe sex 159
saliva pH 71
saliva testing 220
saturated fat 132
seasonings 232
second line of defense 13, **97**
Sex **157**
sex
   anal intercourse 159–160
   antihistamines 158
   Betadine 160
   cranberry juice 160
   Hibiclens 160
   intimacy 158
   lack of 159
   Phisohex 160
   positions 157
   safe 159
   tap water enema 160
   vaseline 160
sexual lubricants
   glycerin 158
shame 163
shopping suggestions 231
SIgA 76
skullcap 183
sleep cycles 147
slippery elm bark (ulmus fulva) 177
Slippery Stuff 158, 160
smoking 91
sodium **97**, 206
   inorganic 206
   organic 206

Solving the Interstitial Cystitis Puzzle

trigger points 293
triggers 34
triglycerides 96, 132
trigone (bladder) 23

U

Understanding Acid-Alkali Balance **49**
urethra 23
urinalysis 23, 27
urination
    frequent 132
urine
    appearance 25
    bilirubin 27
    blood 26
    casts 26
    cloudy 26
    crystals 26
    ketones 27
    milk 27
    pH 26, 69
    protein 26
    sugar 27
Urised 157
UV-B 139

V

vaginal intercourse 160
Vanderbilt Study 32
Vata 274
vegetarian diets 210
victim 165
villi 75
vitamin B-1 102
vitamin B-12 103
vitamin B-2 102
vitamin B-3 102
vitamin B-5 102
vitamin B-6 102
vitamin C 102
vitamin D 139
    adverse affect of dairy consumption 141
    deficiency 139
    dosages 140

Order Form

For additional copies of this book:

Solving the Interstitial Cystitis Puzzle
A Natural Guide to Healing

ISBN: 0-9710869-2-3

For each book, send $28.75 (to cover shipping and handling) to:

Holistic Life Enterprises
9461 Charleville Blvd Ste 198
Beverly Hills, CA 90212-3017

or visit http://www.holisticnurse.com to purchase online.

Name: _____

Address: _____

_____

City: _____

State: _____ Postal Code: _____ - _____

Email: _____

Make cheques payable to Holistic Life Enterprises

MasterCard, Visa, or Discover (Please circle appropriate type.)

_____ _____ _____ _____ exp. ___ / ___

Signature _____ Date _____

(Please photocopy this form if you wish to order books.)

Made in the USA
Lexington, KY
12 December 2009